FEMORAL NECK FRACTURES AND HIP JOINT INJURIES

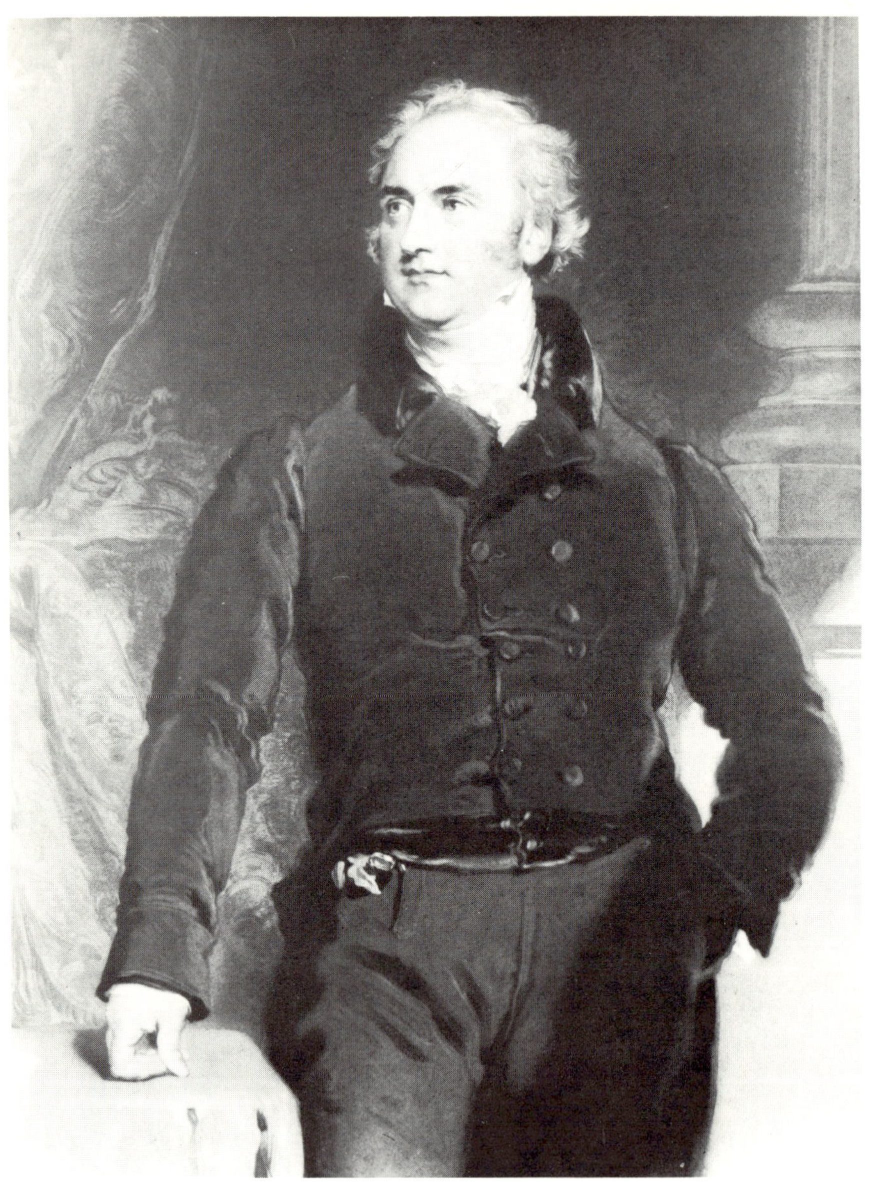

SIR ASTLEY PASTON COOPER (1768–1841)
Guy's Hospital, London (By courtesy of the Wellcome Trustees).

'I have stated it to be a general principle, that the neck of the thigh bone, when it is broken within the capsular ligament, and attended with the usual characters of that fracture, viz. occurring in advanced age, a limb shortened from $1\frac{1}{2}''$ to $2\frac{1}{2}''$, accompanied as it usually is by an everted knee and foot, such fracture does not unite by an ossific process, but by means of a ligamentous substance passing from the capsular to the reflected ligament, and from bone to bone. The main principle upon which this want of union depends, I have endeavoured to show, exists in the lessened nutrition of the head of the bone.'
From: '*A Treatise on Dislocations and on Fractures of the Joints*' (1823) 2nd Edn., p. 570. Longman, Hurst, London.

FEMORAL NECK FRACTURES AND HIP JOINT INJURIES

Edited by

D.S. MUCKLE

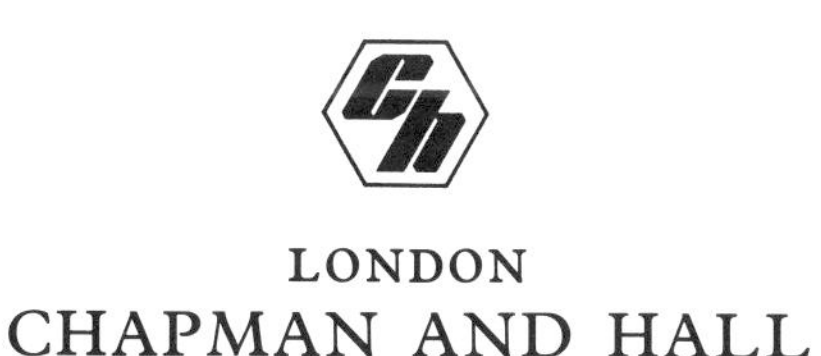

LONDON
CHAPMAN AND HALL

First published 1977
by Chapman and Hall Ltd
11 New Fetter Lane, London EC4P 4EE

Photoset by
Thomson Press (India) Ltd, New Delhi
and printed in Great Britain by
T & A Constable Ltd, Edinburgh

ISBN 0 412 13690 2

CONTENTS

ACKNOWLEDGEMENTS

I would like to acknowledge, with gratitude, the following people who helped in the preparation of this book: Mr J. Cockin, F.R.C.S. (Oxford), Mr J. C. Scott, F.R.C.S. (Oxford) and Professor J. Stevens, F.R.C.S. (Newcastle-upon-Tyne) for their advice on the subject material and its presentation; the Photographic Department of the Nuffield Orthopaedic Centre and Robert Emanuel; the Department of Medical Illustrations, Radcliffe Infirmary, Oxford; Lois Allen, Librarian, Nuffield Orthopaedic Centre, Oxford; Margaret Stevenson, M.A. for checking the proofs; and the secretarial help from Wendy Cox, Joy Taylor, Pat English, Olive Kingsworth, Anne Bayliss, Joan Anderson, Hilda Moore, Annabel Filipowska, Julia Thornton, Janet Lever, June Maliphant, Veronica Dollin, Elsie Boswell and Jean Barclay.

Oxford, November 1976 D. S. Muckle

CONTRIBUTORS

G. Bentley. M.Ch., F.R.C.S.	Professor in Orthopaedic Surgery, University of Liverpool. Formerly Clinical Reader in Orthopaedic Surgery, Nuffield Orthopaedic Centre, Oxford.
H. C. Burbidge. M.R.C.S., F.F.A.R.C.S.	Consultant Anaesthetist, Nuffield Orthopaedic, Oxford.
J. Cockin. M.A., F.R.C.S.	Director, Accident Service, Radcliffe Infirmary, Oxford. Consultant, Nuffield Orthopaedic Centre, Oxford.
G. Deane. M.Sc., F.R.C.S.	Consultant to the Orthopaedic Engineering Centre, Nuffield Orthopaedic Centre, Oxford.
J. W. Goodfellow. M.B., F.R.C.S.	Consultant Orthopaedic Surgeon, Nuffield Orthopaedic Centre, Oxford.
R. A. Griffiths. M.R.C.P., M.R.C.G.P.	Consultant Physician, Geriatrics, Cowley Road Hospital, Oxford.
F. H. Kemp. M.A., M.D., F.R.C.P., F.F.R.	Consultant Radiologist, Oxford Area Health Authority (Teaching).
J. Kenwright. M.A., Ph.D., F.R.C.S.	Consultant Orthopaedic Surgeon, Radcliffe Infirmary and Nuffield Orthopaedic Centre, Oxford.
D. S. Muckle. M.B., B.S., M.S., F.R.C.S.	Consultant Orthopaedic Surgeon, Cleveland Area Health Authority. Formerly Senior Registrar in Orthopaedic Surgery, Nuffield

	Orthopaedic Centre and Accident Service, Radcliffe Infirmary, Oxford.
R. Smith. M.A., M.D., Ph.D., F.R.C.P.	Hon. Consultant Physician, Oxford Area Health Authority (Teaching).
E. W. Somerville. M.A., F.R.C.S.	Consultant Orthopaedic Surgeon, Nuffield Orthopaedic Centre, Oxford.
C. G. Woods. M.B., B.Sc., M.R.C. Path.	Consultant Pathologist, Nuffield Orthopaedic Centre, Oxford.
J. C. Scott. M.A., M.D., M.S., F.R.C.S.	Consultant Orthopaedic Surgeon, Radcliffe Infirmary and Nuffield Orthopaedic Centre, Oxford.

FOREWORD

These relatively common injuries are of great importance not only to the many thousands who suffer them each year and their families, but also to the Health and Social Services because of the enormous demands made on them by those injured. The injuries are of interest to the medical profession for the above reasons and also because they present a challenge through a wide range of subjects from human nutrition to biomechanics. Much has been written on their natural history and the many problems created, but there is still a need for improvement in the general understanding of them and their management. There is a need for a text confined to this subject and, therefore, able to deal with the many important points in some detail. In the present state of knowledge a clinical bias is essential and an authoritative approach to this aspect of the problem will be of most value to the patients and to the many young surgeons called upon to deal with them. The clinical bias will in no way preclude attention to all the relevant fields of research.

These injuries alone or in combination present many practical problems. The principles and methods to be applied to their care will be appraised and discussed in detail along with the results to be expected from proper treatment. In any gathering of experts in this field reference to the 'unsolved fracture' would immediately and generally be recog-zed as the intracapsular fracture of the femoral neck. This is *the* problem in the area, full of interest surrounded by prejudice and conjecture and in urgent need of solution.

'At the beginning of the century, fracture of the neck of the femur was a therapeutic derelict – the futility of conventional treatment demonstrated by Sir Astley Cooper had been accepted as a finality and permanent disability as an inevitable sequence of the injury.' So opened the paper on his method of Abduction Treatment by Whitman in 1925. The clue to this method had come to him in 1890 when he 'identified the fracture of the neck of the femur in a child'. The resultant deformity was corrected by the surgical removal of a wedge from the base of the trochanter to restore abduction and internal rotation. From this success it was reasoned that the treatment of the acute femoral neck injury should be to hold the limb in abduction and internal rotation until the fracture united. From the description there now seems little doubt that he was dealing with slipping of the upper femoral epiphysis. It was soon generally accepted that Whitman's method was worthwhile, but controversy centred around the cause of the considerable number of poor results. Whitman (1930) concluded that 'by far the large proportion of too numerous failures may be attributed not to the fault of the method, but to its faulty application even in the hands of distinguished surgeons and orthopaedic specialists'. This statement was understandably unpopular, partly because of its medico-legal implications and also because Whitman took care never to publish an analysis of his own results.

This was the background to the appointment, in 1929, by the American Orthopaedic Association, of a commission 'to study the true end results of unimpacted fractures of the neck of the femur within the capsule in persons over 60'. The results presented in that report Campbell *et al.* (1930) are similar to those with which we are at present familiar – an early mortality rate of 28.6%; and 30% with proved bony union after 12 months. The commission gained the impression that the results were better 'when the Whitman method was efficiently employed' than by any other of the methods used.

A similar review carried out by the same body in 1930 was of less value because it included fractures in those under 60 years of age. The main point of interest in the second review was that it included 34 cases treated by bone grafting with a new technique described by Albee with '97.4% proved bony union after one year'; and 31 cases treated by open reduction and internal fixation with a triflanged nail. This method introduced by Smith-Petersen was at that time unpublished. Of these 31 cases '83.8% resulted in proved bony union at the end of one year'. Geist (1931) reported 53.8% bony union in 210 intracapsular fractures treated by the Whitman method and remarked on the fact that 'in this particular fracture the percentage of non-union does not compare with any other fracture – non-union in other types of fracture is comparatively rare'.

The purpose of this introductory focus is to try to put the major problem into perspective and to emphasize the fact that there was at that time a turning point in the management of this injury. It was accepted that closed conservative treatment was possible and produced a proportion of excellent results and also that open reduction and internal fixation with nail or graft could yield better results. Finally it was appreciated that for some unknown reason non-union was much more frequent in fractures of the femoral neck than in other fractures. Has 40 years and more of cumulative experience led to the progressive improvement in management and results that we should have been able to achieve? I think not.

By 1939 Whitman's and other methods of conservative treatment were effectively relegated to the history books and the emphasis in practice and investigation was on the mechanics of reduction and the methods of internal fixation. It was at this stage that the relatively common appearance of 'avascularity' in the femoral head after cervical fracture was recognized and given importance as a causative factor in non-union and later disintegration of the head (Urist, 1964).

The great increase in the incidence of the fracture during and after the Second World War, the demonstration of fracture patterns and other studies into the natural history of the 'disease' led to a new emphasis on the quality of the bone. That 'bones become thin in their shell and spongy in texture' as part of the ageing process had been pointed out by Astley Cooper in 1824. That this was not a universal process or equally applicable to both sexes, or all countries, was gradually appreciated. That the changes did not apply to all bones or even to all parts of one bone was also realized. The term 'osteoporosis' crept gradually into common use and its presence in relation to this fracture took on increasing significance. Evidence, such as the increasing incidence of pertrochanteric fracture relative to the intracapsular variety with advancing age indicated that the skeleton was amenable to metabolic and other influences even at this advanced age.

The relationship between relative avascularity and cartilage attrition is one of the important features and these inevitable companions of femoral neck fracture have received little attention. Early weight-bearing may be of value in maintaining synovial circulation and with it the synovial fluid contribution to the nourishment of articular cartilage. Lesser cartilage loading by active exercises may serve this purpose equally well and this type of mobilization may reduce the danger of failure of fixation in the early stages or collapse of the head in the later stage.

The constructive conclusion arising from these observations is that it may be possible, by suitable supporting therapy, to maintain the quality of bone into old age and by so doing to prevent the majority of these fractures.

Apart from identifying and dealing with the acknowledged pathological element in these fractures there are special technical problems in the age group principally concerned. As well as the surgeon, proper management closely involves the anaesthetist and the geriatric physician and these aspects are dealt with in separate sections.

Over the whole field of injuries dealt with and the extremely wide range of problems involved, there is not a single area in which there is room for complacency. A volume such as this should have two main purposes – to improve the understanding of the presenting problems by a clear and accurate assembling of existing knowledge and to emphasize the areas where continuing research is likely to be most valuable. Thereby it will inform and stimulate any student along the right lines.

J. C. Scott
M.A., M.D., M.S., F.R.C.S.
Consultant Orthopaedic Surgeon, Radcliffe Infirmary,
and Nuffield Orthopaedic Centre, Oxford.

CAMPBELL, W.C., WINNETT ORR, H. and OSGOOD, R.B. (1930). *J. Bone Jt. Surg.* **XII**, 966.

GEIST, E.S. (1931). *Lancet* **51**, 230.

URIST, M.R. (1964). *Proc. Conf. Aseptic Necrosis of the Femoral Head.* p. 259. Natn. Inst. Health, U.S. Public Health Service.

WHITMAN, R. (1938). *J. Bone Jt. Surg.* **XX**, 960.

WHITMAN, R. (1930). *Lancet* **50**, 281.

Chapter One

BASIC SCIENCES OF THE HIP

D. S. Muckle, G. Bentley, G. Deane, F. H. Kemp

Surgical and applied anatomy ~ The structure and function of articular cartilage ~ Biomechanics of the hip in relation to hip fractures ~ General radiology of the hip

SURGICAL AND APPLIED ANATOMY

An understanding of the anatomy of the hip region is required to plan reduction and surgical management, and to determine the possible complications after injury. As with all fractures the final position of the bone fragments is dependent upon many interrelated factors including the magnitude and direction of the deforming forces, the restraint of the surrounding soft tissues, and the superimposed muscle pull. In the case of femoral neck fractures displacement may be slight because the forces concerned are of low magnitude and the strong ligaments of the hip apply a restraining action.

The acetabulum

The articular margin of the acetabulum is only a lunate strip (Fig. 1.1) which surrounds the acetabular fossa. The mouth of the acetabulum is directed laterally, distally and anteriorly. A reinforcing buttress of bone is found at its superior and posterior margins to counteract the forces exerted by the femoral head not only in the erect attitude but also during hip flexion. The roughened component, filled with fat, synovial membrane and ligamentum teres, provides a weak surface and predisposes to central dislocations and fractures. The cavity is deepened by the fibrocartilaginous labrum which embraces the femoral head tightly beyond its equator, thus enhancing the stability of the hip joint. The labrum is continued as the transverse ligament across the acetabular notch. The triradiate cartilage which separates the three

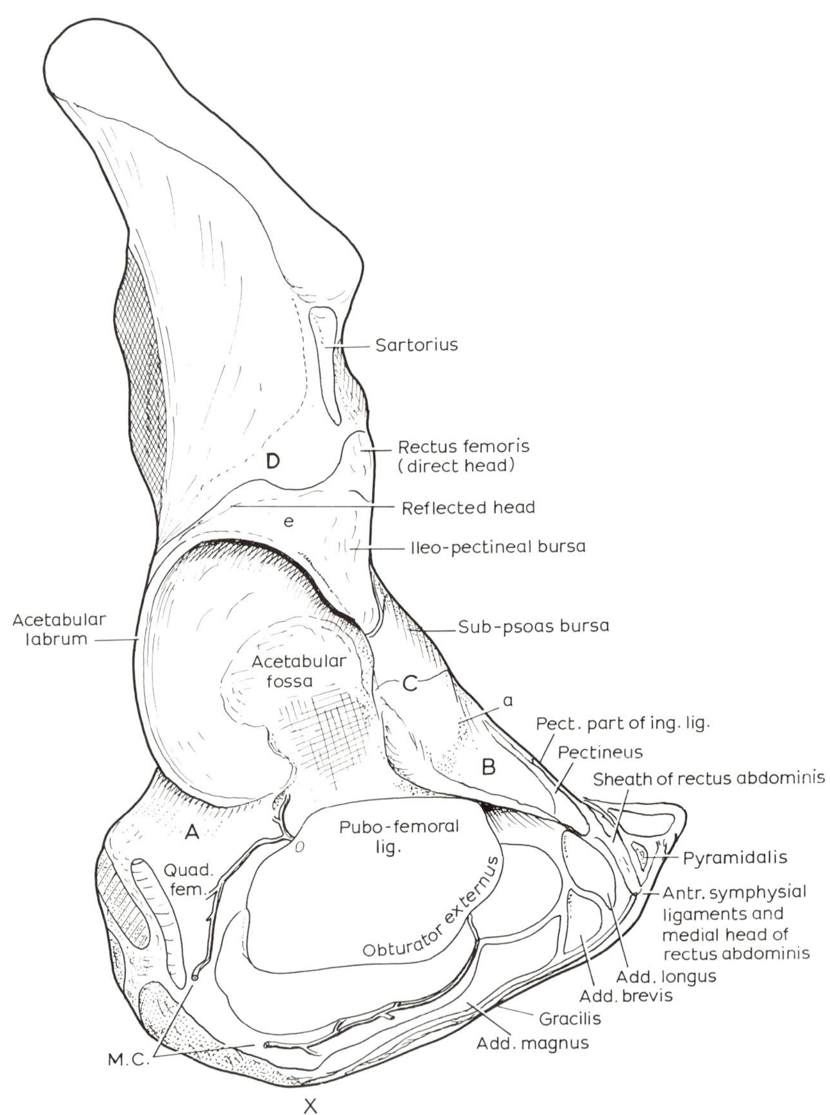

FIG. 1.1*a* Lateral view of the acetabular and ischio–pubic region. (A) is a region on the bone in front of the position of quadratus femoris which is in relation with the tendon of obturator externus. (B) is a sloping area which supports the pectineus, and the covering fascia reaches the bone at a. The psoas lies on (C). (D) is covered by gluteus minimus which arises above the dotted line; below (D) the muscle lies on the reflected head of rectus femoris and the capsule. (O) and (M.C.) are branches of the obturator and medial circumflex arteries. (X) marks an ill-defined depression which indicates where the origin of the adductor magnus passes from the lateral side of the ramus to the lower aspect of the ischial tuberosity. (Reproduced by kind permission from Frazer's Anatomy of the Human Skeleton.)

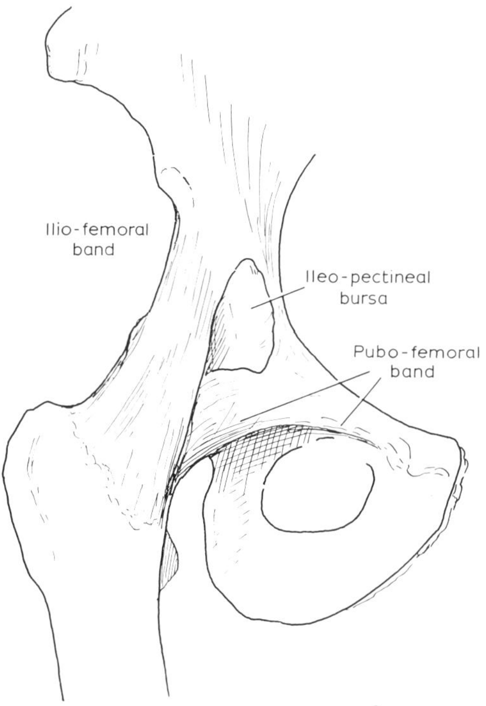

FIG. 1.1*b* Anterior view of the hip joint indicating the structure of the strong ilio-femoral band, and its relationship with the ileo-pectineal bursa. (Reproduced by kind permission from Frazer's Anatomy of the Human Skeleton.)

elements of the pelvis until puberty, may develop a variable number of ossifying centres and they can be confused with fracture fragments. Other extra ossicles may be found at the acetabular margins.

Behind the acetabulum the synovial membrane transgresses the labrum. There is only a slight capsular attachment behind for there are no true transverse fibres posteriorly (Frazer, 1965). This potential weak area is readily traversed by a posterior dislocation of the femoral head. The sciatic nerve is vulnerably adjacent (Fig. 1.2).

The femoral head

This structure forms rather more than half a sphere, but is slightly compressed in an antero–posterior direction. It is entirely intracapsular and the epiphyseal line almost corresponds with the edge of the articular surface (Fig. 1.3). In any joint position only two-fifths of the head occupies the bony acetabulum. There is also an intimate relationship with the femoral artery, with psoas major and the capsule in between;

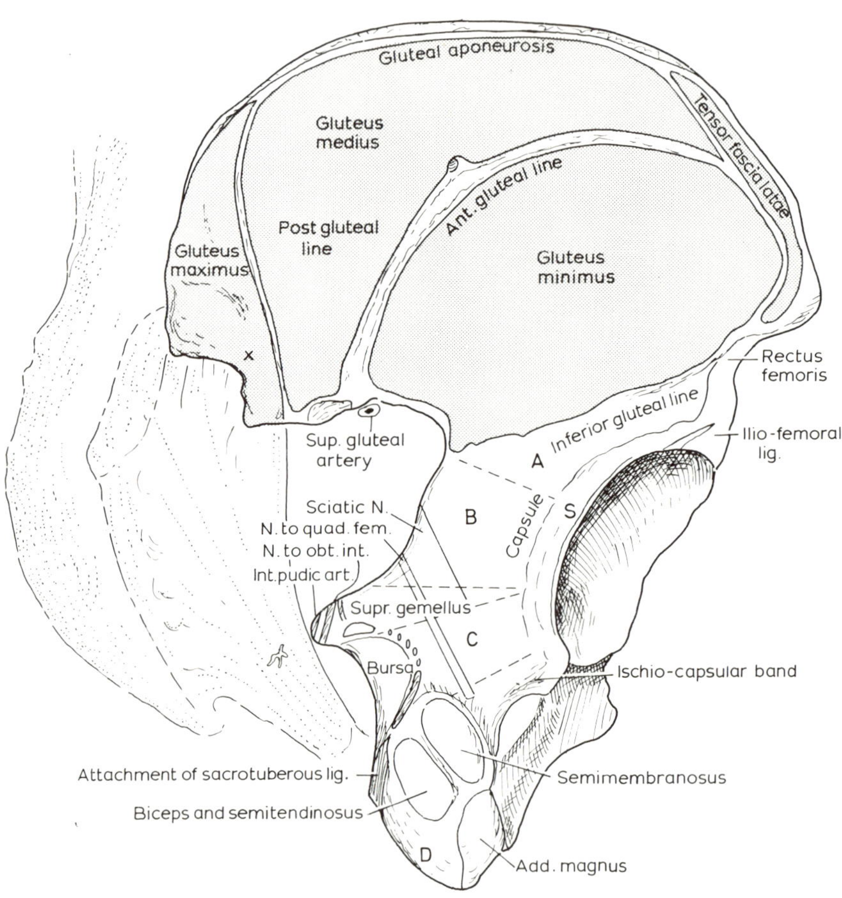

FIG. I.2 Posterior–lateral aspect of the right hip. (A) is the surface below the inferior gluteal line covered by gluteus minimus; (B) the area covered by piriformis, with the sciatic nerve interposed; (C) is covered by obturator the internus and gemelli which lie between the sciatic nerve and the bone, but have nerve to the quadratus between them and the bone. The muscles mentioned are practically in a continuous curved plane, so that the areas (A–C) make a convex surface, curved and smooth, round the acetabulum; the muscles pass to the raised greater trochanter so do not mould the bone by pressure. (Reproduced by kind permission from Frazer's Anatomy of the Human Skeleton.)

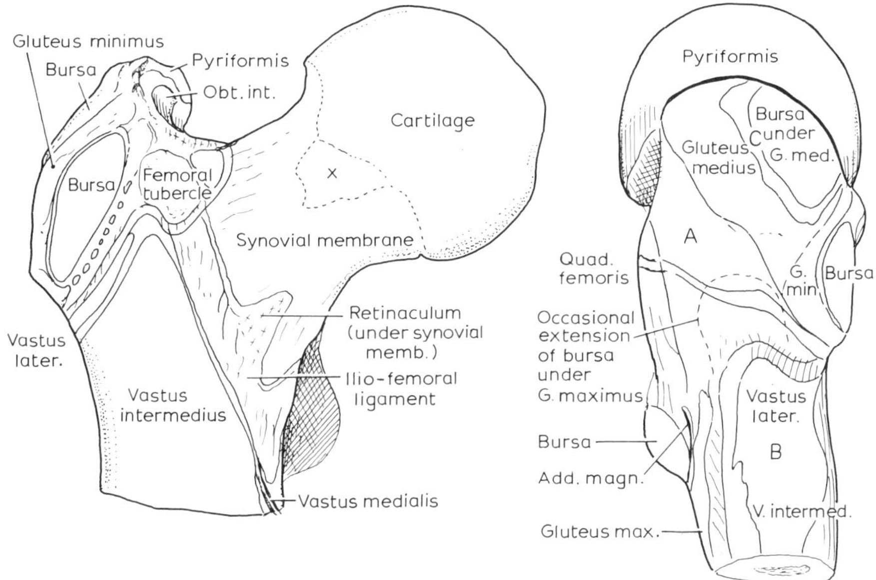

FIG. 1.3*a* The extension of the cartilage on the head on to the neck is shown at x on the anterior view. The oblique insertion of the gluteus medius is continuous below and in front with that of the gluteus minimus, and frequently with that of piriformis above and behind; it divides this aspect of the trochanter into two areas, (C) under medius and therefore bevelled off in the direction of that muscle, and (A) covered and moulded by maximus. The surface at (B) is covered and flattened by the vastus lateralis. The vastus intermedius fuses with the lateralis at a lower level. (Reproduced by permission from Frazer's Anatomy of the Human Skeleton.)

this relationship should be recalled when bone levers are used in this area. The intact ligamentum teres, attached to the fovea, may act as a fulcrum around which the head may twist after a subcapital fracture.

The femoral neck and trochanters

The neck, which is embryologically a continuation of the shaft, joins the latter at an angle which varies from 125 to 135°, but does not lie in the same plane (Fig. 1.4) but is carried forwards. This angle of femoral torsion poses practical difficulties and is often responsible for the plethora of guide wires during internal fixation. In the adult the angle of torsion is between 12 and 15°.

The femoral neck is a 30-50 mm tube which gradually changes shape (Fig. 1.5) (Backman, 1957). It forms an angle opening posteriorly and downwards, leading to the unfortunate area where a reamer may easily

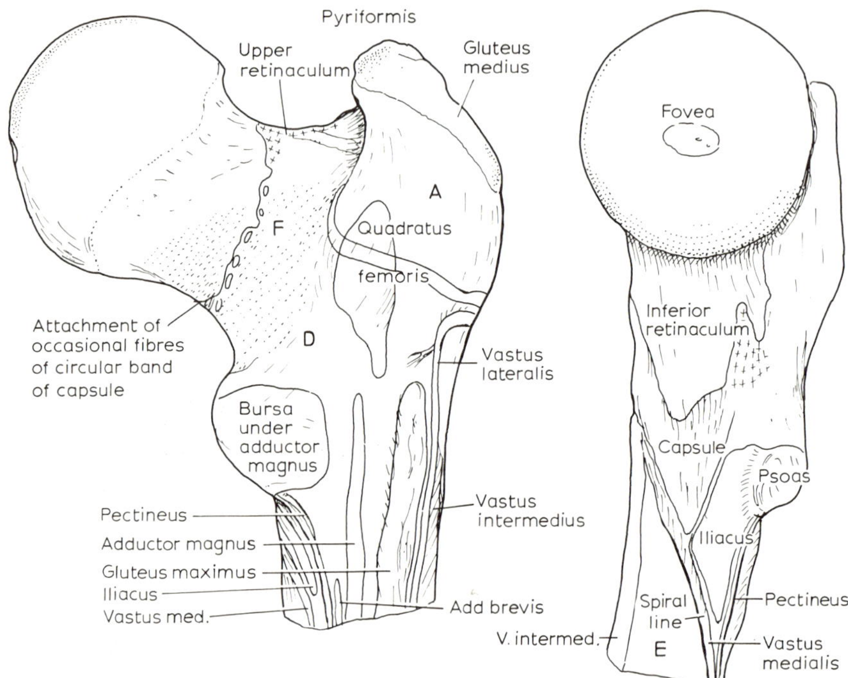

FIG. 1.3*b* The posterior aspect with surface (D) covered by the quadratus femoris. Deep to this muscle, the obturator externus lies against the bone, moulding the back and lower part of the neck in the area (F) as it passes to the trochanteric fossa. The medial aspect shows the surface (E) covered by the vastus medialis but not giving an origin to it; while the vastus intermedius does not transgress the medial border. (Reproduced by the kind permission from Frazer's Anatomy of the Human Skeleton.)

slide through the cortex of the shaft, while preparing the neck for an endoprosthesis. The trabecular arrangement is discussed under the section 'Biomechanics'. The anterior surface of the neck is intracapsular but only half of the posterior. A faint groove crosses the posterior surface. It is produced by the obturator externus tendon as it passes to the trochanteric fossa. This tendon can become impacted in the fracture line. The capsule is reflected along the neck as retinacular fibres, while the synovial membrane is blended with the attenuated periosteum. The paucity of the latter is responsible for the lack of periosteal callus after femoral neck fractures.

The upper border of the greater trochanter lies one hand's breadth below the tubercle on the iliac crest and is on a level with the centre of the femoral head. It forms an important landmark for all surgical

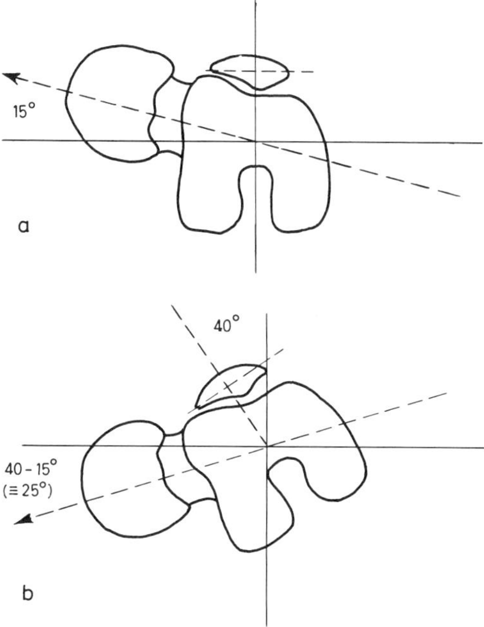

FIG. 1.4 The angle of femoral torsion is shown in the neutral position (a) and with the limb in internal rotation (b).

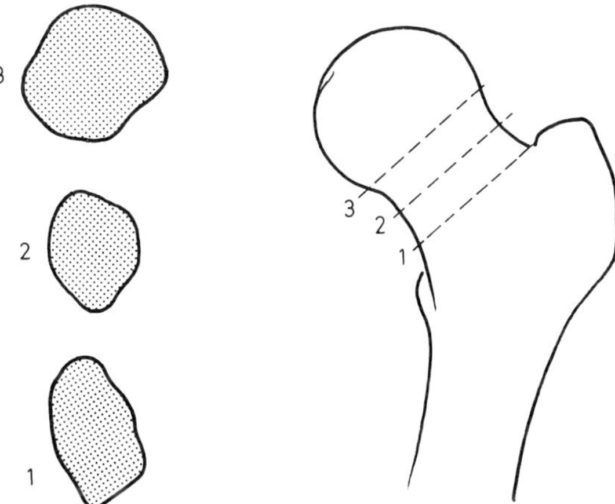

FIG. 1.5 The variations in the shape of the femoral neck are depicted at three levels. (Reproduced by permission of J.M.G. Viera, *Epifiolise Superior do femur*, Medical Faculty, Lisbon, 1972.)

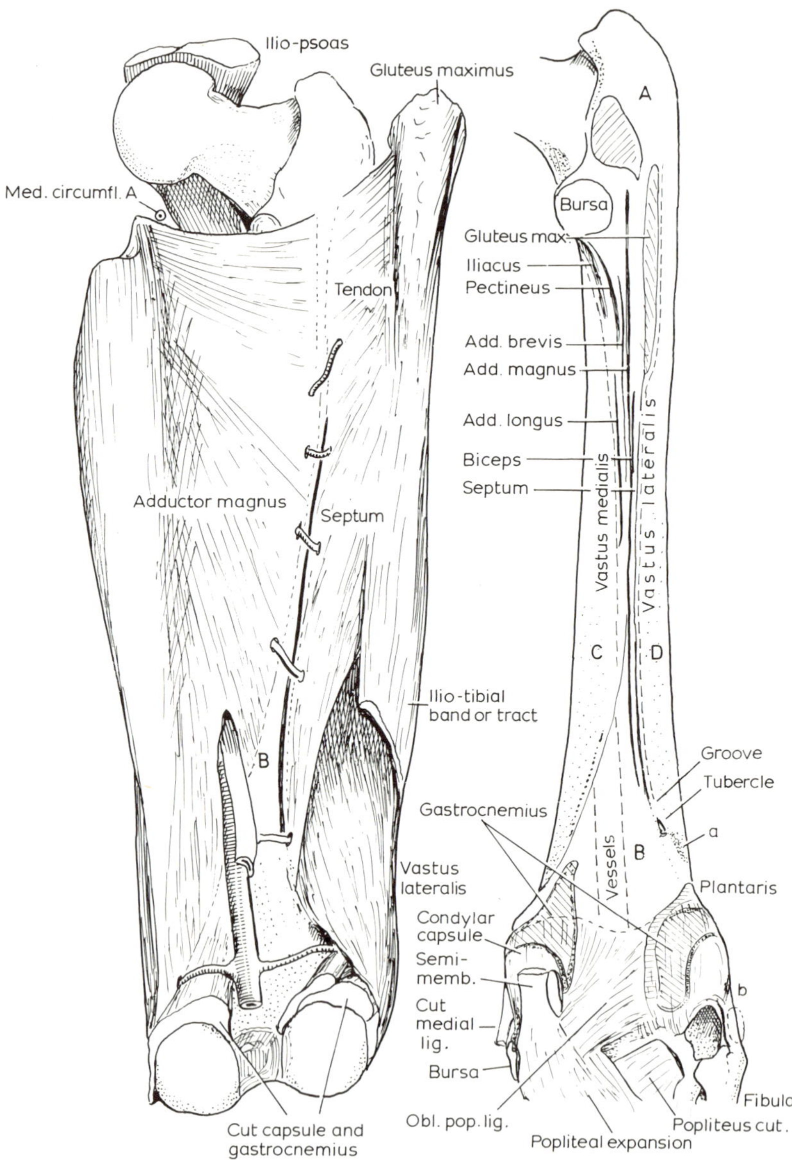

FIG. 1.6 The posterior aspect of the right femur. (A) is covered by the gluteus maximus, (B) by the popliteal surface; (C) and (D) are covered by the vastus medialis and lateralis respectively. (Reproduced by kind permission from Frazer's Anatomy of the Human Skeleton.)

approaches. The greater trochanter provides insertion for most of the muscles of the gluteal region (Fig. 1.3). In the elderly it may have cortical bone so attenuated that it resembles a cyst filled with fat and a few trabeculae.

The lesser trochanter is placed too deeply to be palpated. Its apex and anterior portion are roughened for the insertion of the psoas major tendon, and the base expanded for the iliacus insertion. The shaft is covered, except on the linea aspera, by the knee extensors. The vastus lateralis arises in front of the greater trochanter and follows it to the upper end of the gluteal tuberosity (Fig. 1.6), which receives the lower portion of gluteus maximus. The junction between the vastus lateralis and the abductors of the hip is a triangular area filled with fatty tissue and forms an important access point during the lateral exposure. The vastus medialis, although covering the medial surface of the shaft, does not take its origin from it, but protects the profunda femoris artery which may be traumatized by drills or screws protruding from the medial side of the shaft.

The capsule

Anteriorly this structure reaches the intertrochanteric line, but posteriorly it extends only half-way down the neck. The capsule is made up of dense, fibrous tissue reinforced anteriorly by the sturdy ilio-femoral ligament of Bigelow (Fig. 1.1), below by the pubo-femoral condensation, and posteriorly by the thin ischio-femoral element. The zone orbicularis is a condensed group of deeply placed circular fibres which reinforce the action of the labrum. The femoral attachment of the capsule is reinforced by fibrous extensions into the many vascular foramina at the base of the neck. Some of the innermost fibres are reflected in a medial direction as retinacula on to the neck, along which they pass to the subcapital articular sulcus. Covered by synovial membrane these retinacular fibres are concentrated superiorly, inferiorly and occasionally anteriorly, and they provide a relatively safe passage for the blood vessels of the femoral head.

Fascia

The deep fascia of the thigh ensheathes the muscles like a well-fitting stocking. Distally it blends with the deep fascia of the leg and proximally it is attached to the iliac crest, the inguinal ligament, the ischio-pubic ramus and the sacrotuberous ligament. A thick condensation on the lateral side forms the ilio-tibial band, which splits into two layers at its proximal end to receive the insertion of the tensor fasciae latae and three-fourths of the gluteus maximus. The fascia also passes as intermuscular septa to the femoral shaft; one condensation passing from the anterior margin of the abductors to the ilio-femoral ligament, contains the ascending branches of the lateral circumflex vessels. The aponeurotic insertion for tensor and gluteus maximus slides freely over the greater trochanter as evidenced by a large bursa.

Muscles

Anteriorly the sartorius, adductor longus and the inguinal ligament outline the femoral triangle, with the iliopsoas as part of the floor, separating the femoral vessels and nerve from the hip. The iliopsoas may overlie a bursa which in 10% of cases communicates with the joint. The obturator nerve is not found in the triangle until the adductor longus is artificially separated from the pectineus. The gluteus maximus is a thick, coarse-fibred muscle; all of the superficial layer and the proximal part of the deep layer is inserted into the ilio-tibial tract, while the remaining deep portion joins the gluteal tuberosity (Fig. 1.6). The inferior gluteal nerve breaks up rapidly into smaller branches on entering the muscle and the posterior cutaneous nerve of the thigh adheres to the deep aspect but is separated by fatty tissue from the sciatic nerve and external rotators. Of the latter muscles the piriformis passes through the greater sciatic foramen with the superior gluteal neurovascular bundle above it. In the buttock the gluteus maximus and piriformis cover the sciatic nerve. The gluteus medius and minimus pass from the dorsum ilii to the greater trochanter (Fig. 1.2) and cover the superior and lateral aspect of the joint. The adductors clothe the inferior aspect (Fig. 1.6).

SURGICAL APPROACHES TO THE HIP

There are three basic approaches: anterior, posterior and lateral.

Anterior approaches

Tronzo (1973) lists six main anterior approaches, but the Smith-Petersen approach (sometimes called the antero-lateral approach) (Fig. 1.7) gives excellent access. The incision passes from just below the iliac crest to the anterior superior spine and then vertically for 4–5 inch. The fascia is divided and the muscles innervated by the

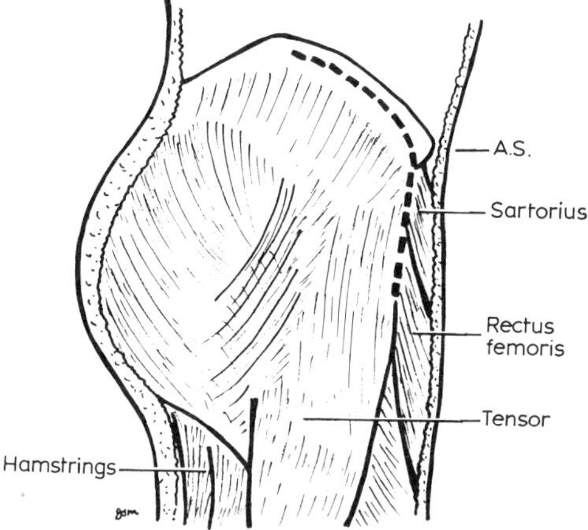

FIG. 1.7 The Smith-Petersen's approach to the hip joint.

superior gluteal nerve (tensor, gluteus medius and minimus) are dissected subperiosteally in a single flap from the iliac crest as far posteriorly as necessary. The periosteal elevator follows the surface of the ilium and bleeding is controlled by packing. The dissection continues in the vertical plane between the tensor laterally and the sartorius and rectus femoris medially. The ascending branch of the lateral femoral circumflex artery is ligated and the lateral femoral cutaneous nerve is retracted medially before capsulotomy of the hip is performed. If required the direct and reflected head of the rectus may be divided.

The true anterior approach is merely this approach without the subperiosteal flap and the incision begins at the anterior superior spine. Thus it is somewhat limited in its application.

Posterior approaches

Eleven posterior approaches have been tabulated by Tronzo (1973). The skin incisions are essentially similar and lie parallel to the fibres of the gluteus maximus, with an extension from the greater trochanter along the lateral proximal shaft of femur. The following approaches are commonly employed.

The Kocher approach, modified by Gibson (1950) causes minimal damage to the soft tissues and has the advantage of providing dependent drainage. The proximal limb of the incision begins 2.5–3 inch in front of the posterior superior iliac spine (Fig. 1.8) and passes downwards

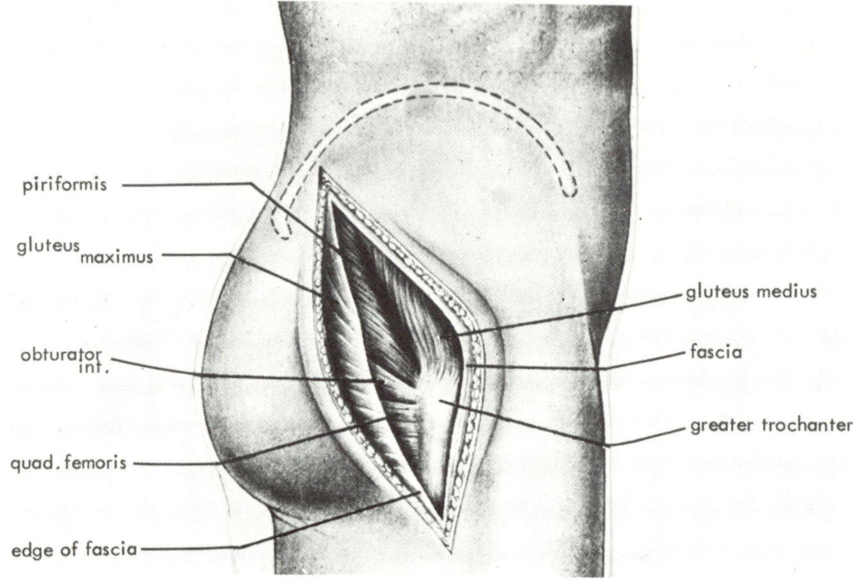

FIG. 1.8 The Kocher approach (modified by Gibson). (After Henry, 1957.)

and laterally to the upper border of the greater trochanter; from there it is carried distally in the line of the thigh. The deep fascia is incised and the upper border of gluteus maximus defined. Flaps are developed by cutting the insertion of this muscle into the ilio-tibial tract and femur. The fleshy and aponeurotic mass is retracted to expose the whole range of subgluteal muscles (Fig. 1.9). The abductors can be detached at their tendinous insertion and retracted anteriorly. The piriformis insertion is cut and, if necessary, the other short external rotators excluding the quadratus femoris. The capsule is clearly exposed and can be incised as required.

The external rotators require repair with interrupted silk or dexon sutures, and it is important to insert stay-sutures in the muscles or their tendinous origins before division, and to mark these sutures with artery clips. Occasionally their insertion can be split with an osteotome, and the thin layer of bone reattached with wires or screws.

Osborne (1930) used an incision from a point 1.75 inch below the posterior superior iliac spine to the postero-superior angle of the greater trochanter and then distally for 2 inch. The gluteus maximus fibres are spread bluntly and the short external rotators divided at their insertion into the femur.

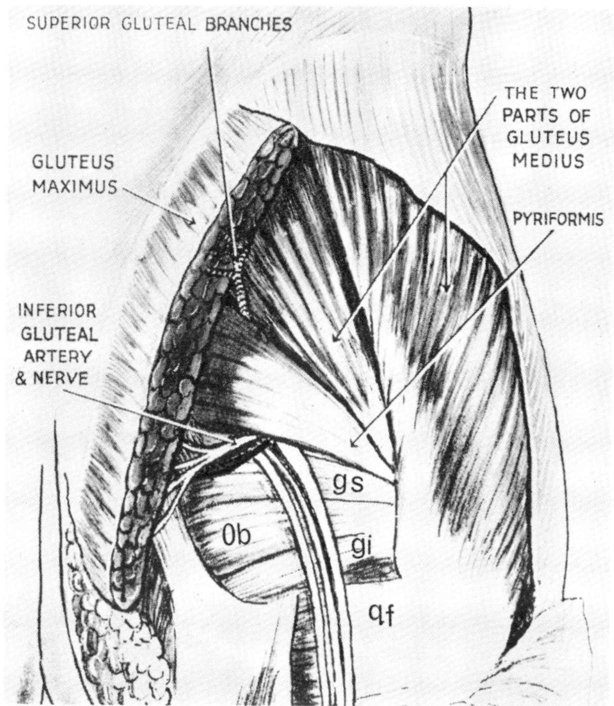

FIG. 1.9 The structures at risk during the posterior approach. Gemellus superior (gs), obturator internus (Ob) and gemellus inferior (gi) are closely related to the sciatic nerve and inferior gluteal vessels. Quadratus femoris (qf), adductor magnus and the origin of the hamstrings are shown. (After Henry, 1957.)

Crenshaw (1971) describes the 'southern exposure' or 'Moore approach' to the hip. The incision begins 4 inch below the posterior superior iliac spine (i.e. lower than the 'Osborne' incision) and extends distally and laterally parallel with the fibres of gluteus maximus to the posterior margin of the lesser trochanter (Fig. 1.10). Then the incision is extended along the femoral shaft for 4–5 inch. The fascia is divided and the fibres of the gluteus maximus split, taking care not to damage the superior gluteal vessels. The upper fibres of gluteus maximus are retracted to expose the greater trochanter, while the lower fibres are split off the linea aspera. The sciatic nerve is exposed and retracted carefully. The external rotators are divided and capsule incised following the long axis of the femoral neck.

Many of thc modifications of the posterior approaches are so slight as hardly to merit the description of a new technique. This approach

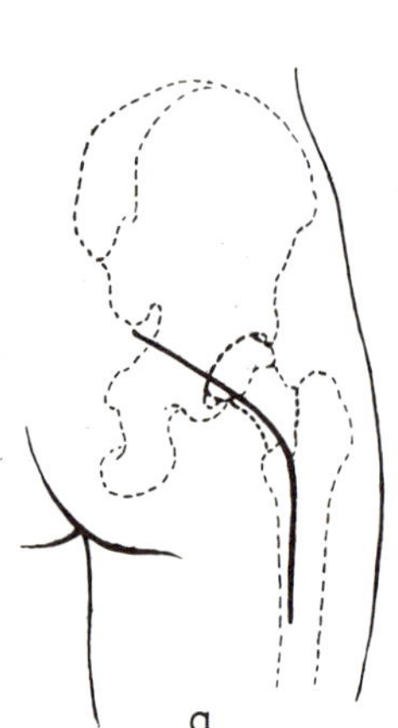

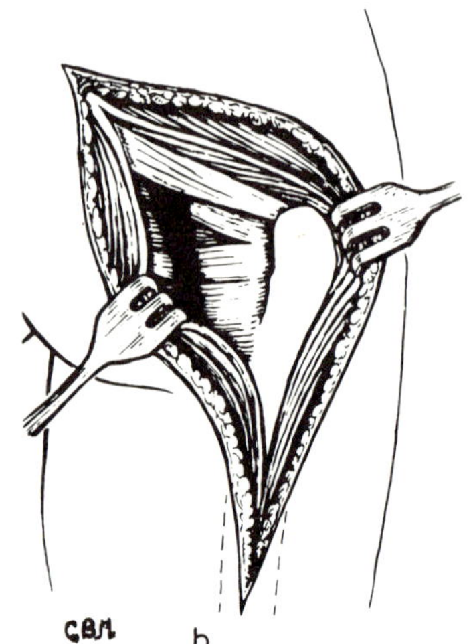

FIG. 1.10 The 'southern exposure'. (The sciatic nerve is identified as the dark structure crossing the external rotators.)

gives excellent access to the femoral head but a restricted approach to the acetabulum. Pressure on the wound area from prolonged recumbency can cause problems, while if the elderly patient sits out of bed too soon dehiscence of the muscle sutures and dislocation of the prosthesis may result.

Lateral approaches

Tronzo (1973) lists eight lateral approaches, many of which are well documented in Crenshaw (1971) and Henry (1957).

The Watson–Jones approach (Fig. 1.11) (or its modifications) is popular and uses an incision beginning 1 inch distal and lateral to the anterior superior iliac spine. It is extended distally over the lateral aspect of the greater trochanter and for a further 2–3 inch along the femoral shaft. The fascia lata is incised in the line of the incision and, if necessary, the interval between the abductors and tensor found. The dissection is carried forward by excision of a pad of fat, thus exposing the anterior aspect of the hip joint. In order to facilitate exposure, the origin of vastus lateralis may be reflected or the anterior fibres of the abductor tendon detached from the greater trochanter.

This exposure is well suited for pin and plate fixation but gives limited access for prosthetic replacement.

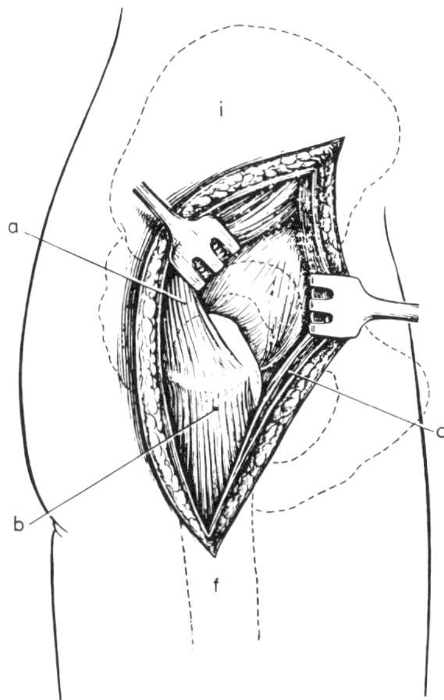

FIG. 1.11 The Watson–Jones approach. A lateral approach exposing (a) the abductors, (b) vastus lateralis and (c) tensor.

The approach described by McKee and Watson-Farrar (1966) gives excellent access to the acetabulum. The incision begins at the anterior superior iliac spine, and extends towards the tip of the greater trochanter and for 2–3 inch along the femoral shaft, with a slight curve anteriorly. The interval between tensor and gluteus minimus and medius is opened to reveal the capsule. The plane of cleavage is easily found distally where, after incision of the deep fascia, it is located by the finger. Proximally, the muscles are intimately blended and need separation by sharp dissection. Once these muscles have been separated the outer aspect of the wing of the ilium is partly cleared of muscle attachments. The capsule of the hip joint is now clearly visible, as is the reflected head of rectus femoris, which is excised with the anterior half of the capsule. Once this has been cleared the head of the femur is dislocated, and the head and neck removed with a Gigli saw.

All the lateral exposures involve a route between the tensor fasciae latae and the abductor muscles. Some approaches require detachment of the abductors by an osteotomy of the greater trochanter (popularized in the Charnley method of total hip arthroplasty). Thc skin incisions also vary considerably, including the U-shaped Ollier incision and the goblet extension of Murphy. However, of the many lateral approaches, the Watson–Jones approach and the McKee–Farrar approach are to be recommended.

BLOOD SUPPLY TO THE FEMORAL HEAD

An interruption in the blood supply to the femoral head is one of the most serious complications of femoral neck fractures; indeed, an understanding of the vascularity of this area is essential to appreciate the problem of avascular necrosis of the femoral head.

Fig. 1.12 outlines the anastomotic arrangement around the upper femur, the vascular loops ensuring an adequate blood supply to the hip during all positions of the joint. There are numerous anastomoses connecting periosteal and endosteal capillaries. The vessels of the femoral neck are disposed along the retinacular fibres of the capsule. Shortly before the articular margin they enter the foraminae in the cortex and reach the interior of the neck. Here they may communicate with the terminal branches of the nutrient artery (Fig. 1.13*a*) which usually arises from the second or third perforating branch of the profunda femoris. However, the nutrient artery does not contribute to the nutrition of the femoral head, (Tucker, 1949).

The following description of adult vessels is based on the work of

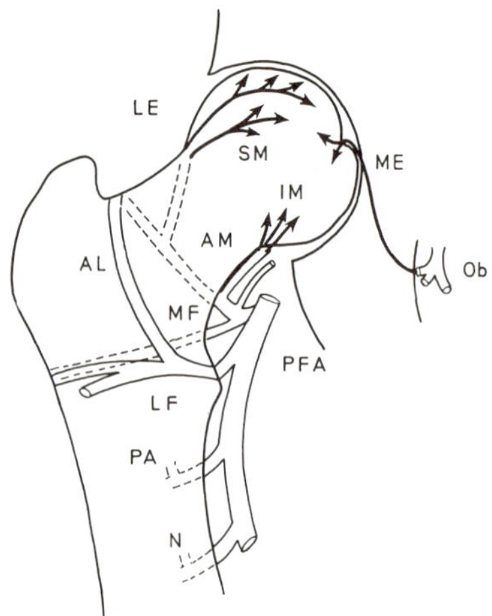

FIG. 1.12 The arterial arrangement around the upper femur. (PFA) profunda femoris; (LE) and (ME) lateral and medial epiphyseal; (Ob) obturator; (SM) and (IM) superior and inferior metaphyseal; (PA) perforating artery; (N) nutrient; (AM) and (AL) ascending branches of circumflex vessels; (MF) medial circumflex femoral and (LF) lateral circumflex femoral.

Trueta and Harrison (1953) which is a classical monograph on the subject. Since the vascular pattern established during the phases of growth is not replaced at maturity, but largely persists throughout life, the basic arrangement is one of an epiphyseal and metaphyseal circulation, even when the growth plate has disappeared. By reference to the site of entry (Fig. 1.13*b*) the epiphyseal arteries are named lateral and medial; and the metaphyseal arteries superior and inferior. The lateral epiphyseal and both metaphyseal arteries arise from the medial circumflex artery; the medial epiphyseal is usually a continuation of the artery of the ligamentum teres (which arises from the acetabular branch of the obturator artery).

The lateral epiphyseal arteries are the most important. They supply two-thirds of the femoral head, and since they are intimately applied to the posterior and superior aspects of the femoral neck, they are commonly torn in displaced subcapital fractures.

The medial epiphyseal vessels run laterally on the same level as the fovea through which they have entered, until they meet and anastomose with the lateral epiphyseal vessels.

The inferior metaphyseal arteries supply that part of the femoral head derived from the metaphysis. They enter the bone close to the inferior margin of the articular cartilage.

The superior metaphyseal vessels enter the superior aspect of the femoral neck some distance from the femoral articular margin. Before they enter the bone the metaphyseal vessels show frequent anastomoses in the subsynovial tissues.

The metaphyseal vessels are only ruptured when the displacement of the capitate fragment is quite marked. However, their rupture places the femoral head at risk since it may have to depend on the arteries of the ligamentum teres (medial epiphyseal) should the lateral epiphyseal vessels be involved.

The small arteries in the ligamentum teres are usually unable to maintain the viability of the femoral head. Sevitt and Thompson (1965) were unable to produce filling of the capital vessels after retrograde injection into the foveal vessels. Catto (1965) showed that when a greater part of the femoral head was rendered necrotic by ischaemia a small segment of bone remained viable close to the fovea. It seems, therefore, that the vessels in the ligamentum teres are seldom large enough to maintain the whole of the capitate fragment; if they were, ischaemic necrosis of the femoral head would not occur after subcapital fractures.

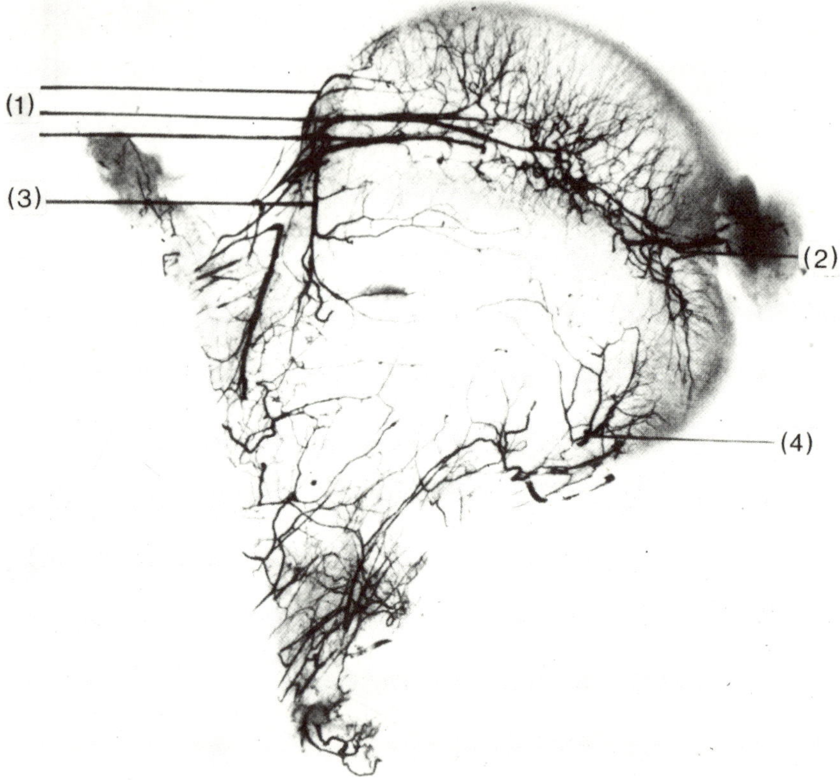

(1)

(3)

(2)

(4)

(*a*)

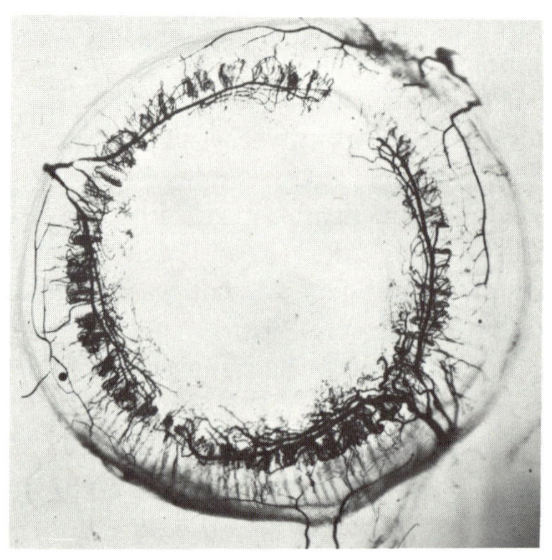

(*b*)

Trueta and Harrison (1953) were unable to find any decrease in patency of the vascular tree of the femoral neck with advancing years.

The venous outflow from the femoral head and neck has been described by Phillips, (1966). Limino-capsular veins consisting of a double or single channel course infero-medially along the trochanteric line and then towards the obturator foramen where they drain into the obturator vein. The circumflex group are found as a diffuse plexus in the basal portion of the femoral neck and greater trochanter, and pass medially to leave the femur at the level of, or just proximal to, the lesser trochanter. These veins enter the common femoral vein. Groups of smaller veins arising in the posterior aspect of the neck and greater trochanter course to plexuses in the region of the ischial tuberosity and greater sciatic notch. Slight venous drainage occurs through the veins of the linea aspera but none through the ligamentum teres.

HIP JOINT INNERVATION

The hip joint is densely innervated by primary and accessory articular nerves. The former are direct articular branches of adjacent nerve trunks, and the latter are articular twigs arising from nerves within the muscles related to the joint (Dee, 1969)

The three primary articular nerves have been called:

(a) posterior articular nerve;
(b) medial articular nerve;
(c) nerve to the ligamentum teres.

The posterior articular nerve consists of a varying number of short articular branches (approximately 6 mm long) of the nerve to quadratus femoris. These branches represent the most prolific supply of the hip joint. They pass laterally on the surface of the ischium, beneath the obturator internus tendon and gemelli muscles, to enter the posterior capsule of the joint.

The medial articular nerve usually arises as a single branch from the anterior division of the obturator nerve through its lateral branch to

---

FIG. 1.13(*a*) A coronal section of the femoral head after an injection of barium constrast medium. (1) Lateral epiphyseal arteries; (2) medial epiphyseal artery; (3) superior metaphyseal artery and (4) inferior metaphyseal artery. (From Trueta and Harrison, 1953.) [N.O.C. Photographic Dept.]

(*b*) Section across femoral neck showing retinacular vessels perforating cortex and anastomosing with medullary vessels.

pectineus and adductor muscles. This branch is distributed to the antero-medial and inferior aspects of the joint capsule (the region medial to the iliopsoas tendon).

The nerve to the ligamentum teres arises from the posterior division of the obturator nerve which supplies the obturator externus. Having passed through the acetabular notch with the articular vessels, it breaks up into fine filaments which ramify along the surface of the ligament, a few being distributed to the fat pad. Thus, the hip joint resembles the knee joint (Freeman and Wyke, 1967) in that its intra-articular ligament is provided with an independent articular nerve (as are the cruciates in the knee).

Only a very small proportion of the hip joint is innervated through accessory nerves, mainly from the femoral nerve. No primary articular nerve arises from this nerve (Dee, 1969) and the only constant femoral innervation is provided by the accessory articular branch from the nerve to pectineus.

The articular nerves contain a mixture of myelinated and unmyelinated fibres, commonly ending in fine nerve-plexuses or special end-organs. A few unmyelinated fibres end in the walls of the blood vessels and the subsynovial tissues.

THE STRUCTURE AND FUNCTION OF ARTICULAR CARTILAGE

Although a hip fracture is usually clearly seen on radiological examination, the associated articular cartilage damage has to be surmised. The exploration of injured joints has revealed minute articular cartilaginous flakes or small loose bodies. This cartilage damage is the precursor of degenerative arthorosis which may, in the long run, be more disabling than the original injury. Acute cartilage necrosis can follow slipping of the capital femoral epiphysis, with areas of denuded bone and extensive granulation tissue being formed (Maurer and Larsen, 1970).

Hyaline articular cartilage covers the femoral head and acetabulum. The cartilage on the head thins towards the periphery and terminates at the subcapital sulcus. The cartilage consists principally of long chain molecules of proteoglycan interspersed with collagen fibres. These form the matrix in which the cells (chondrocytes) are relatively sparse. Histological examination shows that there are four zones of chondro-

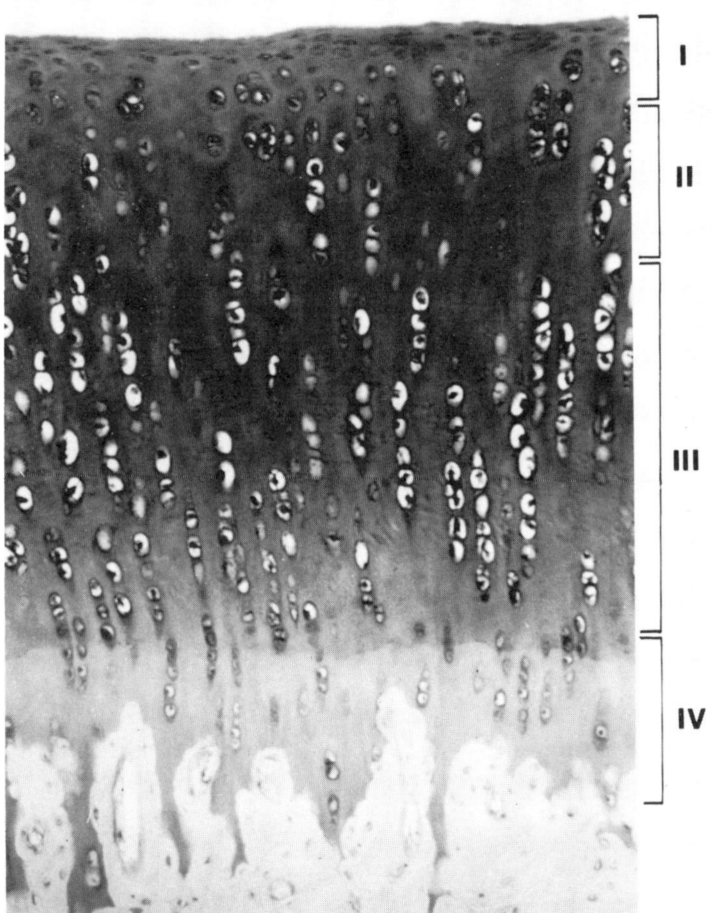

FIG. 1.14(*a*) Normal adult articular cartilage. Tangential zone (I) has oval or round cells with their long axis parallel to the surface. The transitional zone (II) has randomly arranged ovoid cells, whilst the radial zone (III) has smaller cells, basophilic and arranged in columns perpendicular to the surface. The calcified zone (IV) has irregular cells with pyknotic nuclei in lacunar spaces surrounded by calcium salts, probably hydroxyapatite. Between zones III and IV (on haematoxylin and eosin staining) is a thin, basophilic wavy line, named the 'tide mark' which is probably a calcification front. x 20

cytes (Fig. 1.14 I-IV) and there are differences in spatial arrangement and cellular morphology in each zone.

Articular cartilage has a structure similar to a sponge. There is a collagen meshwork of fibres supported by proteoglycan and water, which, together with the cells, fill the interstices of the mesh. There is

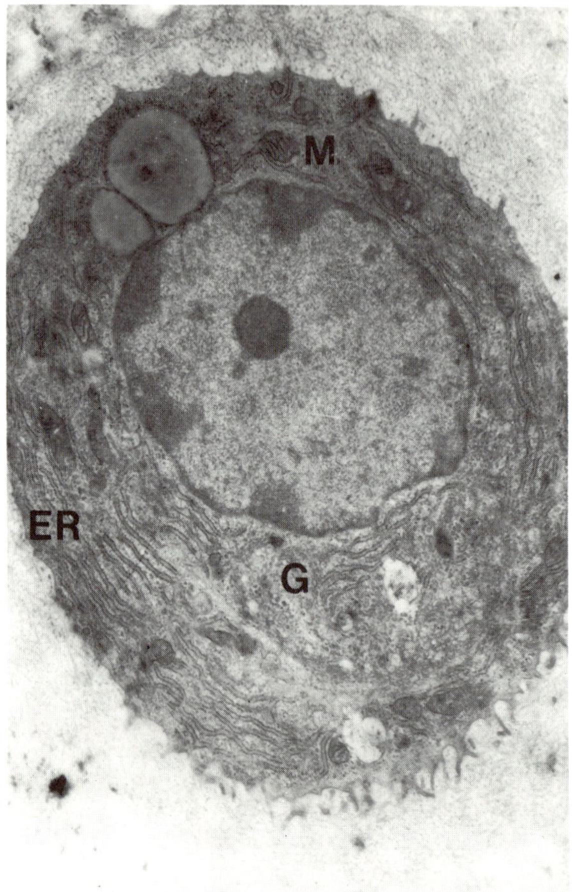

FIG. 1.14(*b*) Electron micrograph study of a typical chondrocyte from zone II. The endoplasmic reticulum (ER), mitochondria (M) and Golgi apparatus (G) indicate an actively synthesizing cell.

an oblique criss-cross pattern of fibres running from the calcified zone through the cartilage to a tightly-packed superficial layer of finer fibres at the surface, which corresponds to the 'lamina splendens' seen in histology (Fig. 1.15). In normal situations a layer of hyaluronic acid is bound to the surface of the articular cartilage and is essential for lubrication. Living cartilage, capable of absorbing and losing fluids, displays a temporary swelling in response to exercise. The elastic behaviour of cartilage is largely dependent on the water content and, indirectly the glycosaminoglycan content because the latter component of the proteoglycan holds the water in a gel by the presence

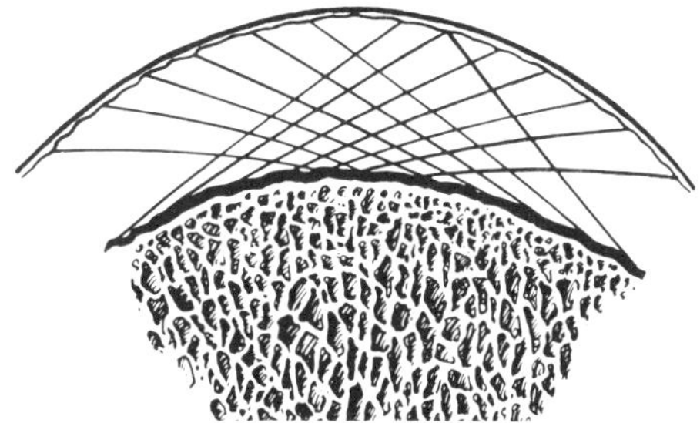

FIG. 1.15 The criss-cross arrangement of collagen fibres in articular cartilage is shown. The fibres of the superficial layer are only 40–120 Å in diameter and have a protective function. They overlie closely-packed bundles of collagen fibres 350 Å thick in zones II and III. The fibres become more parallel as they are embedded in the calcified zone.

of a strong negative charge. Thus the collagen fibres are inflated into a tense meshwork by the osmotic pressure of the glycosaminoglycans and resiliency is maintained. The amount of water declines with increasing age, so that the elasticity declines also, thus predisposing to cartilage breakdown. The pattern of the collagen is ideal for withstanding the compression and shearing stresses during hip movements; most are absorbed in the criss-cross zone II.

NUTRITION IN ARTICULAR CARTILAGE

In immature articular cartilage nutrients enter via both vascular channels from the subchondral bones and via the synovial fluid. After maturity it appears that in the majority of species the nutrient route is via the synovial fluid only (McKibben, 1968). There has been a demonstration of channels between the subchondral bone and the basal zone of articular cartilage in the adult human femur and this may be another route for nutrients in the hip which is not present in other joints (Greenwald and Haynes, 1969).

METABOLISM OF ARTICULAR CARTILAGE

The inability of mature cartilage to repair after injury had been attributed to the low metabolic rate of this tissue. This assumption is false. With the advent of radioisotope studies it has been demonstrated that chondrocytes are not metabolically inert but carry out synthetic activities (e.g. the synthesis of proteoglycans and glycosaminoglycans) as well as the maintenance and degradation of the extracellular matrix components. Mankin (1968) has shown that the rates of synthesis of these constituents are more rapid in immature cartilage, declining at maturity, when the half-life of glycosaminoglycans is between 150 and 200 days (Maroudas, 1973). Synthesis is inhibited by cortisone derivatives, nitrogen mustard and by antimetabolites. It is moderately increased for a short period of two or three weeks by lacerative injury of the cartilage. Mankin has suggested that the matrix turnover maintains the hygroscopic nature of the proteoglycan and hence the water content of cartilage.

LYSOSOMES IN ARTICULAR CARTILAGE

The presence of a system within cartilage capable of splitting proteoglycan at or near the protein–sugar bond was detected by Fell and Dingle (1963). Subsequently the nature of this system was revealed with a demonstration of enzymes from the intracellular lysosomes named Cathepsin B and Cathepsin D, which produce an effect on proteoglycans alone, and not on collagen, of articular cartilage. Under the influence of compression-shearing stress in the hip, damaged cells in zone II release cathepsins from lysosomes. This causes loss of glycosaminoglycans and water, and hence produces loss of resiliency of the cartilage. Thus fissures occur with continued load-bearing, and this results in further cell damage and cathepsin release, in a continuing cycle (Fig. 1.16). The extent of breakdown is related to the extent of

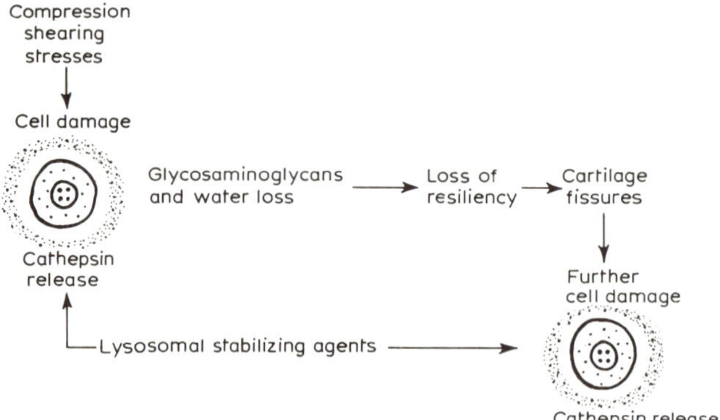

FIG. 1.16 A scheme illustrating the probable mechanism of matrix breakdown occurring after injury to articular cartilage and the potential role of lysosomal-stabilizing agents in its prevention.

damage to the articular surfaces, and will be maximal after comminuted fractures of the femoral head and acetabulum.

LYSOSOMAL-STABILIZING AGENTS

An obvious way of preserving articular cartilage from the damaging effects of lysosomal enzymes following injury would be to inhibit their release. Various agents have been shown to stabilize lysosomes although the extent of their effect on articular cartilage is as yet unknown. These agents are glucocorticoids, chloroquine, inorganic gold salts, indomethacin, colchicine, phenylbutazone and acetylsalicylic acid. The most interesting and potentially useful therapeutic agent is aspirin which appears to inhibit breakdown of cartilage following experimentally-induced damage (Simmons and Chrisman, 1965; Forney *et al.*, 1973).

REPAIR OF CARTILAGE

The repair of articular cartilage in the hip is limited. Mature chondrocytes divide infrequently, if at all, and although they can be induced to do so for short periods by matrix damage such as that produced by laceration, compression, exposure to the enzyme papain or osteoarthrosis, the effect appears to be too small and ill-sustained to repair any but the smallest defects. Yablon *et al.* (1974) found an apparent stimulation of chondrocyte division and matrix collagen production in experimental situations after administering a growth hormone. It is important to realize that if cartilage damage is deep enough to involve subchondral bone then the repair of the surface may occur by filling the defect with granulation tissue from subchondral marrow. This may undergo metaplasia to fibro-cartilage, and in the case of a small defect, to hyaline cartilage. Thus good results can accrue from the accurate reduction of an intra-articular fracture as distinct from widely-separated fragments.

CARTILAGE GRAFTING

Allografts of articular cartilage and subchondral bone have been used experimentally to replace damaged joint surfaces. Such grafts have been moderately successful in the hips and knees of animals but failed in the human situation because of fixation problems, rejection and

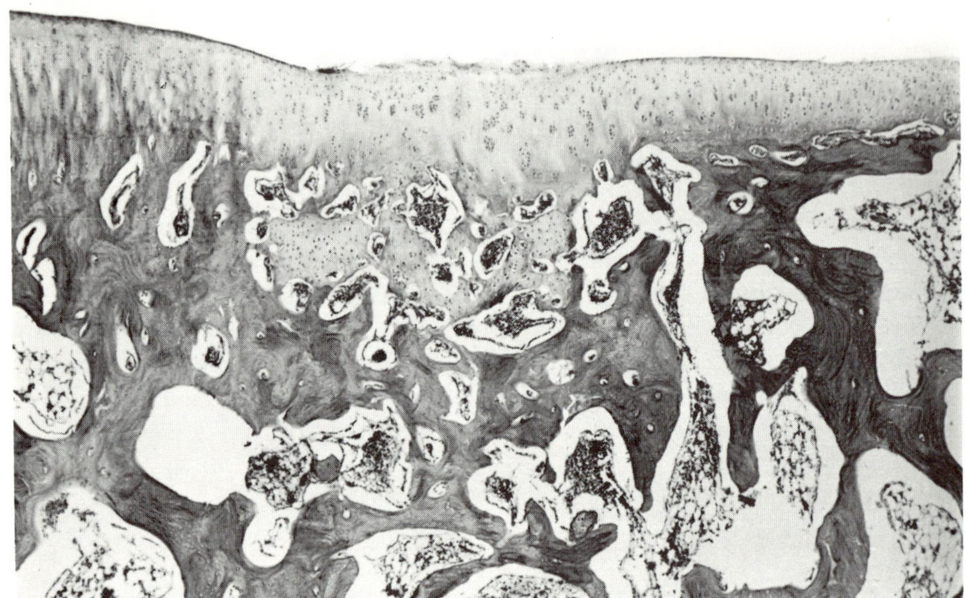

FIG. 1.17 Photomicrograph of the articular surface of a mature rabbit 8 weeks after an allograft of freshly isolated epiphyseal chondrocytes into a drill hole in the surface. The filling of the defect by cartilage and incorporation into the host tissue is apparent. (H and E x 10)

mismatching. Another approach has been carried out by Chesterman and Smith (1968), Bentley and Greer (1971) and Bentley (1972). Cartilage cells were isolated from the epiphyseal growth plate of animals and transplanted, in suspension, to defects in the articular cartilage of recipient animals and the defects were filled without host rejection (Fig. 1.17). This method may have clinical applications if long term storage of chondrocytes becomes feasible.

Conclusions

After a hip injury one must be aware of the associated articular cartilage damage (Fig. 1.18). Isolated lesions of the cartilage have been described without bone damage (Crock, 1964). Also trauma may aggravate a primary degenerative condition which is not yet radiologically apparent. Accurate reduction of disrupted surfaces is needed to achieve maximum function, and early non-weight-bearing exercises will help to prevent stiffness and aid cartilage nutrition.

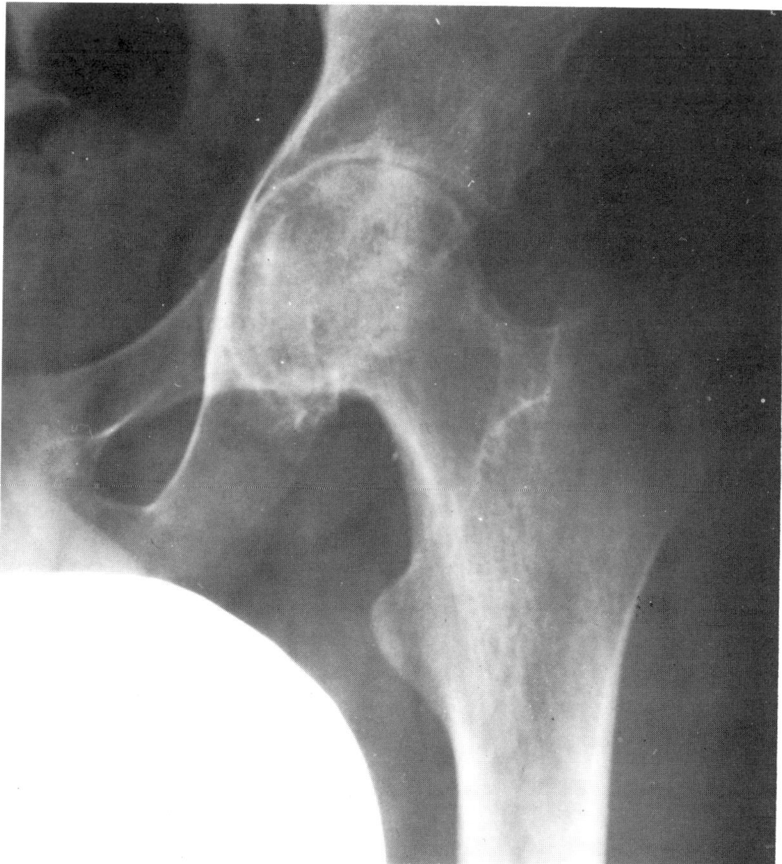

FIG. 1.18 Radiograph of the left hip in a man of 18 years who 10 months previously sustained a degloving injury of the lower leg and a fracture-dislocation of the ankle. Despite the absence of symptoms and signs at the time of injury, 10 months later pain and stiffness persisted in the hip due to articular cartilage damage.

BIOMECHANICS OF THE HIP IN RELATION TO HIP FRACTURES

The hip is a ball and socket joint and thus has inherent structural bony stability, relying less on the ligaments and muscles than in other joints, such as the knee. A ball and socket provides multiaxial freedom of movement, which in some measure provides protection from sudden stresses. However, the bony constraint means that forces will be transmitted directly to the skeleton thus producing a variety of injury patterns. The advantage of this bony constraint is the stability gained for walking and transferring from a standing to a sitting posture.

A fracture disrupts the supporting structures and therefore eliminates the functional performance of the hip joint. The aim of all treatment is to provide support and anatomical realignment of the skeletal parts while healing takes place and function can be restored.

BASIC STRUCTURE

Bone

Bone has a vital role to play in providing the essential supporting framework and locations for muscle attachments. It consists of cortical and cancellous parts, each of which has distinct mechanical properties. The cortical bone is a more solid and rigid structure, and it is anisotropic, a feature which makes the analysis of physical properties difficult.

In 1867 Von Meyer and Culmann, an anatomist and an engineer, compared the trabecular arrangement of the cancellous bone within the neck of the femur to a Fairbairn crane and from this developed the stress trajectorial theory of bone formation (Fig. 1.19). There are differing proportions of cortical and cancellous bone in the trochanteric region compared with the neck region. It is generally regarded that

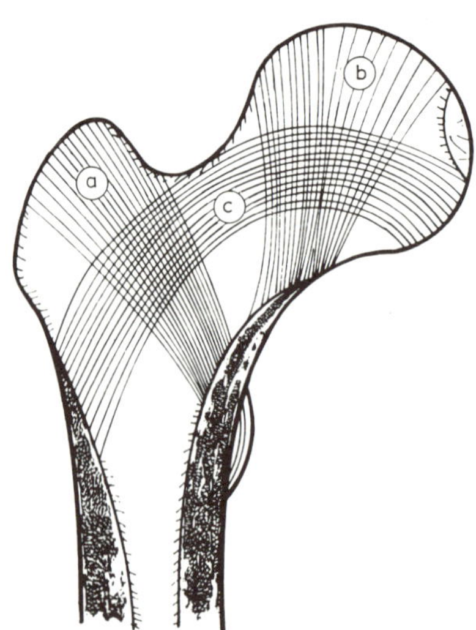

FIG. 1.19 The principal trabeculae in the femoral neck are arranged into three distinct bundles, (a) the lateral; (b) the medial and (c) the arcuate system. (From '*Studies on the Anatomy and Function of Bones and Joints*' ed. F. Gaynor Evans, p. 55.)

95% of bone tissue in the neck is of the cortical variety whereas the ratio is reversed in the trochanteric region.

The work of Paul (1965) on calculations of the direction and magnitude of forces passing through the femoral head during walking, using standard gait analysis techniques, and the more direct measurement of an instrumented Austin Moore prosthesis by Rydell (1966), which produced similar figures, determined for the first time that the trabecular pattern within the head and neck of the femur did correspond to the calculated loading. The medial trabecular system has always been regarded as a compression system in response to the maximum resultant compressive load. The lateral trabecular system was originally thought to have been laid down in accordance with Woolf's law (1870) as a result of tensile stresses. However, more recent work shows that the cortical shell of the femoral neck is in fact entirely in compression, the maximum compression being on the medial aspect, corresponding to the medial trabecular pattern, diminishing down to a very low compressive stress on the lateral aspect of the femoral cortical neck (Frankel, 1960).

Under normal physiological conditions, there is no tension in the femoral neck, and the original neutral axis of the neck of the femur as proposed by Koch (1917) does not exist. Only if the loading of the head and neck is in an unphysiological position, for instance increased varus, will an element of tension be occurring in the lateral and superior aspects of the femoral neck (Fig. 1.20). Thus, compression is the major loading configuration of the bone of the upper end of the femur with tension only in abnormal situations. Because of the multiaxial freedom in a low friction system within the joint, torsion of the femoral neck is negligible.

Articular cartilage

Cartilage is important in load transmission and energy absorption through the joint and in lubrication. Greenwald (1970) has demonstrated the contact areas in the hip joint, and the importance of incongruence between the articular surfaces has been stressed by Bullough *et al.* (1958).

The coefficient of friction between two bearing articular cartilage surfaces is in the range of 0.005–0.01 (Linn, 1967). In order to achieve this most advantageous level, which reduces wear to an absolute minimum, a number of theories have been put forward. A summary of the likely mechanisms is in Fig. 1.21. The low friction between the

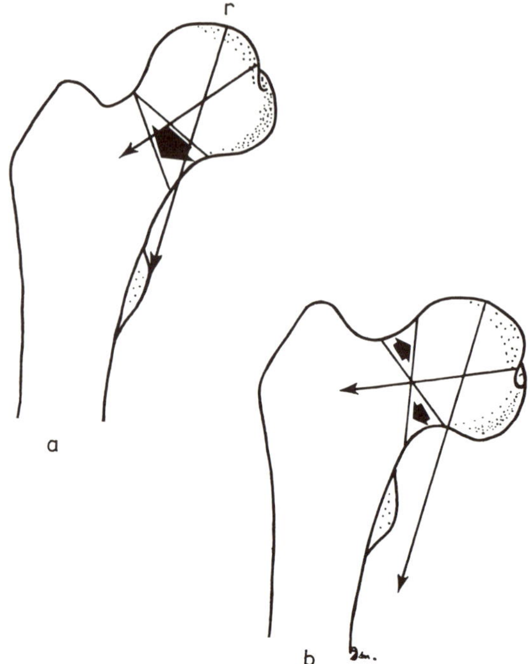

FIG. 1.20 (*a*) A diagram illustrating that in the physiological situation, the neck of the femur is normally in a state of compression, maximal medially.

(*b*) Only in non-physiological situations, such as coxa vara, does the loading on the femoral neck exhibit tension on the lateral side.

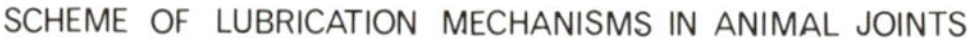

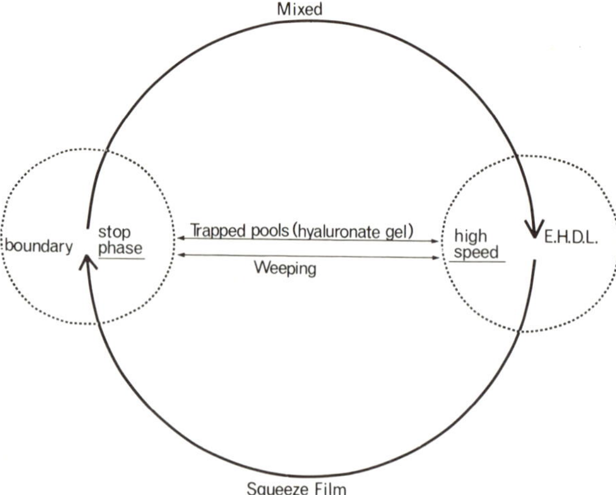

FIG. 1.21 A suggested summary of the likely lubrication mechanisms that are occurring in human synovial joints. (From Duthie and Ferguson '*Mercer's Orthopaedic Surgery*', 7th edn., p. 82.)

bearing surface means that little energy can be absorbed here and this will increase the demand for energy absorption in the bone itself.

Muscles and ligaments

The complex arrangement of the muscles and ligaments around the hip have been detailed in the section on anatomy. As well as providing voluntary movements these structures have a very important function in preventing abnormal movements, providing proprioceptive information and absorbing energy after a fall.

The initial position of the hip joint has a marked influence on the action of adjacent muscles. Starting from extension the glutei medius and minimus produce abduction of the hip, although the anterior fibres may aid in internal rotation and the posterior in external rotation; and the obturator internus is an external rotator. However, commencing in flexion, the same glutei now produce internal rotation and the obturator internus has become an abductor with the gluteus maximus, normally a powerful extensor. The external rotators are practically three times more powerful than the internal rotators but internal rotation is reinforced by hip flexion. The short pericapsular muscles are more important as postural muscles and stabilizers, reinforcing the ligaments and capsule to which they are often attached, than as prime movers of the joint.

The longitudinal fibres of the capsule are relaxed during hip flexion but become twisted and taut when the hip is in full extension, limiting that movement by torsional impaction of the femoral head into the acetabulum and producing close apposition.

Hip joint forces

When the hip joint is considered as a whole, it is seen that the forces involved are generated from two main sources, the body weight on the hip joint itself, and the muscles acting across the joint. The movements produced by muscle action during normal activities such as walking are quite considerable, and provide a large magnification factor to the body weight applied directly on the joint.

The magnitude of the hip joint force can be seen in Fig. 1.22 taken from Paul's work. It is seen that in level walking, peak loads as much as 5-6 times weight are occurring in the hip. This high level of loading accounts for many of the problems associated with hip fractures.

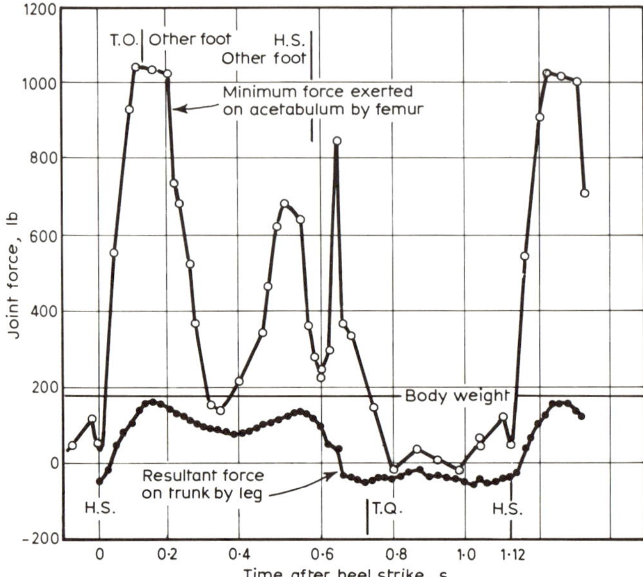

FIG. 1.22 Graph of the variation in hip joint force during level walking, showing peak loadings of over five times body weight. (From Paul in '*Biomechanics and Related Bioengineering Topics*', ed. R.M. Kenedi, p. 379.)

THE MECHANICS OF HIP FRACTURES

The mechanism of bone failure

A structure will fail if it suffers an overload situation. An overload situation will occur if the system is unable to absorb the energy that is applied to it. In the hip joint area this overload situation can occur as a result of a number of independent but often interrelated factors, the following being important:

(a) Falling;
(b) Impairment of energy absorbing mechanisms;
(c) Bone weakness.

Falling

In a standing position, the body possesses a considerable amount of potential energy. In falling, the potential energy changes to kinetic energy which, upon impact with the floor, must be absorbed by the structures of the body if a fracture is not to occur. There is sufficient potential energy in the standing body which, if unabsorbed on falling, could break any bone in the body. In an average sized woman, the amount of potential energy to be absorbed in a fall would be approximately 4000 kg cm, and the energy absorbing capacity of the upper end of the femur is only 60 kg cm approximately. Thus, if a bony injury is not to occur energy absorbing mechanisms must operate.

Impairment of energy absorbing mechanisms

The principal dissipation of energy is performed by active muscle contraction. This dissipation requires time and in the event of high speed trauma, there is not a sufficient period for the muscular contraction to absorb energy before overloading of the bone has occurred, and failure results. In the elderly, the neuromuscular response may be slower and thus the energy absorption may not be rapid enough to prevent a fracture. It is interesting that fractures of the neck of the femur are more common in patients with rheumatoid arthritis or diabetes mellitus, who are likely to have a neuromuscular defect (Alffram, 1964). In the elderly the normal protective muscle contraction in the event of a slip rather than a fall, may lead to an uninhibited muscle contraction around the hip joint, and produce sufficient force (i.e. more than 600 kgf) to fracture the neck of the femur without implicating any other factor.

Bone weakness

In the presence of osteoporosis, or osteomalacia, there is a reduction in strength to approximately three-quarters of normal, healthy young bone (Frankel, 1974), and a lower energy absorbing capacity to failure. Griffiths *et al.* (1971) showed that fatigue fractures can occur in elderly necks of the femur if cyclically loaded within the physiological range. Senile subcapital fractures in osteoporotic patients due to fatigue, preceded by an accumulation of isolated trabecular fatigue fractures, have been demonstrated by Freeman *et al.* (1974). Thus, fatigue of elderly bone can occur without a fall.

The patterns of femoral neck fractures

The pattern of femoral neck fracture is influenced by the resultant line of force which is applied at the moment prior to fracture. If the normal resultant line of force under physiological conditions is considered, it can be seen that this force can be resolved into one perpendicular to the axis of the femur (a bending component) and one in the line of the axis of the femoral neck (a compressive component) (see Fig. 1.23).

If the resultant line of force acting at the moment before fracture is altered from the physiological position, then the relative size of these two components will be altered. Frankel (1960) has shown experimentally that if the bending component is increased relative to the compressive component, then a transcervical fracture is likely. If the bending component is reduced relative to the compressive component a subcapital fracture with a spike, and finally a subcapital fracture, are produced. The resultant line of forces from muscle contraction alone produces a subcapital fracture experimentally; a pattern of fracture seen after an electric shock. Basal and intertrochanteric fractures have not been explained satisfactorily since they cannot be reproduced experimentally.

If a direct external force from an accident is applied along the line of the neck of the femur, then it is likely that the acetabulum will be fractured.

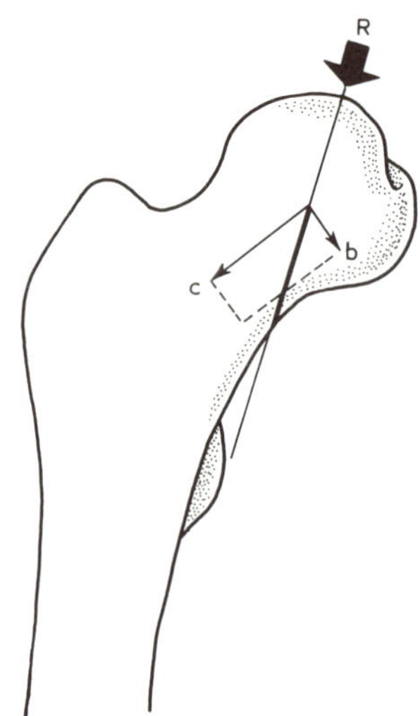

FIG. 1.23 The resultant force through the femoral head and neck can be resolved into a compressive component (*c*) in the axial line of the femoral neck, and a bending component (*b*) perpendicular to it. If the *c*/*b* ratio is less than 1.6 then a transcervical fracture is likely to occur, but if over 1.7 a subcapital fracture will occur (Frankel, 1960).

THE MECHANICS OF SURGICAL TREATMENT

When a fracture occurs the supporting role of the affected bones is lost. The general aim of any treatment is to establish an anatomical reduction which can be maintained while the bone is healing, which may be three months or more. In the hip region this presents a number of different problems, which will be amplified in relation to specific treatment for hip fractures.

Traction

Traction may be applied to the injured leg in fractures involving the acetabulum for two reasons. Firstly, by means of traction, certain fractures of the pelvis involving the joint surfaces themselves, will be aided in their anatomical reduction by this means, and following this reduction, the purpose of the traction will be to maintain load relief across the joint, thus allowing the fracture to unite without deforming forces being applied. It will also allow mobilization of the hip joint at an earlier stage, which is important if the articulating surfaces are involved. If open reduction and fixation of fragments with screws has been performed, then for protection of the screw fixation, some load relief must be achieved, as simple screws would not be able to stand the loading occurring during the normal walking cycle. Nor would they be able to stand the load across the hip joint on straight leg raising from a supine position, which is in the order of twice the body weight.

The nail and nail-plate

Fracture of the neck of the femur produces many mechanical problems. Because of the age group mostly being considered here, it is very desirable to reduce and fix the fracture to allow early mobilization out of bed, and generally to ease nursing management. In addition, it is desirable to allow weight-bearing, as many elderly patients do not find it possible to mobilize on crutches without weight-bearing. All these factors dictate a need for adequate fixation.

In the use of a nail or nail-plate, the points of fixation that have to be relied upon are the femoral head itself and the lateral cortex of the upper femur. The femoral neck itself provides very little support for any device, and thus in this method, the nail is bridging the fracture site with its support being almost entirely at each end. There must be adequate strength in the construction of the nail, as it is subjected to a considerable bending moment. The three and four-finned type of construction is generally adequate in strength and few failures occur; unless the fracture fails to unite and a true fatigue situation exists with cyclic loading over an extended period leading to fracture of the implant. This situation is seen if fixation by means of multiple Moore's or Knowle's pins is undertaken, as each of these pins does not have the strength of support and quite often one or two pins are seen to break within the normal period of bone healing at the femoral neck. This demonstrates the magnitude of the cyclic loading which is occurring

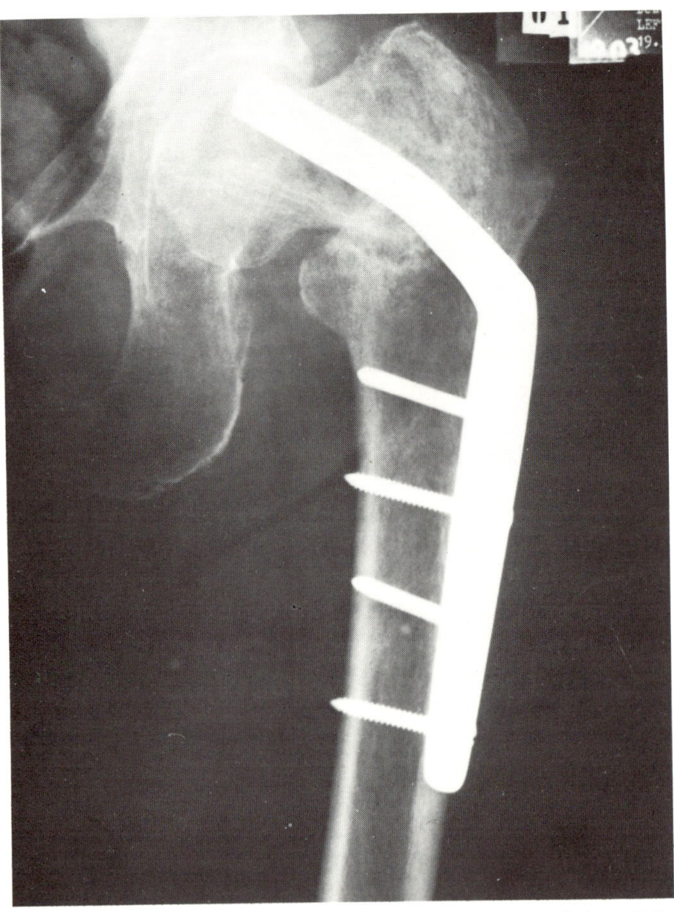

FIG. I.24 Radiograph showing bending of a nail-plate due to fatigue failure, in a situation when the fracture has failed to unite and the nail has been subjected to the entire cyclic loading of normal weight-bearing.

when a patient is mobilized at an early stage and is reliant on the fixation entirely (Fig. 1.24).

The other problem of the fixation nail is that it can back out from the lateral femoral cortex as the fracture compresses down, particularly if, at the time of operation, this compression was not achieved and the correct selection of nail length made. The backing out of the nail can be prevented by providing a plate fixed to the outer cortex of the upper femur. This is an arrangement which is standard in the treatment of inter-trochanteric type fractures, where a nail by itself would not give sufficient fixation to the distal fragment. The provision of a plate in attachment to a nail leads to some other potential mechanical problems. Firstly, if the fracture settles down and compresses on the nail, then the end of the nail may protrude through the femoral head and score the acetabulum. Some nail plate designs do provide for a collapsing or telescopic segment in the nail to prevent this eventuality. Secondly, the fixation of the nail to the plate itself, usually by means of a nut, is a potentially weak point in the entire fixation. It is here where the construction of each component is at its weakest and where failures do occur through fatigue, or simply that nut fixation becomes loose. In order to try and avoid this, single piece nail-plates, such as the Jewett or Holt, have been designed, but even these can fail if the fracture does not unite.

Thus, although more problems are likely to occur if fracture fixation is not adequate, a completely rigid fixation may also lead to problems. As the normal slight flexibility of the upper end of the femur is reduced with rigid fixation, then with cyclic loading an 'anvil' effect on the femoral head occurs which may produce collapse of the superior segment. This is just one of a number of potential difficulties which lead to late surgery being required following femoral neck fractures.

Prosthetic replacement

The earliest type of prosthetic replacement to be used on a wide scale was the Judet prosthesis, an acrylic femoral head surrounding a small metal pin. A majority of these prostheses broke in service because at the time of design the magnitude of the forces across the hip was unappreciated. Also the problems of manufacturing an integral metal and plastic one-piece prosthesis were not fully understood.

The all-metal prostheses of Austin Moore and Thompson have provided adequate strength and have largely eliminated breakages of the prosthesis in use. The transference of load through the prostheses distributed down the upper part of the femoral shaft is much more satisfactory. In the case of the Austin Moore prosthesis the fenestrations in the stem are designed so that bone will grow across and lock the prosthesis firmly into the femur. This, in most instances, does occur. However, the relative rigidity of the metal stem compared to the bone that it is within, does lead to some stress raisers at points of contact and the possibility of fracture of the bone occurring around the prosthesis (see Fig. 1.25). With the Thompson prosthesis, since the introduction of methyl methacrylate bone cement, the fixation of the femoral stem to the bone has been both immediate and more sure. This has two

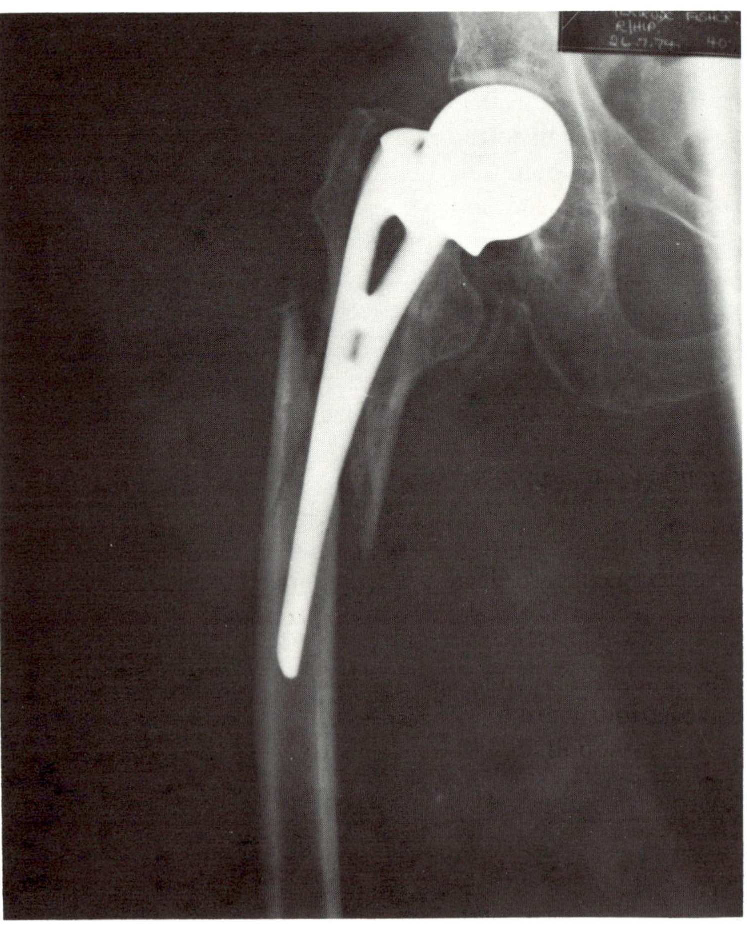

FIG. 1.25 Radiograph of a fracture of the upper end of the femur, in the subtrochanteric region with an Austin Moore prosthesis *in situ*.

advantages. Firstly, the distribution of load is taken much more evenly throughout the interface between the prosthesis stem, the cement and the bone, rather than in point contacts; and secondly, because the fixation is more sure and immediate, the possibility of movement of the prosthesis within the femoral shaft which may cause pain or incorrect placement in relation to the hip joint, is reduced.

The coefficient of friction between a metal femoral head prosthesis and articular cartilage is still very acceptable, but that between metal and subchondral bone is not. In addition, metal against bone produces pain which may be a late complication following prosthetic replacement in the fractured neck of the femur. It is fortunate that it is rare for the joint to be suffering degenerative osteoarthrosis in patients with a fractured neck of the femur, and therefore a metal upon articular cartilage articulation usually occurs, and this is likely to give a satisfactory long-term result provided the activity of the patient is not too great.

If any damage has occurred to the acetabulum, as a result of collapse of the femoral head resulting in an irregular articulation or scoring by a nail, then a simple replacement of the femoral head is not likely to produce good long-term results. In this instance, with the high mechanical efficiency of total hip replacement as well as a good predictability of the result, a total hip arthroplasty would be a more acceptable alternative.

GENERAL RADIOLOGY OF THE HIP

Accurate diagnosis of injuries in the vicinity of the hip joint is not difficult in the majority of cases provided that the radiographic examination is related to the history and clinical features.

SEVERE INJURIES

Under these conditions it is possible to miss a dislocation or a fracture/dislocation of the hip especially if there are other fractures in the affected limb. Such patients can be radiologically examined in two ways: (*a*) they can be placed on a radio-lucent stretcher over a floating-top radiography table with a movable grid which can be adjusted so as to cover all parts of the body or (*b*) the injured patient may be received on to a Kifa-type table with facilities for television fluoroscopy. This

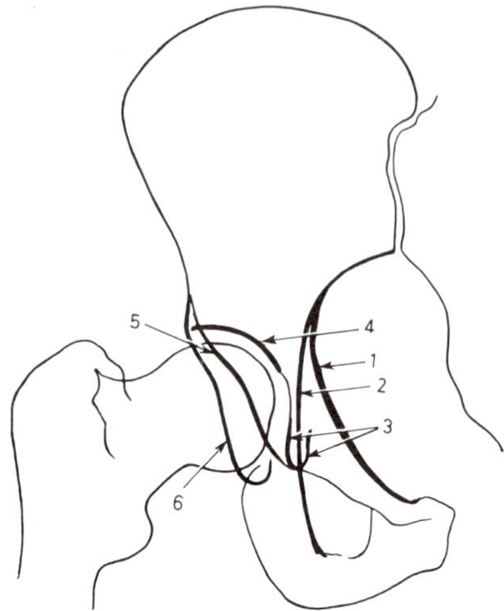

FIG. 1.26 Standard antero–posterior X-ray of the hip showing the main landmarks: (1) superior channel, the arcuate or ilio-pectineal line; (2) ilio-ischial line; (3) the tear drop; (4) the roof of the acetabulum; (5) the anterior lip of the acetabulum; and (6) the posterior lip of the acetabulum.

latter method must not be used to diagnose relatively trivial injuries and is not reliable for minor fractures.

Antero–posterior films are inspected first (Fig. 1.26) and then lateral or supplementary projections taken. A badly injured patient must not be moved unnecessarily during radiography and only essential views are required. The time factor is important and the skilled radiographer will need at least 30 min to take and process adequate films of skull, chest, abdomen, pelvis and one limb of a badly injured patient.

Dislocation of the hip

Most dislocations are easily appreciated in an antero–posterior film, unless it is associated with a fracture of either the acetabulum or femur; the confirmatory lateral film may have to be deferred until the patient is under anaesthesia when there is severe trauma involving both limbs.

Fractures of the acetabulum

Cracks in the acetabulum are easily missed in standard antero–posterior projections of the pelvis. The initial examination should comprise a standard antero–posterior projection of the whole pelvis. This may be all that is required for comminuted fractures unless the patient is very fat or muscular; then other projections (Chapter 7) are needed. The soft tissues must not be forgotten and the presence of air, foreign bodies or a large haematoma are noted. It is worth recalling that the radiological signs of a fracture are a radiolucency due to separation of fragments, a radio-density due to compression and angulation of microfragments, or a step in the anatomical contours. The extent of the radiological survey of the hip joint should conform with the surgeon's policy for

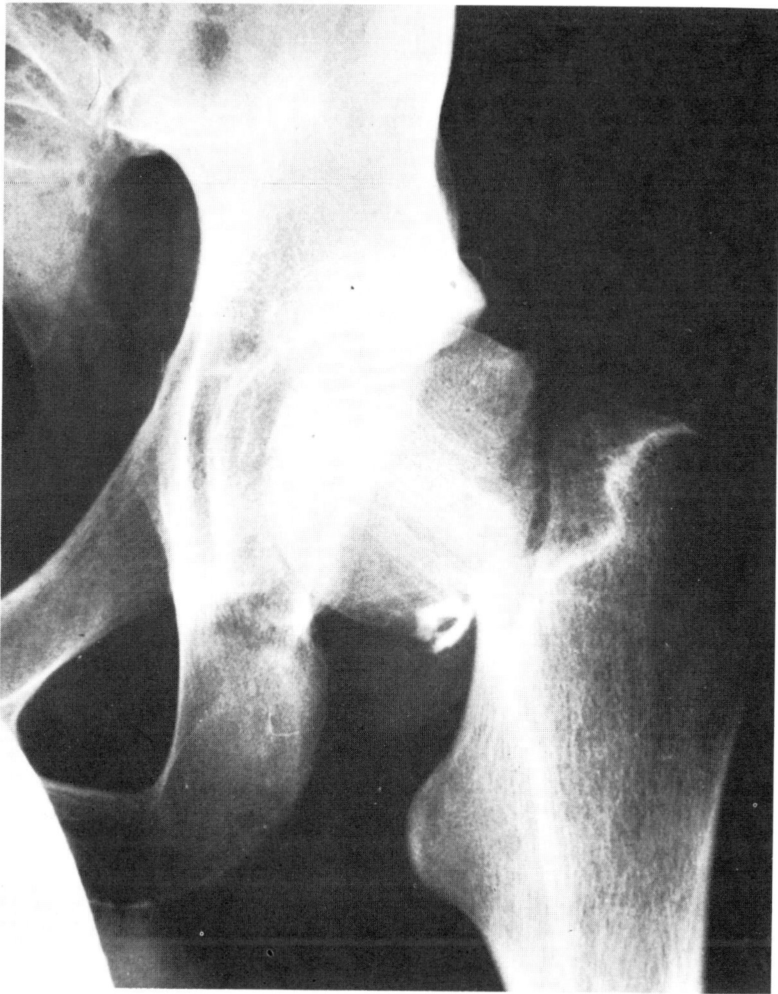

FIG. 1.27 A fracture of the femoral neck in a woman aged 65 years, the bone showing no radiological evidence of gross osteoporosis.

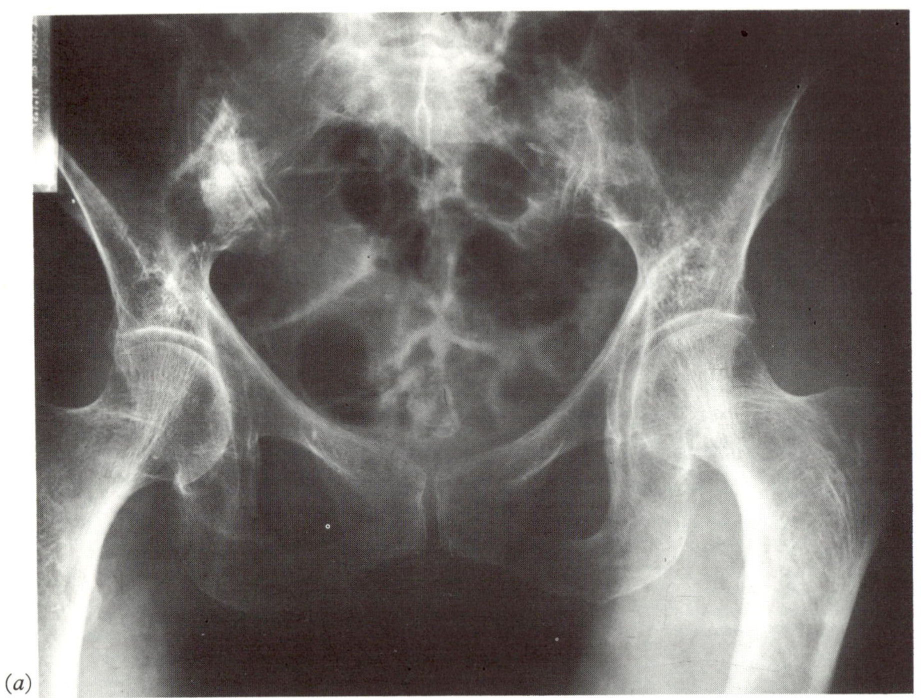
(a)

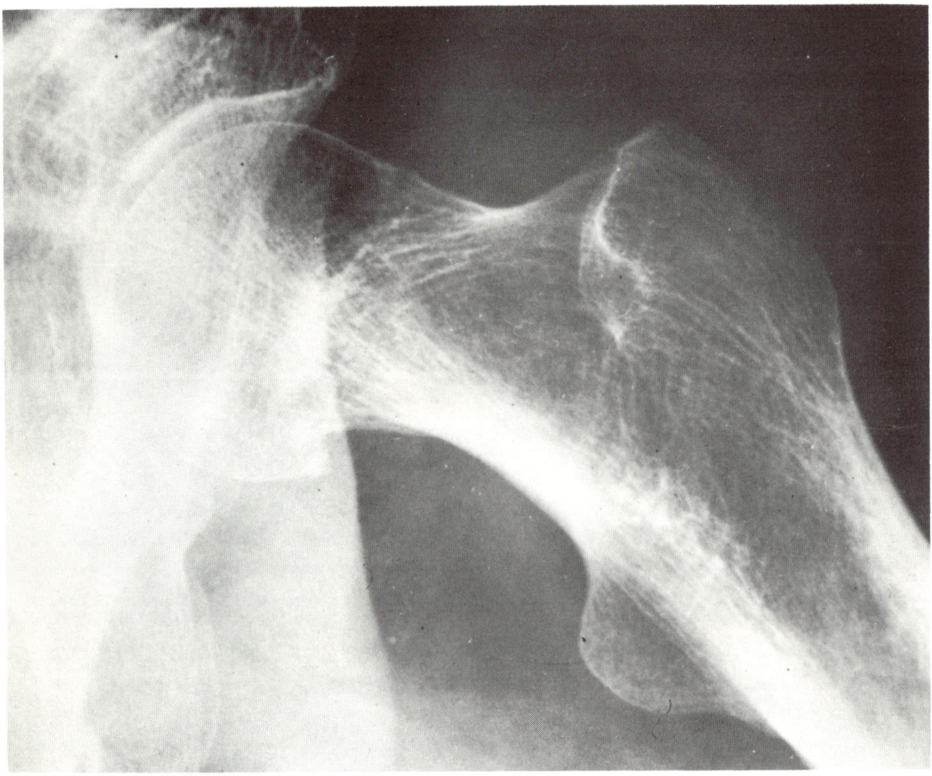

(b)

treatment, for if there is to be no attempt at radical reconstruction there is little point in submitting a patient to a protracted and perhaps painful examination.

Fractures of the upper end of femur

Femoral neck fractures usually occur in patients with osteoporosis, but often the femoral neck region may not show any clear evidence of loss of either cortical or cancellous bone (Fig. 1.27). Radiographs of the muscles around the hip frequently show fatty infiltration. In many instances a suggested diagnosis of malignant disease based on an apparent radiotranslucency of the femoral neck proves to be unfounded. Paget's disease is often present in other bones but such pathological fractures in the upper femur are rare. It is also unusual for the femoral neck to be broken in patients suffering from gross arthritic changes of the hip joint but patients with unilateral disease may break the opposite side. Fractures of the femoral neck in children are detailed in Chapter 6.

Patients with femoral neck fractures may present with the limb externally rotated. If they are radiographed in this position then the femoral neck is foreshortened and is obscured by the overlapping greater trochanter: a fracture may be concealed. It is therefore necessary to rotate internally the lower limb to bring the femoral neck parallel to the X-ray table top, and to fix the leg with a sandbag. When a fracture is suspected and it is still impossible to achieve adequate internal rotation it is better to take a film with the limb in external rotation with a beam angled at 30–40° or with the other limb raised upon a pillow (Fig. 1.28). Patients with the limb flexed, adducted and externally rotated are very difficult to examine radiologically. Fortunately, in most instances, the adductor spasm will subside if the patient is rested for several hours and sedated. Portable examinations should be restricted to patients who are too ill to move. If the radiological examination is negative and a femoral neck fracture is still suspected then additional films can be taken at 24 h, and at 1 or 3 weeks. After fracture it remains

FIG. 1.28 Fractured femoral neck with minimal displacement: missed at initial examination.

(*a*) Adducted thigh. Fractured (L) femoral neck suspected.

(*b*) Patient rotated by placing a pillow under the contralateral thigh: it shows a band of radio-density across the femoral neck due to compression of microfragments, a break in cortex of the junction of the head and neck superiorly and a step in the contour of the neck inferiorly. Lateral film confirmed fracture.

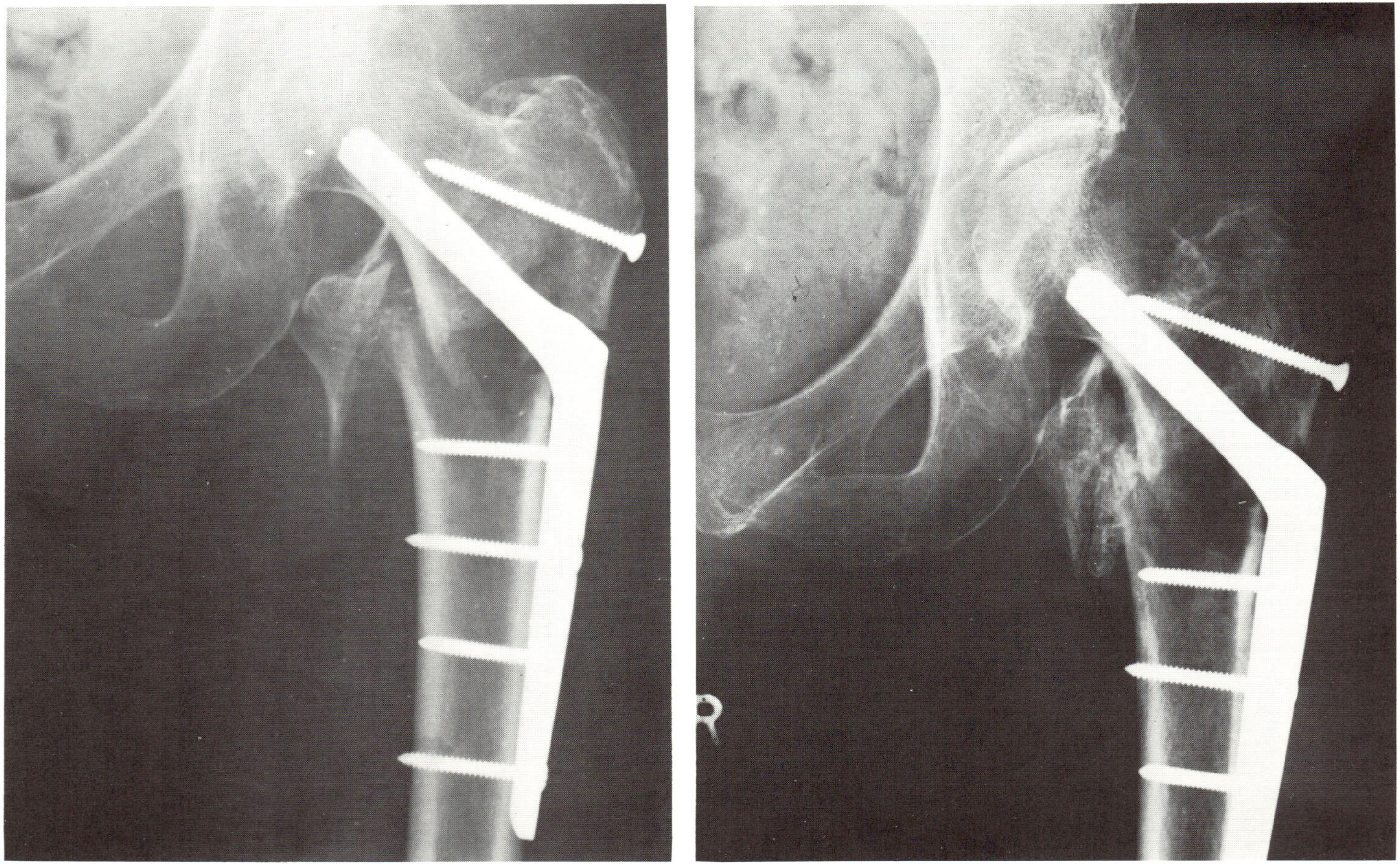

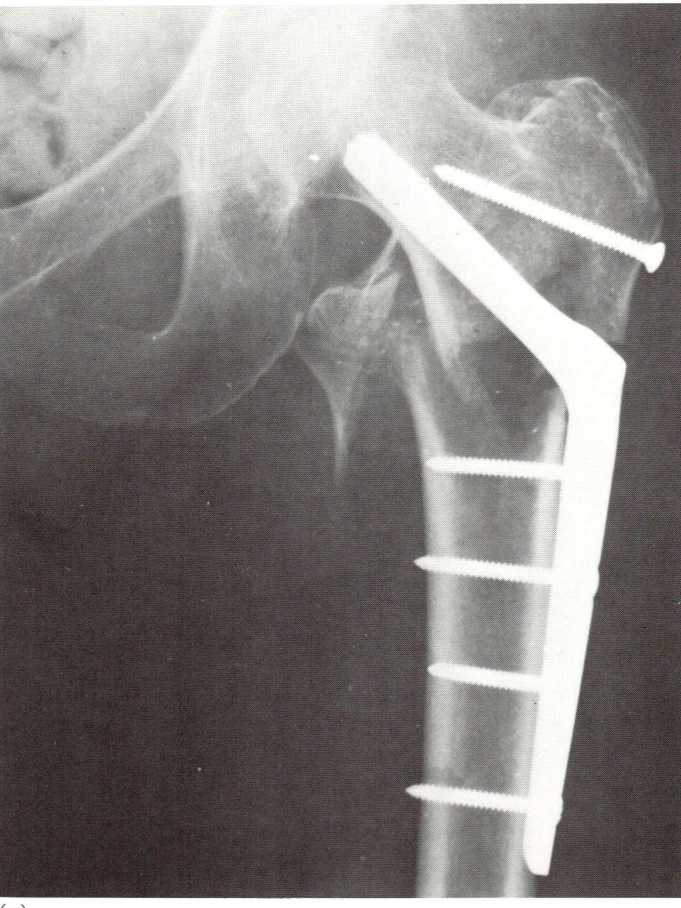

(a)

(b)

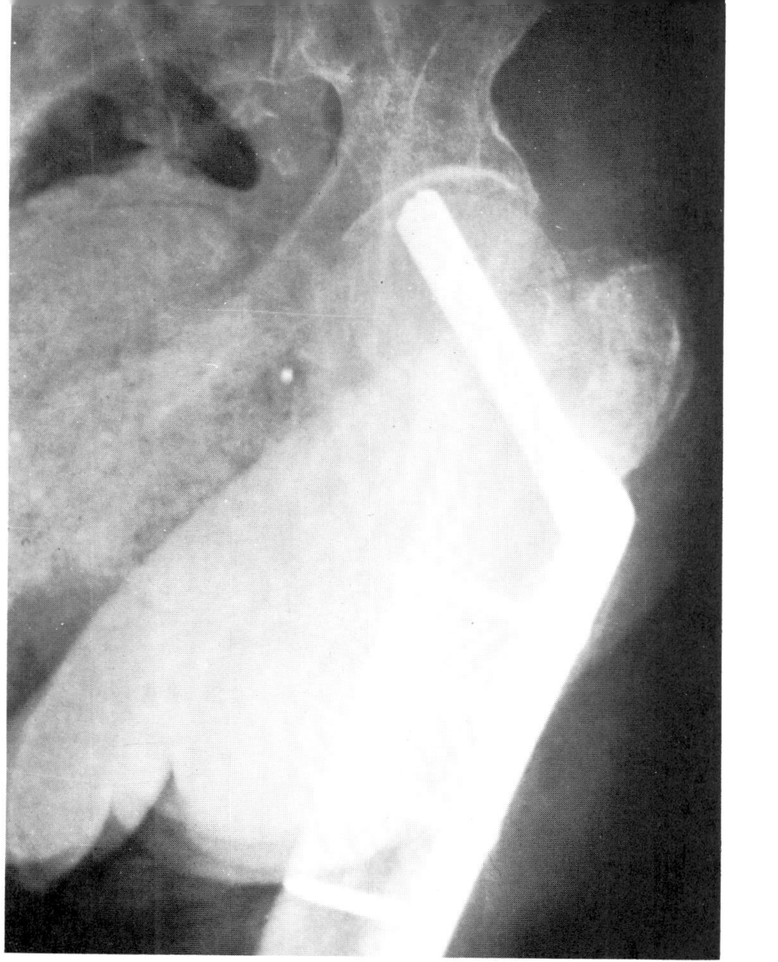

FIG. 1.29 (*a*) Fixation with a fixed-angle Jewett nail-plate (*a*) with little stability at the medial cortex. (*b*) Four months later there is collapse of the upper fragment (note close approximation of screw and nail) with demineralization and the patient is unable to take full weight-bearing. (*c*) Collapse of the fracture site in this patient has led to the pin protruding through the femoral head with subsequent scoring of the acetabulum.

impossible to be sure that avascular necrosis will not supervene unless the patient is followed for at least 2 years.

UNION OF FRACTURES OF THE ACETABULUM AND UPPER END OF THE FEMUR

In most cases union of a fracture in the vicinity of the hip joint must be presumed from indirect evidence. Radiological evidence of union based on restitution of the normal architectural pattern is difficult to establish with certainty in less than 18 months from the date of injury. Bridging callus is seldom a useful feature except for certain fractures of the acetabular margins or trochanter. The disappearance of the fracture line, if it can be shown that this is not due to altered projection, constitutes evidence that healing is occurring. However, removal of microfragments of dead bone may result in some loss of definition. A clearer outline of the fracture after some weeks of immobilization suggests delayed union. Loss of position indicates inadequate fixation and non-union (Fig. 1.29). Failure of union is found after distraction of the fragments and fixation in this position, with soft tissue interposition, or when infection is present. Union may break down on attempted mobilization or when there is limited hip movement. Abduction/adduction films can be taken to demonstrate movement at the fracture site and non-union.

THE SIGNS OF AVASCULAR NECROSIS

There are always avascular fragments in the plane of the fracture or on the surface of the cortex where the periosteum has been detached. These fragments are normally absorbed before the granulation tissue crosses the gap and in consequence the fracture may become unstable unless it is held by organization of the haematoma around the bone, (i.e. bridging callus), or by operative fixation. Some degree of shortening usually results. If one of the fragments is relatively avascular, absorption of the dead micro-fragments comprising the edge may be delayed until a gap between the major fragments has been bridged. A femoral capital fragment may not be wholly deprived of its blood supply and may not die in part or whole until it is subjected to stress. Union of the fragment with the neck may occur.

Recognition of dead bone depends upon the reaction of the living tissues. When bone is viable it will lose calcium content. Within ten

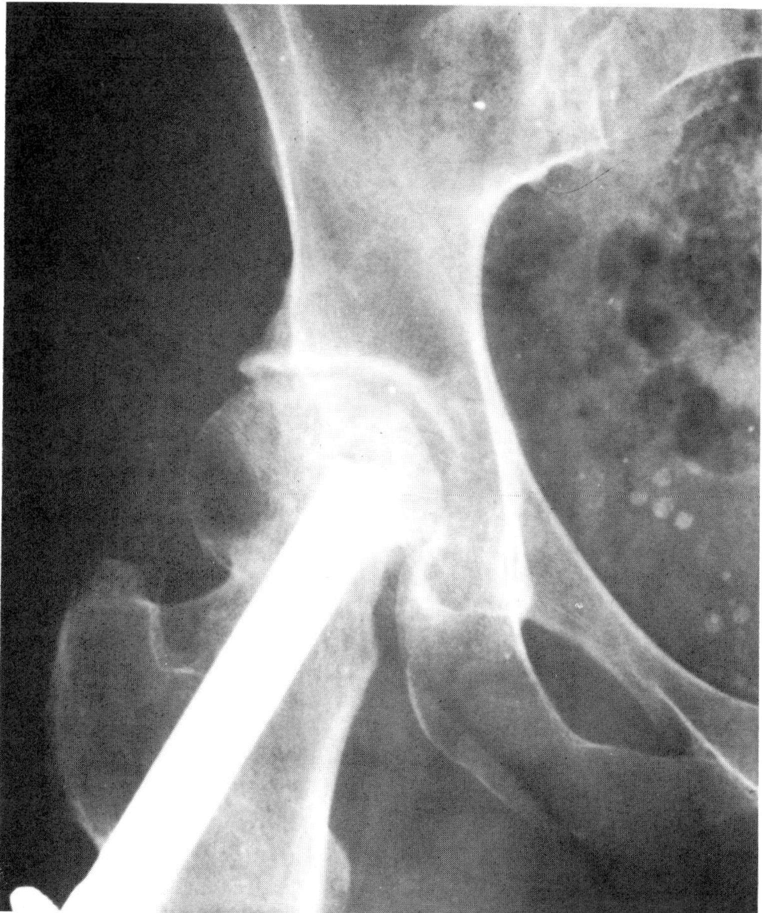

FIG. 1.30 Male aged 60 years. Pinned fracture in exaggeration of valgus position. Recurrence of pain 7 years later. Sound union of fracture. Deformity of dome of the head due to fracture, a large fragment of sequestrated bone lies just above the tip of the pin. Areas of radio-lucency surrounded by lines of demarcation comparable to those shown in Fig. 1.31. The lateral part of the head which is not subjected to significant weight-bearing shows a large area of bone absorption converting it to a shell.

days to three weeks after the injury the affected bone is more radio-lucent and definition of the bony trabeculae is impaired. When many fragments of dead bone in the line of fracture and those beneath the detached periosteum are being removed there is impaired definition of the fracture and of the cortical edge of the adjacent bone. In some instances when the ends of the fracture have been impacted the absorption of

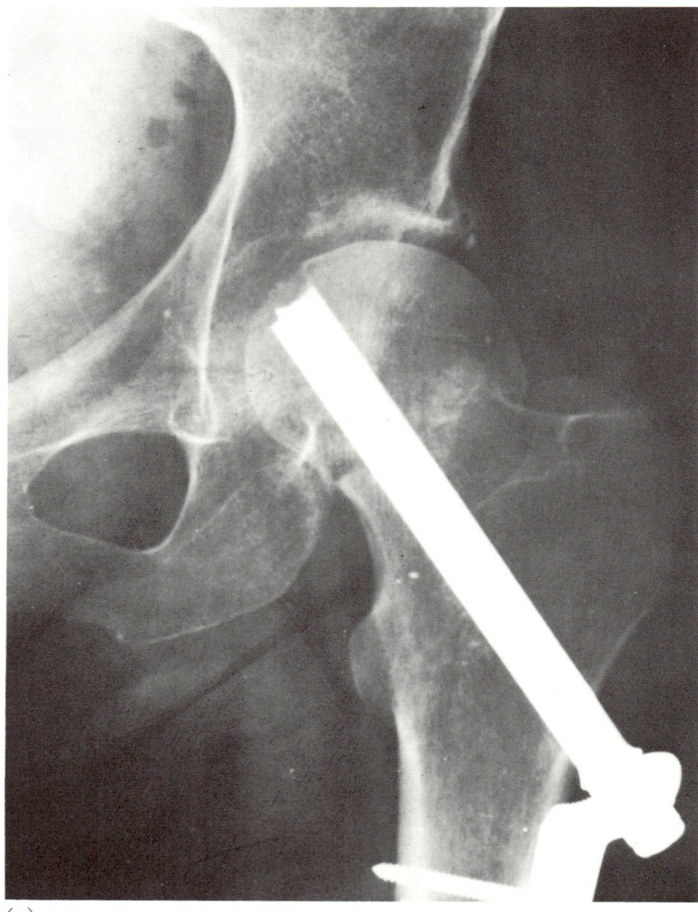

(a)

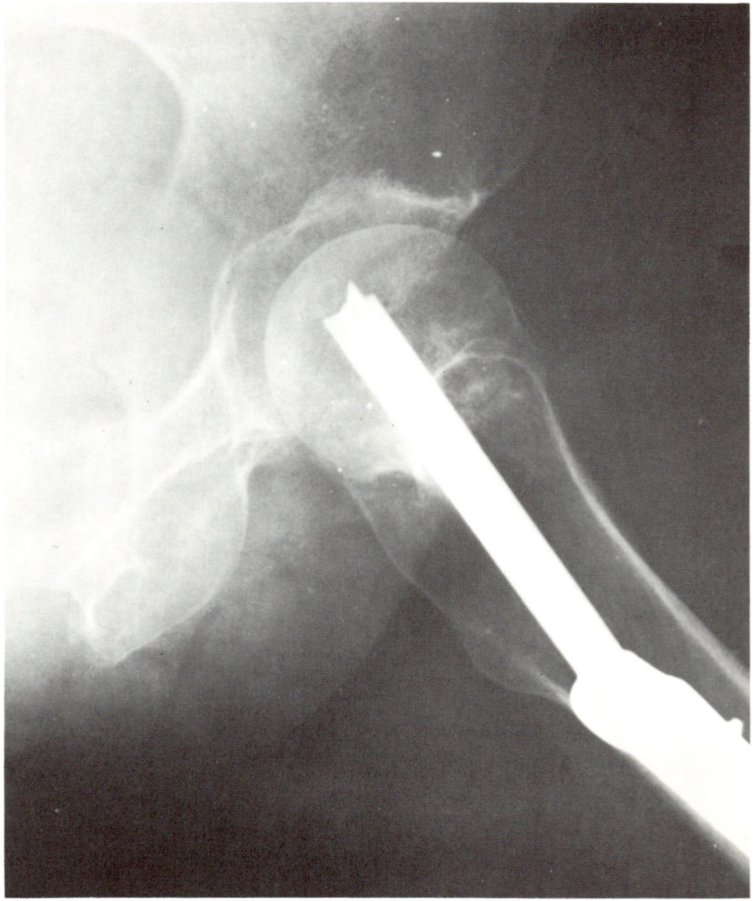

(b)

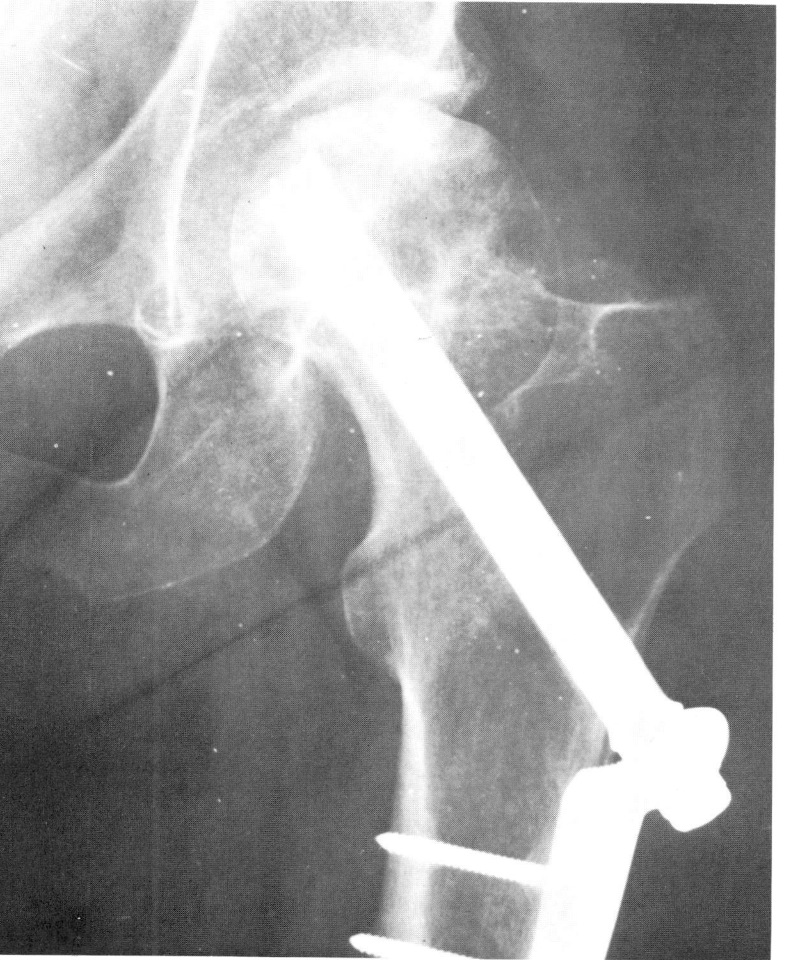

FIG. 1.31 The development of avascular necrosis. (*a*) Three months after injury with osteoporosis in all situations except for a large part of the femoral head which is normally calcified: the radio-lucency of the lower part of the capital fragment emphasizes the relative radio-density of the sub-articular bone. Inference: most of the sub-articular bone is dead. (*b*) Although sound union of the fracture clinically, a lateral X-ray showing a normal shaped dome of head indicates a zone of relative radio-lucency in the neck. This radio-lucency outlines the relative radio-density of the sub-articular bone. Antero-posterior projection shows appearance almost identical with (*a*) taken 3 years before. (*c*) Six months after (*b*), and 3.5 years from the injury, there was a recurrence of pain and limitation of movement. The dome of the head has fractured and shows segments of collapse: these have occurred in the areas of radio-density shown in (*a*). Neck shows circumscribed areas of radio-lucency indicating areas of dead bone or cavities, or areas filled with fibrous tissue: these are surrounded by demarcation zones.

the dead fragments frees the ends. A gap between the fragments may result and the fracture surfaces may move relative to each other. Longitudinal stress may bring the bone ends together with some resultant shortening and muscular imbalance may cause angulation of fragments.

If the vascular supply is impaired the bone's density and definition remains normal for a much longer time in striking contrast with the decalcified viable bone. The fracture surface may remain sharp until a gap is crossed by granulation tissue originating in the living tissues. Subsequent changes depend upon how much of the blood supply of the capital fragment is impaired and the stresses to which it is subjected. Dead bone is unable to withstand normal stress: the whole or part of the head may crush and crumble into fragments. One of the earliest signs of relative avascularity is a fracture of the dome of the head which may be recognized by angulation and disalignment of a segment of the articular surface relative to the normal contour. Crushing increases the relative radio-density of the dead fragment.

Another response to avascularity is the removal of some of the dead bone without collapse of the bony shell: this change may take place in one or more areas of the cancellous bone: the radiological changes are decalcification and blurring of the trabeculae in the affected area. They usually occur in areas of the sub-articular bone in a region not subjected to stress. As the changes progress the bony trabeculae in the affected area disintegrate, the resulting cavity may collapse, become filled with fibrous tissue which may ossify, or form a cyst (Fig. 1.30).

There are three factors concerned in the production of a so-called dense avascular fragment. Firstly, the dead bone is only relatively dense i.e. normal in contrast with the surrounding decalcified or living tissue (Fig. 1.31). Secondly, the dead fragment is compacted by crushing. Thirdly, the dead tissue may be thickened by the deposition of new bone consequent upon vascular permeation of the spaces of the dead cancellous tissue.

Fractures of the femoral head

A fracture of the femoral head is very rarely seen without preceding pathological change. It is a common sequel to avascular necrosis. It may be found in association with a hip dislocation (Fig. 1.32). The diagnosis may be made with confidence when the radiograph shows an angular deformity of the dome of the femoral head. Good contrast

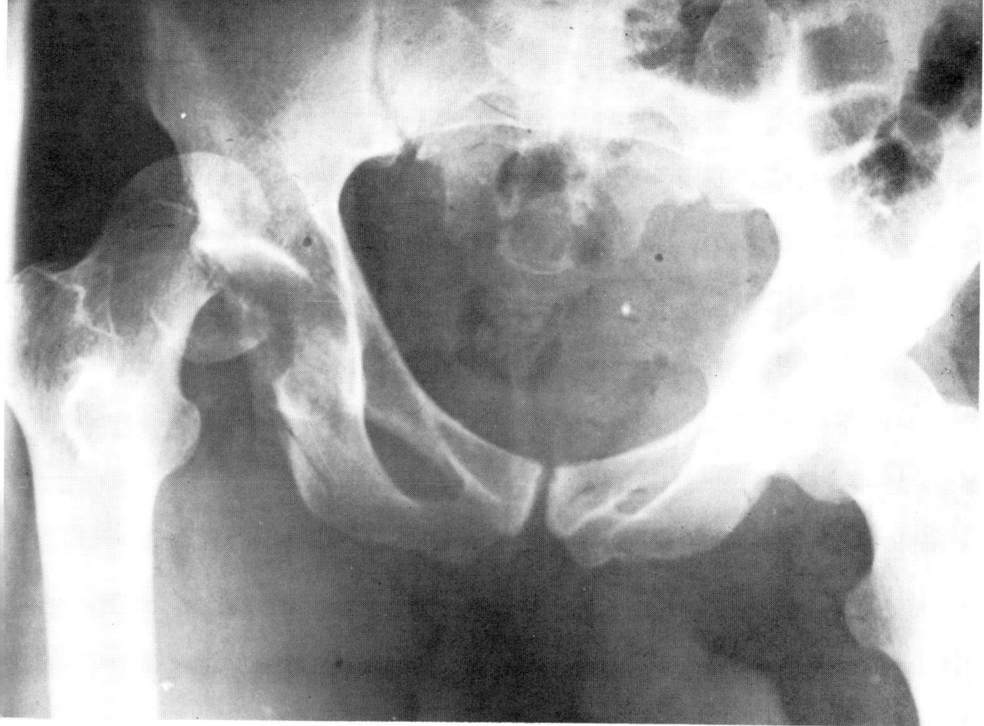

FIG. 1.32 Fracture of the dome of the femoral head with a hip dislocation.

radiography may be needed especially when injury has occurred in the acetabulum, and tomography may be required to clinch the diagnosis.

Slipped epiphysis

This condition is described in Chapter 9.

SKELETAL REACTIONS TO MATERIALS USED FOR FIXATION PURPOSES

All materials inserted into bone under tension tend to cause a layer of necrosis of adjacent bone; this layer varies in thickness depending upon the stresses involved, the quality of bone and its blood supply.

With rigid fixation the amount of bone absorption may be small and remain undetected radiologically. With poor fixation, such as obtained with a flanged nail, the necrosis may be greater and a radiolucent zone may be detected around the nail. A circular core may be observed around the nail which is then free to rotate within the capital fragment or within the bone of the neck and shaft if a plate has not been used. The result is also influenced by comminution of the avascular fragment of the femoral head or by a thin osteoporotic cortex of the femur.

It does not follow that loosening of fixation consequent upon absorption of bone is necessarily followed by non-union. Vascular granulation tissue may fill the space and become dense fibrous tissue; many years later this tissue may necrose and become fluid.

If the layer of radio-lucency around the implant is relatively wide, one should suspect that it is loose, and if the width is greater at one end than the other it is almost certainly loose, especially if there is an oval or circular cavity surrounding the nail. A change in position of the nail relative to the bone which cannot be explained by an alteration in limb position or projection indicates loosening. Similar considerations apply to the stem of a prosthesis. A control film followed by gentle traction to the limb may reveal movement of the fixation device. When television fluoroscopy is available these films may be taken under fluoroscopic control. The development of round, oval or fusiform cavities close to foreign material strongly suggests infection; cavity formation around the end of a pin or plate is not so significant and can be due to mobility of the pin.

Implant fracture

Wires, pins, plates, nails and cement may fracture (Fig. 1.33). The fracture indicates that stresses are still being applied to the part. The most important local factor is absorption of bone thus freeing the screws which fix the plate. The implant fracture may also result from angulation of the bones consequent upon absorption at the fracture site of an avascular segment. Many weeks may elapse before the bone crumbles and the pin or plate snaps.

Fracture of the bond between radio-lucent cement and bone constitutes a special problem and is not visible radiologically unless an opaque component has been added to the cement. In some instances it may be justifable to demonstrate the fracture by injecting a water soluble contrast medium in the area and stressing the parts.

Bone thickening due to the insertion of foreign material may induce periosteal reaction which may surround and cover wires, screw heads and a plate. There may be thickening of the endosteal layers of the

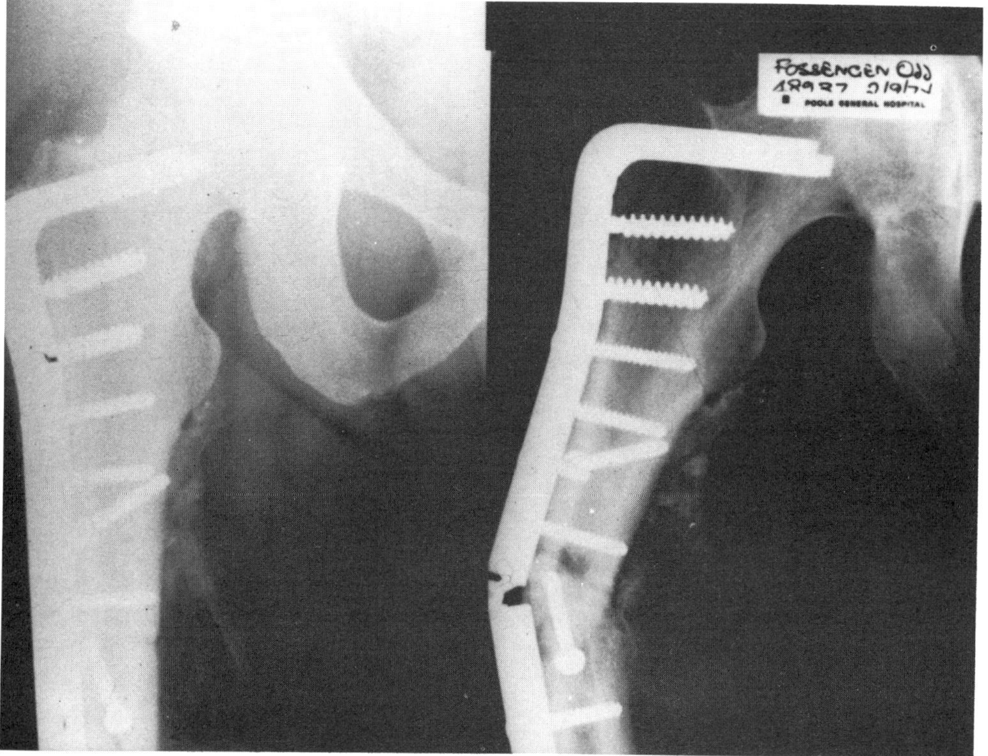

FIG. 1.33 Although the fracture was judged to be united radiologically, weight-bearing proved this assumption to be incorrect.

cortex, sometimes restricted to the level of the screws but at other times spreading far beyond the level of fixation; it is of the nature of buttressing.

Other features of the radiology of the hip region are included in the appropriate chapters.

REFERENCES

ALFFRAM, P.A. (1964). *Acta Orthop. Scand. Suppl.* 65.

BACKMAN, S. (1957). *Acta radiol. Suppl.* p. 146.

BENTLEY, G. (1972). *Degradation, Repair and Replacement of Articular Cartilage.* Ch. M., Thesis. University of Sheffield.

BENTLEY, G. and GREER, R.B. (1971). *Nature* **230**, 385.

BULLOUGH, P., GOODFELLOW, J.W., GREENWALD, A.S. and O'CONNOR J.J. (1968). *Nature* **217**, No. 5135, p. 1290.

CATTO, M. (1965). *J. Bone Jt. Surg.* **47B**, 749.
CHESTERMAN, P.J. and SMITH, A.U. (1968). *J. Bone Jt. Surg.* **50B**, 184.
CRENSHAW, A.H. (Ed.) (1971). *Campbell's Operative Orthopaedics.* 5th Edn, Mosby, St. Louis.
CROCK, H.V. (1964). *J. Bone Jt. Surg.* **46B**, 530.
DEE, R. (1969). *Ann. R. Coll. Surg. Engl.* **45**, 357.
FELL H.B. and DINGLE J.T. (1963). *J. Biochem.* **87**, 403.
FRANKEL, V.H. (1960). *The Femoral Neck: Function, Fracture Mechanics, Internal Fixation.* Charles C. Thomas, Springfield.
FRANKEL, V.H. (1974). In: *Surgery of the Hip Joint*, Chap. 5, (Tronzo, R. G). Lea & Febiger, Philadelphia.
FRAZER, J.E. (1965). *Anatomy of the Human Skeleton.* Churchill, London.
FREEMAN, M.A.R. and WYKE, B.D. (1967). *J. Anat. Lond.* **101**, 505.
FREEMAN, M.A.R., TODD, R.C. and PIRIE, C.J. (1974). *J. Bone Jt. Surg.* **56B**, 698.
FORNEY, H.J., MATHEWS, R.S. and BENTLEY, G. (1973). *Orthopaedics.* Oxford, **6**, 19.
GIBSON, A. (1950). *J. Bone Jt. Surg.* **32B**, 183.
GREENWALD, A.S. (1970). D. Phil. Thesis, University of Oxford.
GREENWALD, A.S. and HAYNES, D.W. (1969). *J. Bone Jt. Surg.* **51B**, 747.
GRIFFITHS, W.E.G., SWANSON, S.A.V. and FREEMAN, M.A.R. (1971). *J. Bone Jt. Surg.* **53B**, 136.
HENRY, A.K. (1957). *Extensile Exposure.* Livingstone, Edinburgh.
KOCH, J.C. (1917). *Am. J. Anat.* **XXI**, 177.
LINN, F.C. (1967). *J. Bone Jt. Surg.* **49A**, 1079.
MANKIN, H.J. (1968). *Bull. N. Y. Acac. Med.* **44**, 545.
MAROUDAS, A. (1973). *Symposium on Normal and Osteoarthrotic Articular Cartilage.* Stanmore, November 5–7, 1973. (In press.)
MAURER, R.C. and LARSEN, I.J. (1970). *J. Bone Jt. Surg.* **52A**, 39.
MCKEE, G.K. and WATSON-FARRAR, J. (1966). *J. Bone Jt. Surg.* **48B**, 245.
MCKIBBEN, B. (1968). *The Nutrition of Articular Cartilage in Relation to its Development.* M.D. Thesis, University of Leeds.
PAUL, J.P. (1965). In: *Biomechanics and Related Bioengineering Topics*, (Ed. R. M. Kenedi) Pergamon Press, Oxford.
PHILLIPS, R.S. (1966). *J. Bone Jt. Surg.* **48B**, 280.
RYDELL, N.W. (1966). *Acta Orthop. Scand. Suppl.* 88.
SEVITT, S. and THOMPSON, R.G. (1965). *J. Bone Jt. Surg.* **47B**, 560.
SIMMONS, D.P. and CHRISMAN, O.D. (1965). *Arthritis. Rheum.* **8**, 960.
TRONZO, R.G. (1973). *Surgery of the Hip Joint.* Lea & Febiger, Philadelphia.
TRUETA, J. and HARRISON, M.H.M. (1953). *J. Bone Jt. Surg.* **35B**, 442.
TUCKER, E.R. (1949). *J. Bone Jt. Surg.* **31B**, 82.
VON MEYER, H.D. (1867). *Arch. Anat. Physiol.* **34**, 615.
WOOLF, J. (1870). *Virchows Arch. Orth. Anat.* **50**, 389.
YABLON, I.G., FRANZBLAU, C.J. and LEACH, R.E. (1974). *J. Bone Jt. Surg.* **56A**, 322.

Chapter Two

FRACTURES OF THE FEMORAL NECK: PART 1

D. S. Muckle

Classification ~ Diagnosis ~ Displacement and reduction ~ Surgical technique ~ Internal fixation of subcapital fractures ~ Internal fixation of trochanteric fractures

CLASSIFICATION

Femoral neck fractures can be divided into intracapsular and extra-capsular (Fig. 2.1). This convenient division (first noted by Sir Astley Cooper) allows further subdivisions:

Intracapsular: subcapital;
transcervical;
basal.

Extra-capsular: intertrochanteric;
pertrochanteric;
subtrochanteric;
comminuted.

Often all intracapsular fractures are called 'subcapital' and all extra-capsular fractures called 'trochanteric'. Such a simple arbitary division is necessary to rationalize reduction, fixation and the possible complications of therapy, while the prognosis of the two types of fracture is entirely different. Trochanteric fractures nearly always unite after correct fixation since a wide area of cancellous bone is involved. However, subcapital fractures are complicated by damage to the blood supply of the femoral head. A detailed classification is given in Table 2.1.

Since Linton's classic paper in 1949 the distinction between adduction and abduction subcapital fractures has not been made, since both may arise from lateral rotational strains applied to the lower limb, with the fracture spiral in nature and prising a beak of bone from the back of the femoral neck (Fig. 2.3). In the first degree of displacement

TABLE 2.1 Forms of classification of femoral neck fractures

Classification		
Subcapital		
Pauwels (1935) (Fig. 2.2)	Type I	Angle to 30°
	Type II	Angle to 50°
	Type III	Angle to 70°
Garden (1961)	Type I	Incomplete fracture
	Type II	Complete without displacement
	Type III	Complete fracture with partial displacement
	Type IV	Complete fracture with full displacement
Trochanteric		
Bohler (quoted Stuck, 1949)	Type I	Base of neck, minimal displacement
	Type II	Through trochanters with wide separation
	Type III	Base of neck driven into spongy trochanter
	Type IV	Trochanteric fracture with comminution
Evans (1949)	Type I	Undisplaced inter-trochanteric fracture, with or without lesser trochanter, stable
	Type II	As above but irreducible or unstable due to comminution
Boyd and Griffin (1949)	Type I	Linear inter-trochanteric fracture
	Type II	As above with split in lateral cortex of greater trochanter
	Type III	Subtrochanteric
	Type IV	Trochanteric fracture involving spiral fracture down the shaft

the fragments are impacted but as displacement occurs (Fig. 2.4) the head is pushed downwards and backwards on the posterior aspect of the femoral neck.

GARDEN'S CLASSIFICATION–SUBCAPITAL FRACTURES (FIG. 2.5)

Stage I is the so-called abducted or impacted injury in which the fracture of the inferior cortex is greenstick in nature, and a minimal degree of lateral rotation of the neck creates a radiological illusion of impaction. The medial lamellae of the neck lie in abduction as compared with those in the head which appear adducted. Normally (in the antero–posterior view) the medial trabeculae lie at an angle of approximately 160° with the medial femoral cortex. In the lateral view the medial and lateral trabeculae converge and decussate upon a straight line axis in the centre of the neck.

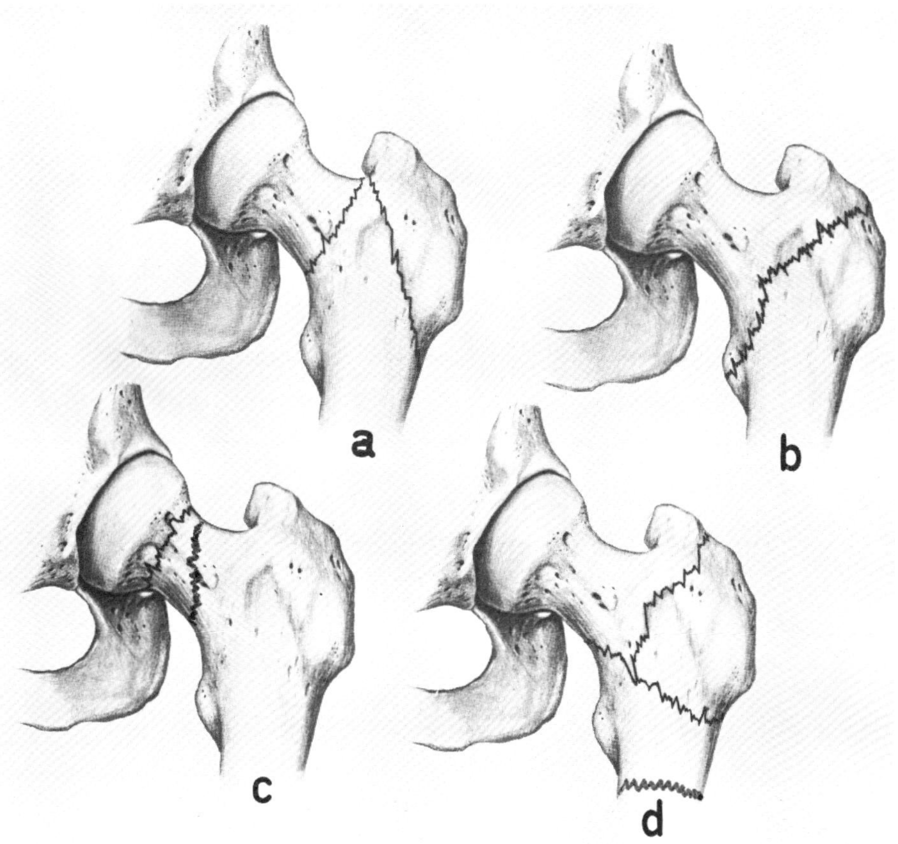

FIG. 2.1 Classification of femoral neck fractures. (*a*) basal, pertrochanteric; (*b*) intertrochanteric; (*c*) subcapital, transcervical; (*d*) comminuted, subtrochanteric.

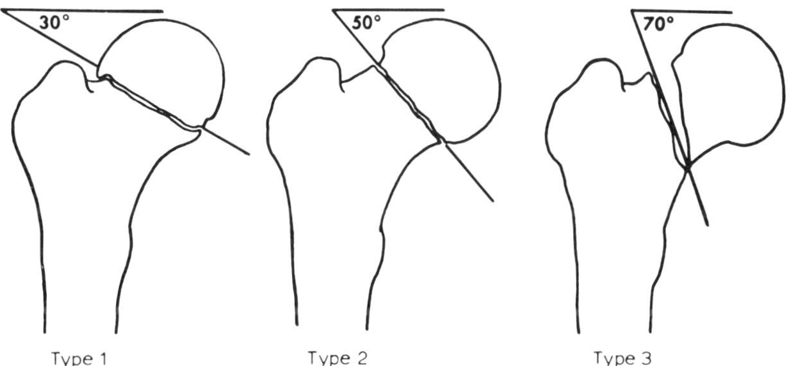

FIG. 2.2 Pauwels' classification based on increasing obliquity of the fracture line; indicating the potential severity of injury.

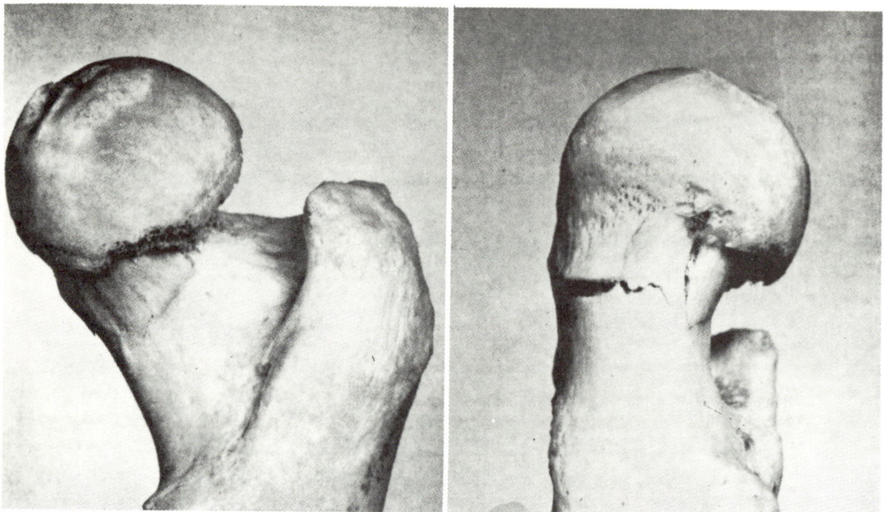

FIG. 2.3 The appearance on radiographic examination suggested an abduction type of fracture; but there was no impaction and it represents no more than one stage of movement terminating in the displacement of an adduction fracture (Linton, 1949).

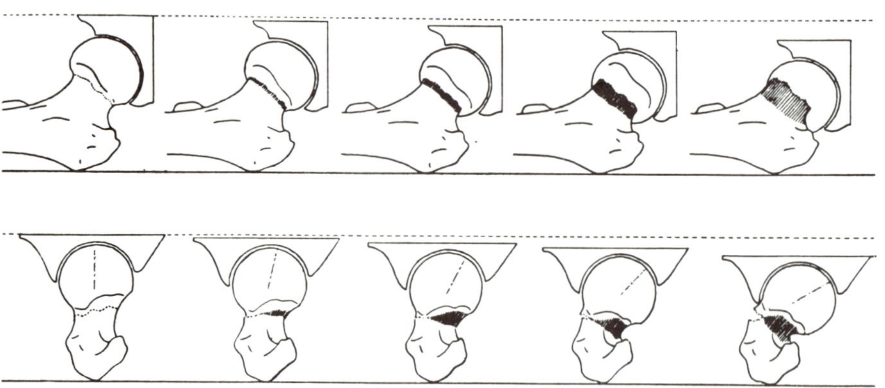

FIG. 2.4 The stages in migration of the femoral head and posterior cortical collapse after a subcapital fracture (Linton, 1949). The capital fragment tends to displace into varus with axial rotation on the neck; the distal fragment rotates laterally, particularly when there is comminution (shaded) of the posterior neck.

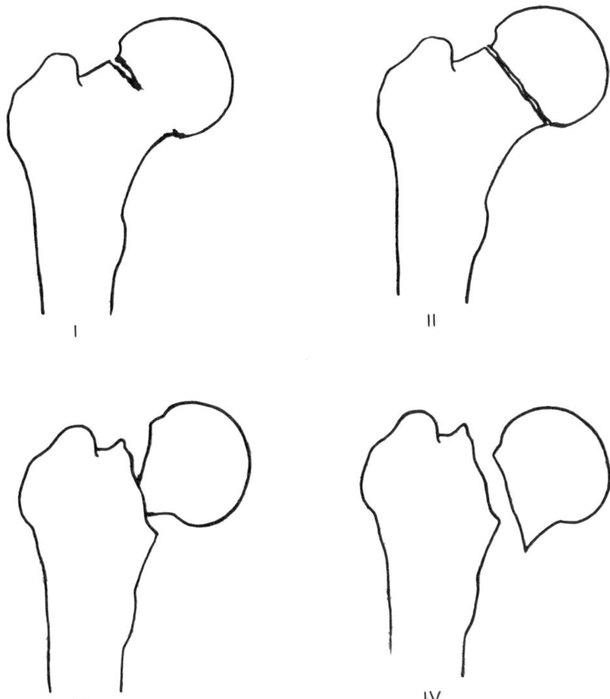

FIG. 2.5 Garden's classification. Stage I is incomplete or abducted or impacted fracture; Stage II complete without displacement. Stage III shows partial displacement, the fracture surfaces are still opposed postero–inferiorly and the fragments have rotated in opposite directions like two cog-wheels in mesh. Stage III fractures show medial tilting of the head (as shown by the trabeculae) with lateral rotation of the neck and shaft. Contact is lost in stage IV and the teeth of the cog-wheel, as it were, have become disengaged. The distal fragment lies anterior to the proximal fragment (head), and the trabeculae in the head lie in normal alignment with their projections in the pelvis.

Stage II is a complete subcapital fracture without displacement. The inferior cortical buttress is broken but there is no tilting of the head.

Stage III is a complete subcapital fracture with partial displacement. The two fragments retain their posterior retinacular attachment but crushing of the posterior cervical cortex (Fig. 2.4) has not taken place. Lateral rotation of the distal fragment tilts the capital fragment into abduction and medial rotation as shown by the direction of the medial trabeculae in the femoral head.

Stage IV is a complete subcapital fracture with full displacement.

If the tendency for the limb to rotate laterally is not resisted by internal or external splinting, stripping of the retinacular attachments and crushing of the thin posterior cortex allows full displacement to occur, and stage III becomes a stage IV subcapital fracture. As the fragments become divorced from each other the head returns to a more normal position in the acetabulum. Then the medial trabeculae of the femoral head lie in alignment with their fellows in the pelvis. Initially the strong retinaculum of Weitbrecht in the posterior capsule (Fig. 2.6) may resist the tendency to lateral rotation of the neck. Gradually this ligament becomes torn and stretched.

Stage II fractures are rare, and many stage III fractures have become displaced (i.e. stage IV) when surgery is undertaken. Thus it is reasonable to have also a broad definition of subcapital fractures as 'undisplaced' and 'displaced' (Fig. 2.7), the former having an excellent prognosis.

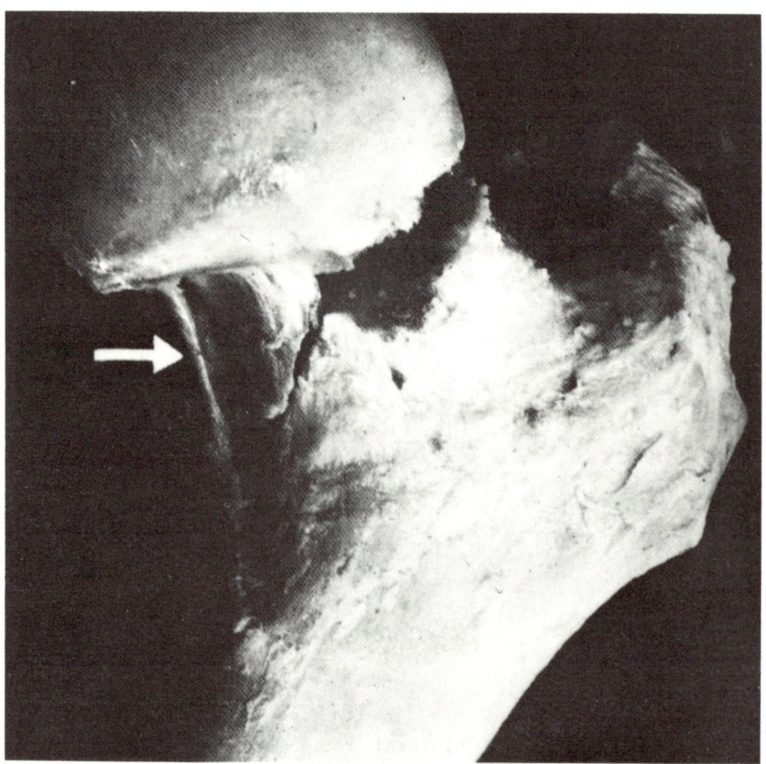

FIG. 2.6 The retinaculum of Weitbrecht in the posterior capsule exerts a hinge effect.

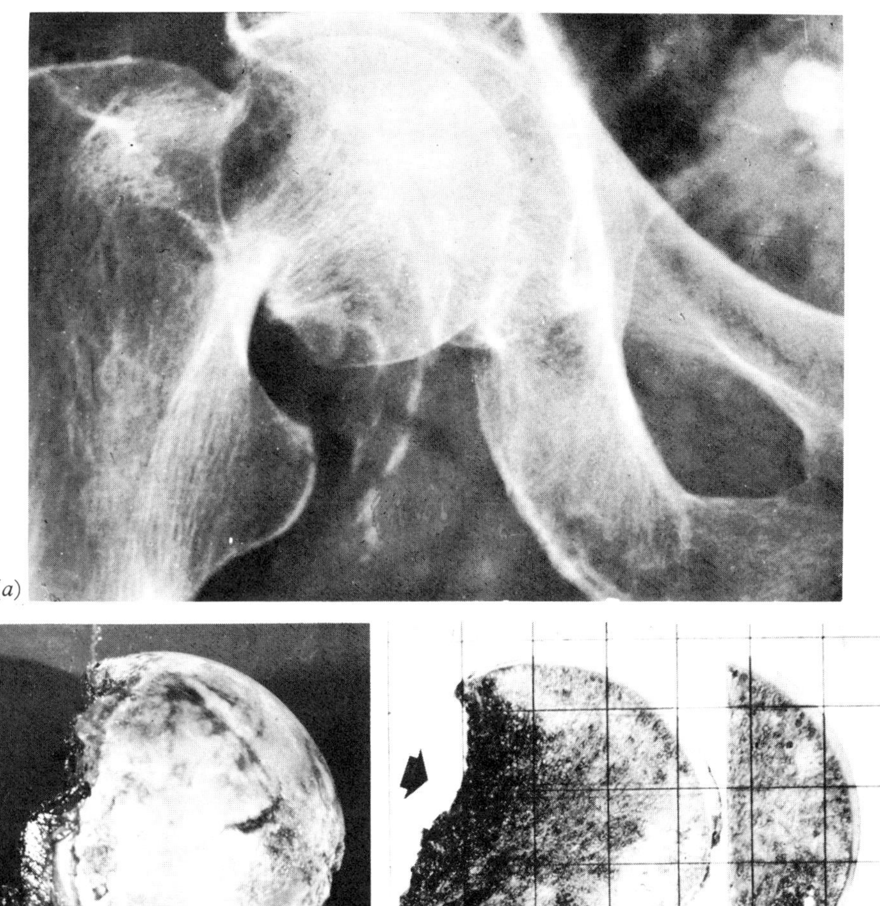

FIG. 2.7 Displaced subcapital fracture (stage III) found to be disengaged at surgery. The characteristic spike of bone is seen on the inferior aspect of the femoral head. Infarction is arrowed in the distribution of the lateral epiphyseal and inferior metaphyseal vessels.

BOYD AND GRIFFIN'S CLASSIFICATION (FIG. 2.8)—TROCHANTERIC FRACTURES

Type 1. Extending along the intertrochanteric line, this fracture is simple and easily maintained.

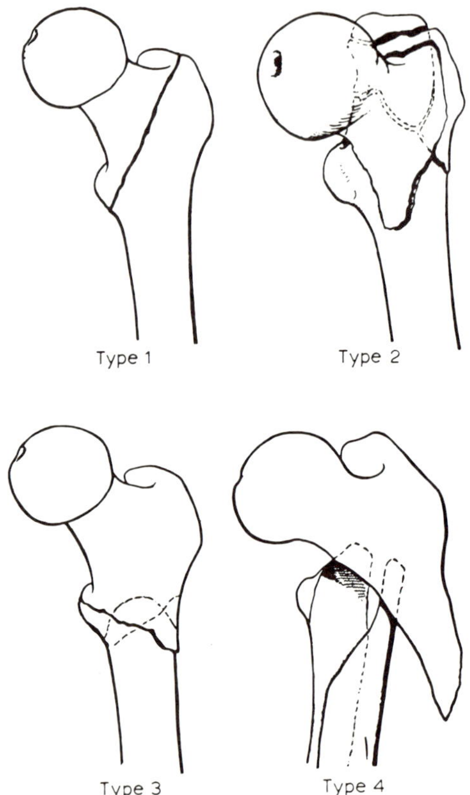

FIG. 2.8 Boyd and Griffin's classification.

Type 2. A comminuted fracture, the main displacement is along the intertrochanteric line with multiple fractures in the cortex.

Type 3. This fracture is basically subtrochanteric, varying degrees of comminution are found.

Type 4. These are fractures of the trochanteric region in two planes, and internal fixation is needed in both planes.

DIAGNOSIS

The underlying aetiological factors are dealt with in later chapters. About 80% of femoral neck fractures occur in persons over 60 years old, and are approximately four times commoner in women than men.

The diagnosis is based on the classical triad of painful hip, limb shortening and external rotation deformity at the foot reflecting this rotation at the hip. Often there is little pain, and the only clinical sign is external rotation and a provisional diagnosis should be made on this evidence alone. Impacted fractures may allow weight-bearing and a full range of movement, but tenderness may be found on springing the pelvis or by pressure over the greater trochanter.

The clinical differentiation between the two main groups of femoral neck fracture is based on the fact that while contact remains at subcapital levels, lateral rotation deformity is limited by the anterior capsule to about 40° or less; whereas when the fracture is trochanteric the deformity often amounts to 90°.

Although closed methods of treatment can be employed in trochanteric fractures, if some factor (such as local infection) makes surgery impossible, all complete femoral neck fractures require surgical intervention because:

(a) Untreated the mortality rate may be as high as 35% compared with 17% after internal fixation (Horowitz, 1966);

(b) Complications such as bronchopneumonia, deep vein thrombosis and sacral ulceration can be reduced by early mobilization;

(c) Avascular necrosis of the femoral head is more likely to supervene if fixation is delayed.

The extent of the problem is outlined by Seal (1972) who found an initial mortality of 16%, a one year mortality of 25%, and that only 34% of patients returned home, the remainder going to long-stay hospitals.

DISPLACEMENT AND REDUCTION

The key to successful and simple surgery is adequate reduction; and the key to successful and simple reduction is an understanding of the displacing forces.

After a subcapital fracture the femoral shaft is pulled into external rotation by the psoas and external rotators, while the psoas and related muscles actively shorten the limb. Thus the femoral head comes to lie postero-lateral to the neck. In order to reduce a subcapital fracture a series of opposing forces have to be brought into play, namely traction, abduction and internal rotation.

With trochanteric fractures the technique of reduction depends upon the level of the fracture. Fractures proximal to the attachment of the short external rotators allow rotation of the shaft but not the

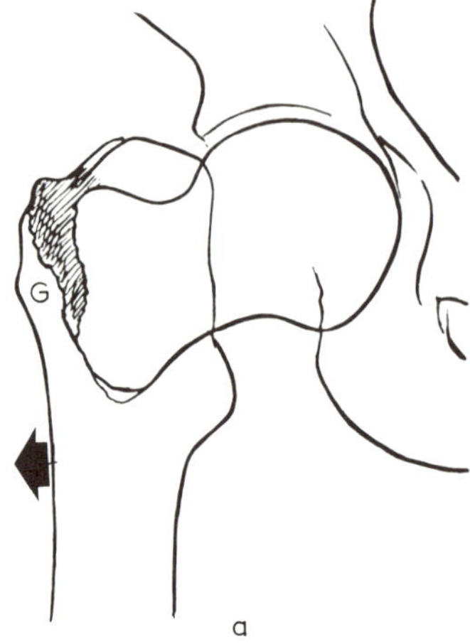

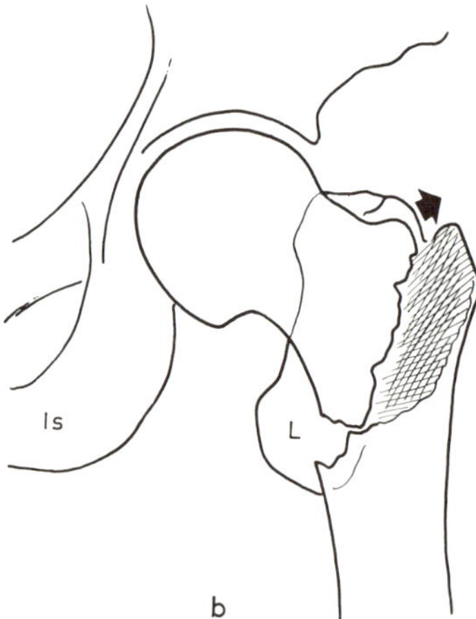

FIG. 2.9 (*a*) The fracture lies proximal to the external rotators and the shaft and trochanters are in full external rotation, with the head and neck in neutral. (G) Greater trochanter.

(*b*) The fracture is distal to the external rotators. The upper fragment which includes the trochanters is externally rotated, as shown by the prominent lesser trochanter (L); (Is) ischium. (After Horn and Wang, 1964.)

upper fragment (Fig. 2.9*a*) and reduction is achieved with the lower limb in the mid-position or with slight internal rotation. Conversely, fractures distal to the insertion of the external rotators lead to external rotation of the trochanteric component and in these instances the femoral shaft may have to be rotated externally for accurate reduction (Fig. 2.9*b*).

With trochanteric fractures the success of closed reduction can be palpated during surgery and fine adjustments made. Many junior doctors still believe that all femoral neck fractures require full internal rotation for accurate reduction and are puzzled to find a wide gap between the components of the trochanteric region at operation, with the limb in this position.

When there is comminution, the hamstrings and gluteus maximus shorten the limb and the upper femoral fragment becomes flexed due to the unopposed action of the psoas. Gentle flexion of the shaft is needed for reduction (Horn and Wang, 1964).

The following principles must be followed to permit accurate reduction of subcapital fractures (Fig. 2.10), bearing in mind the subtle variations in technique required for trochanteric fractures. The original Whitman method required traction on both limbs, with disimpaction of the subcapital fracture by outward traction on the thigh, and the limb internally rotated and abducted once disimpaction had occurred. The Leadbetter method produced a separation of the fragments by flexing the hip to a right-angle and exerting pressure in the calf region by the operator's shoulder, the knee also being at a right-angle, while exerting lateral leverage on the thigh. The limb is then extended, internally rotated and abducted (Wilson, 1938).

The following method of reduction is simple and gives excellent results:

(a) Absolute muscle relaxation is the basis of successful reduction and nothing should be attempted until the patient is fully anaesthetized, with the uninjured limb secured to the orthopaedic table and the perineum against the centre post. The pelvis is steadied by an assistant by light pressure over the iliac crests. A common fault at this stage is not to have the perineum firmly centred against a post so that the patient is too high up the table. Abduction of the leg then causes tilting of the pelvis.

(b) The surgeon stands beside and just below the knee of the injured leg (for example the right) facing obliquely towards the patient's opposite shoulder (left). The knee is grasped from behind with the left hand, the right hand supporting the ankle. The thigh is flexed to 15° and gently abducted, the limb falling into any position of external rotation it wishes to assume. The knee is flexed so that the ankle is supported in comfort.

(c) The surgeon then exerts steady traction through the thigh, taking all the force through the hand above the knee, so that ligamentous

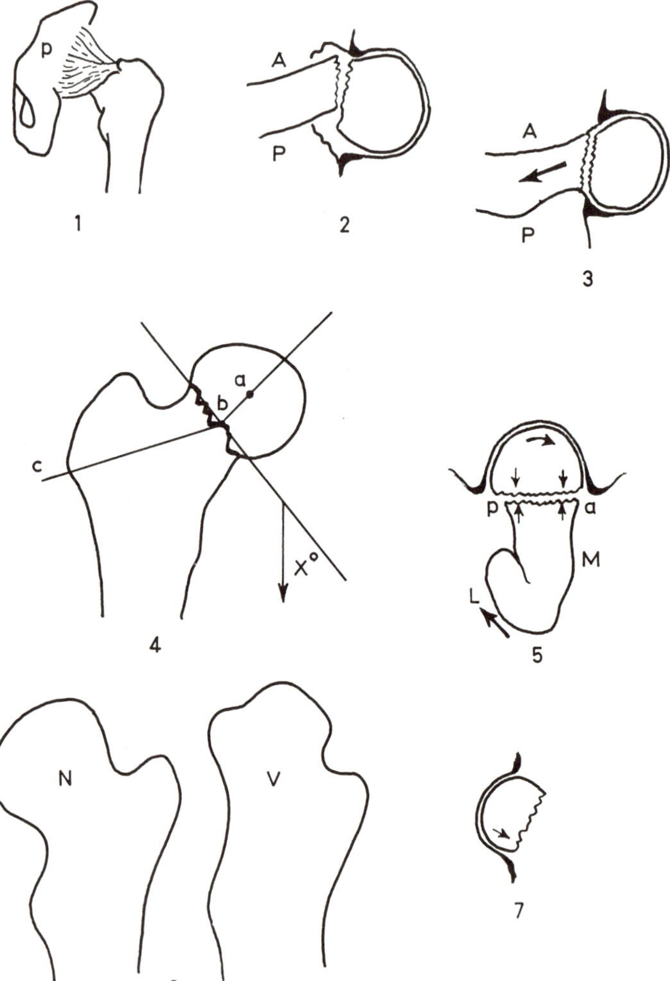

FIG. 2.10 (1) The posterior aspect of the hip capsule shows the spiral fibres that approximate the femoral head into the acetabulum when the hip is in extension and medial rotation. (2) A lateral view of the femoral neck before traction (3) exerted in the line of the long axis of the neck with the hip in flexion and slight abduction. Once the hip is reduced the limb is placed in extension, whilst maintaining traction in the long axis of the neck and slight medial rotation (Flynn, 1974). (4) Tracing to show the measurement points abc, and the angle abc and the shearing angle $\times^{\circ}$. a is the centre of the femoral head; b the midpoint of the fracture line of the distal fragment and c is the ridge at the base of the greater trochanter. The ratio bc:ab provides an index of the fracture level; angle abc shows the apparent upward or downward shift of the distal on the proximal fragment when reduction is incomplete, angle $\times^{\circ}$ is the shearing angle, an angle between the fracture line and

stretching does not occur. Traction is maintained for half a minute or so.

(d) Without disturbing either grip, the thigh is swung from the knee with a gentle deliberation through an arc towards internal rotation. The knee travels through a circle of 9–12 inch in diameter and almost 150–180°. Movement through this arc is essential because internal rotation with a straight limb will not carry the spike on the femoral neck clear of the femoral head. Thus accurate reduction is impossible because the head simply rotates within the acetabulum.

(e) When reduction is complete the extended limb can be easily rotated so that the foot, while resting on the palm of the hand, gently rolls into external rotation and then can be easily returned to full internal rotation. An unreduced limb springs back into external rotation when allowed to rest freely on the palm.

(f) The legs are abducted to produce an angle of 90° between them, this angle allows the image-intensifier to operate successfully. Slight abduction locks the fragments. The degree of traction should be such as to overcome shortening and not to cause excessive distraction of the fracture.

(g) Once the injured limb is secured, the uninjured limb can be abducted to allow optimum siting for the image-intensifier. The level of the pelvis should be checked because internal rotation of the injured limb may tilt the pelvis from the horizontal.

SURGICAL TECHNIQUE

The following operative technique is the basis of many differing procedures designed for the internal fixation of femoral neck fractures, e.g. the fixed-angle plate, sliding nail, compression screw etc.

A lateral incision is usually used once reduction has been achieved. The guide wire is inserted through the lateral femoral cortex, this is facilitated by a 3/16 inch drill hole midway between the anterior and posterior cortices, 3/4 inch distal to the bony ridge where the greater trochanter joints the shaft. The hole, being slightly larger than

---

a line drawn parallel to the femoral cortex (medial). None of these measurements are precisely accurate, and angular variations of less than 10° are not valid (Barnes *et al.*, 1976). (5) Equilibration of forces on a reduced subcapital fracture.
(6) Subcapital fracture reduced (N), and in valgus (V) which is extreme, and a precursor to avacular necrosis (Garden, 1964). (7) Congruity of head and acetabulum after accurate reduction.

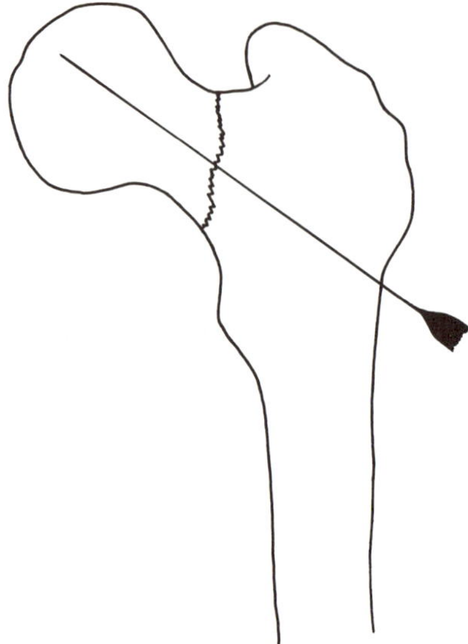

FIG. 2.11 The guide wire is inserted to within 1/4 inch of the articular margin. It should lie almost centrally in the neck.

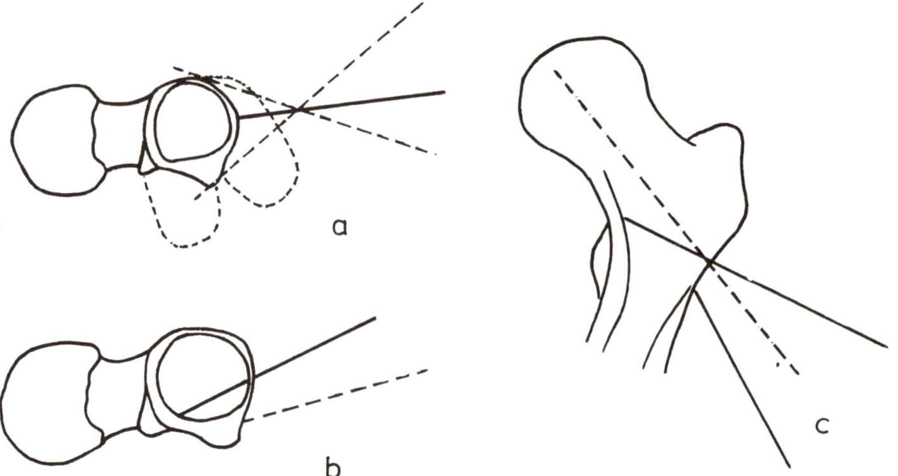

FIG. 2.12 The correct position of the guide wire in relation to the lateral cortex (*a*); (*b*) the wire is too posterior and too transverse; (*c*) the wire is too distal and posterior.

the wire, allows for fine adjustments in angulation. The guide wire is inserted towards the opposite anterior superior spine, usually at about 45° with the shaft. Bent or scored wires should be discarded since they may become impacted in the nail and then driven into the acetabulum. Hand pressure or a power tool can be used, but in either case the wire should not encounter much resistance as it traverses the femoral neck, fracture site and cancellous centre of the head. The wire should be placed in the exact centre of the neck and head (Fig. 2.11); slightly off-centre in the posterior and lower part is acceptable. However, if the wire is in the upper part of the femoral neck the head will tilt into varus and late extrusion of the pin occurs. When the pin engages the anterior part of the head fixation is poor.

When the guide wire is inserted allowance must be made for the angle of femoral torsion and the anterior surface of the patella can be observed to estimate the amount of internal rotation (less 15° gives the angle of insertion). If contact is made with hard bone when less than 3 inch of the guide wire has been inserted then the posterior cortex of the neck or the calcar femorale has been engaged (Fig. 2.12).

Once the surgeon is satisfied with the apparent position of the wires the first X-rays are taken (antero–posterior and lateral) and if necessary a new wire inserted using the position of the other wires to obtain exact alignment. In general up to four should be enough. When many wires have to be used and are unsuccessful then the fracture reduction should be checked; an incomplete reduction, especially in the lateral view, is often found, the wires passing beyond the femoral head although apparently looking satisfactory in the antero–posterior view. A common error is to have the tips of the guide wires protruding through the head; they should stop 1/8–1/4 inch short of the articular surface. The depth of the guide wire inserted, and thus the length of pin required, is estimated by comparison with another wire. If the fracture is unstable a second wire can be inserted 1/4 inch distal to and parallel with the first to steady the femoral head while the pin is being driven home.

The pin, nail or screw is threaded along the guide wire, the lateral cortex of the femur being weakened first. It is often useful to drill this area with a 3/16 inch drill in a trefoil manner. This procedure prevents splitting of the cortex (Fig. 2.13). Each time the fixation device advances the wire is observed for movement, and, if necessary, gently spun to make sure that it is not impacted. Once the device reaches the correct position, the wire is removed and a check film taken.

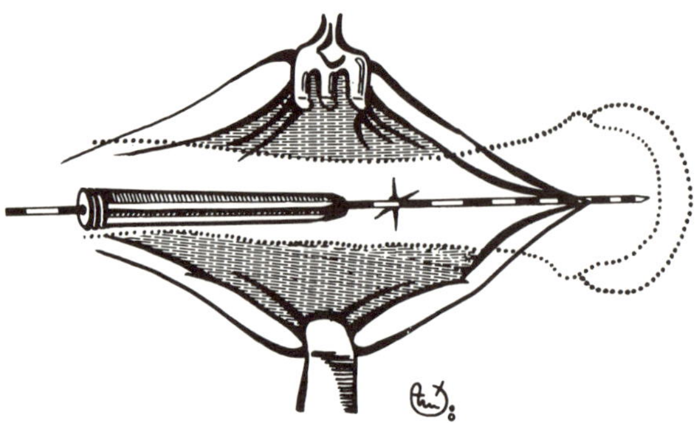

FIG. 2.13 Small cuts or several small drill holes can be used to facilitate the insertion of the Smith-Petersen nail, which is placed over the guide wire and driven into position with a special driver.

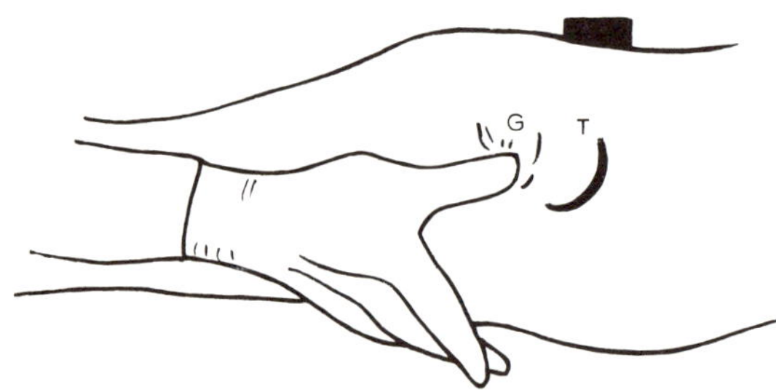

FIG. 2.14 The lateral limit of the femoral neck is identified, and the position of the greater trochanter is outlined.

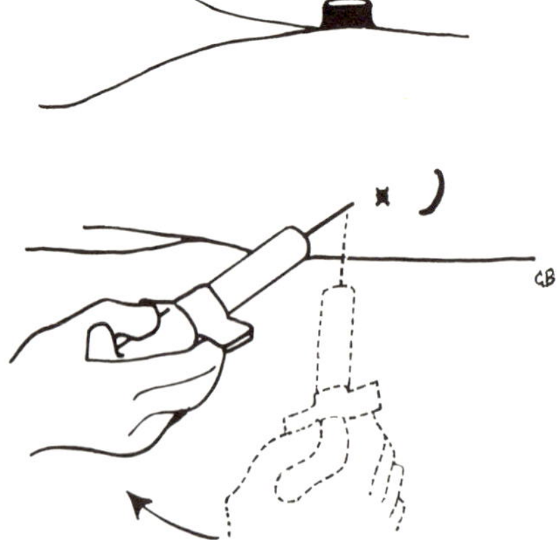

FIG. 2.15 The guide wire can be introduced by a percutaneous technique. The left hand can be used to palpate the opposite anterior superior iliac spine, or towel clips can be used as a marker over the femoral triangle and their position in relation to the head and neck determined by X-ray. The skin is incised but only a small stab incision made through the muscles and fascia. This small incision allows the Smith-Petersen or related nail to be driven along the guide wire and into the femoral head as described in the text.

If due to errors in parallax or the incorrect selection of pins, nails etc. the device is driven through the femoral head, then the whole procedure should begin again especially when it is not possible (as in the case of a blade-plate) to correct the mistake by simply withdrawing the pin. The surgeon should not gain false confidence from the belief that there is a 'good covering of cartilage over the protruding tip'.

If a guide wire jams within a nail and has not penetrated the hip joint, it can be cut flush with the lateral cortex; if penetration of the joint has occurred then the fixation device plus wires must be removed.

Finally, the results will be poor if the head is pinned in varus; this state is the precursor to non-union, delayed collapse of the femoral head and extrusion of the pin.

Figs. 2.14 and 2.15 indicate a method of inserting guide wires through a percutaneous technique, which is used for 'closed' Smith-Petersen pinning.

INTERNAL FIXATION OF SUBCAPITAL FRACTURES

The following methods of fixation of subcapital fractures of the femoral neck will be discussed:

(a) A trifin nail placed centrally in the head and neck;
(b) A long, low nail or screw resting on the calcar femorale;
(c) Multiple pins or screws, which are sometimes crossed;
(d) A sliding or telescoping nail-plate;
(e) A pin and plate or a fixed-angle nail-plate.

Trifin nail

The trifin nail (Smith-Petersen, 1937) is the least effective method of fixation (Barnes, 1967) although many varieties are still popular because of the ease of insertion (Fig. 2.16). This nail has some control over rotation but is dependent on the stability of the fracture surfaces for support and is thus quite unsuitable for grade IV fractures. Although it could be successfully used in impacted fractures there is a danger of disimpaction of fragments during its insertion. Frangakis (1966) showed that in types III and IV fractures the incidence of both ischaemic necrosis and non-union were higher in cases treated by a Smith-Petersen nail. The total failure rate, the aggregate of non-union and union with

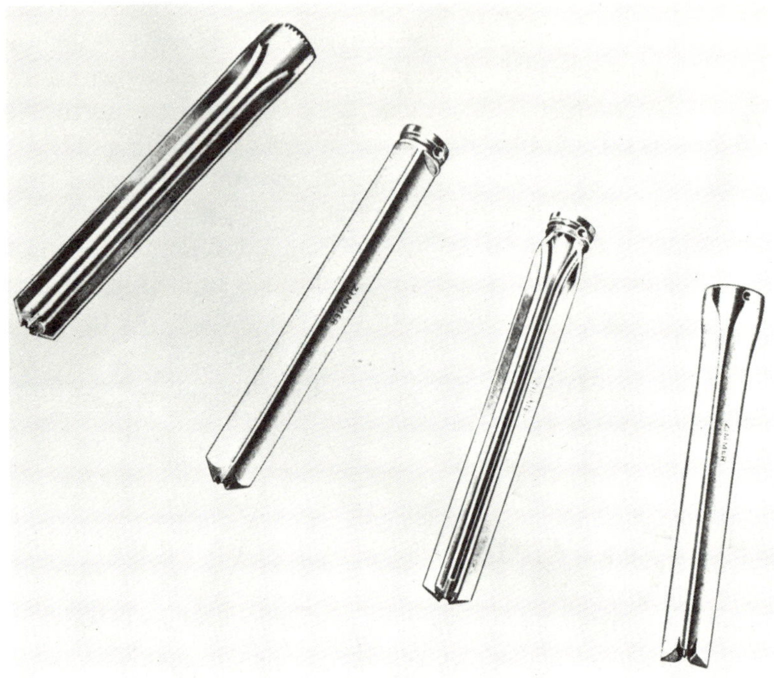

FIG. 2.16 A selection of nails used for fixation of subcapital fractures–left to right: Smith-Petersen, Watson–Jones, Watson–Jones modified Smith-Petersen, Liverpool.

subsequent ischaemic necrosis, was 70.9% after a trifin nail compared with 36.5% after a nail-plate.

In a long-term investigation of 1503 subcapital fractures (Barnes *et al.*, 1976) the Smith-Petersen nail was found to be the least effective form of fixation in displaced fractures (III and IV) (Fig. 2.17) as compared with the sliding nail, cross screw fixation and 'triangular' fixation methods. Just over 50% of displaced fractures united after Smith-Petersen nailing compared to 70% with other methods. However, the method of fixation used bore no relation to the incidence of late segmental collapse.

Makin (1965) advocated a Smith-Petersen nail for intra-acetabular fixation of the femoral head, especially when comminution of the head prevented firm impaction of the nail. By driving the nail through the acetabulum, union of the fracture was achieved at the expense of hip movement. There is no doubt that the Smith-Petersen nail (or its modifications) have proved a major surgical advance in the treatment of femoral neck fractures, but with the advent of other and more rational methods of fixation, this form of treatment is the least effective (Fig. 2.17), and by inference the least recommended.

Low nail or screw resting on the calcar femorale

Garden (1961) advocated the low-angle fixation method (Fig. 2.18). It was also possible to supplement the nail with short transverse nails or screws in unstable fractures thus embodying the principle of triangular nailing. These methods have now been superceded by the following techniques.

Multiple pins or screws (crossed)

Multiple pins

The impacted fracture usually unites readily and it is better to accept the valgus tilt rather than attempting to disimpact the fracture and risk non-union. Under these circumstances 3–5 pins (Knowle's or Moore's) can be used (Fig. 2.19) and the fracture has little likelihood of being disturbed. These pins are inserted in much the same way as a guide wire. Arnold *et al.* (1974) used percutaneous pins as a safe and effective means of treating subcapital fractures, with a low rate of complications (Table 2.2).

The Deyerle plate can be used with 7–12 pins in displaced subcapital fractures (Deyerle, 1965; Metz *et al.*, 1970). This method consists of a valgus reduction at 140°, with multiple pins inserted parallel through a side plate fixed to the femoral shaft. These pins act as a gripping force at the periphery of the femoral neck. Impaction is imperative and is facilitated by pre-drilling the pins holes. If the fracture is not impacted then loosening can occur within a few weeks. The Deyerle method is said to allow immediate weight-bearing and to give thirteen times the fixation of a trifin nail.

The disadvantage of multiple pins is that they provide less stable support at the lateral cortex and femoral neck than crossed screws and nail-plates, and thus may bend or fracture on weight-bearing. However, they are easily inserted under local anaesthesia in frail patients. Strange (1969) reported 50 patients treated in this manner using Moore's pins,

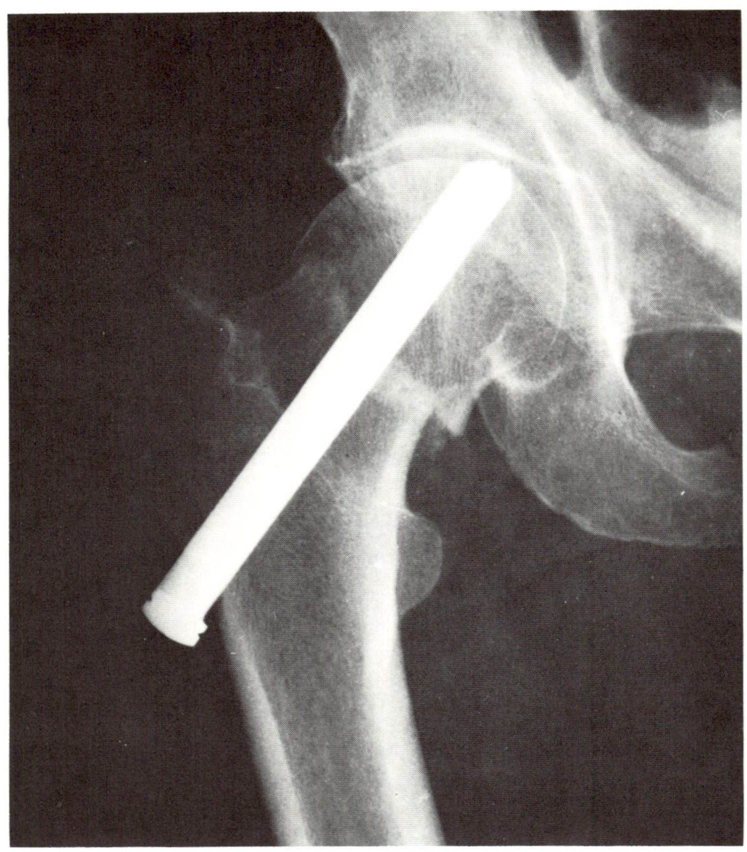

(a)

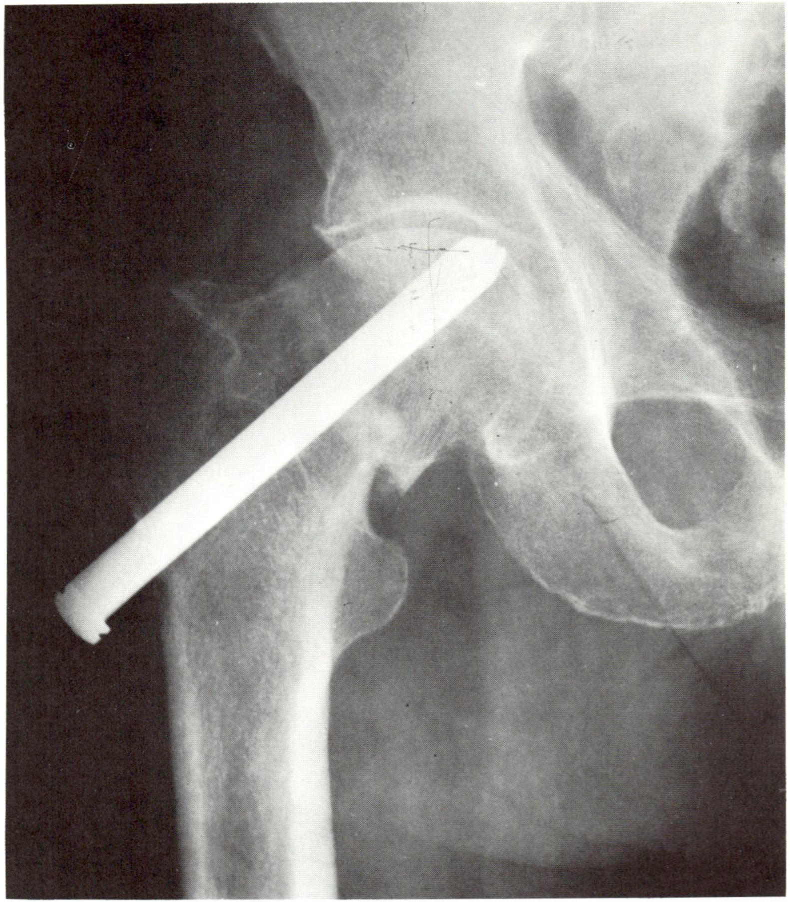

(b)

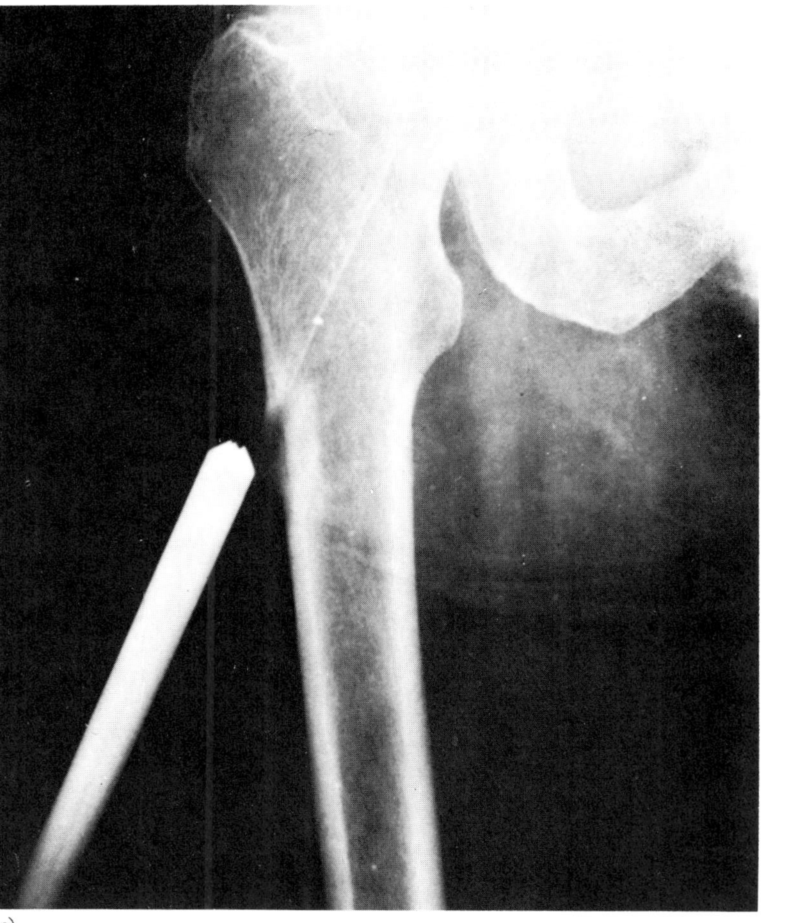
(*c*)

FIG. 2.17 (*a*) The tip of the nail is incorrect and protrudes through the femoral head; (*b*) four months later the head has collapsed; (*c*) nine months later the pin lies in the soft tissues.

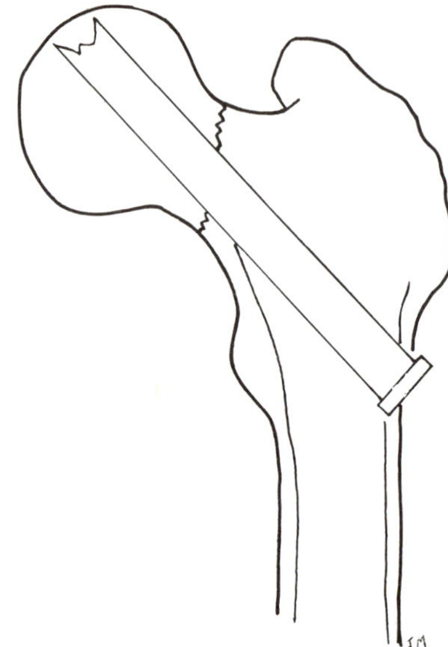

FIG. 2.18 Three point fixation, Garden technique.

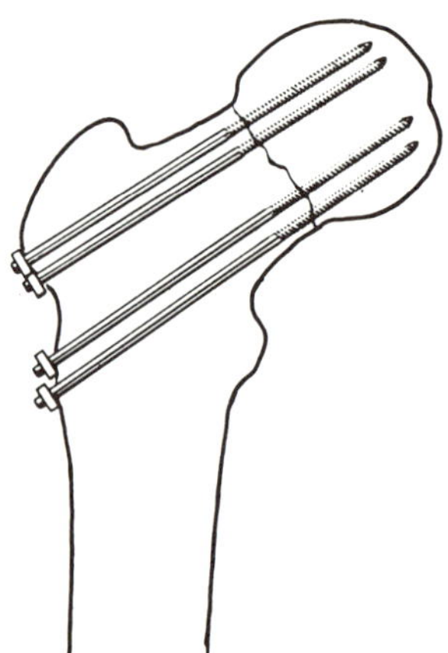

FIG. 2.19 Knowles pins, multiple pins can be used with a Deyerle plate.

11 patients were able to return home the next day and the average stay was 6–8 days.

Arnold *et al.* (1974) reviewed 754 cases of subcapital fracture treated with percutaneous Knowle's pins. The mortality was 1.3% compared with 11.3% in those patients treated by prosthetic replacement, while the infection rate was 0.5% and 16% respectively. In the undisplaced fractures there was a 93% good result, with only 7% non-union. In

TABLE 2.2 Major series of intracapsular hip fractures treated by various methods of internal fixation

FIXATION	AUTHOR	CASES	MORTALITY (%)	INFECTION (%)	NON-UNION (%)	AVASCULAR NECROSIS (%)
M.U.A and POP	St. Lukes (1930–35)	38			76	78
Smith-Petersen nail	St. Lukes (1952)	63			22	25
	Boyd and Salvatore (1964)	400	2.6		11.2	36.8
	Boyd and George (1947)	300	7		13.5	33.6
	Garcia *et al.* (1961)	105	4	3.8		
Low angle nail	Garden (1961)	60			25	16
Crossed screws	Garden (1971)	406			25	21.3
Fixed-angle nail-plate	Jewett (1956)	124			16	10.5
	Frangakis (1966)	41			17	29.2
Triangular fixation	Smyth and Shah (1974)	78			18	40
Deyerle pins	Deyerle (1965)	35				6
	Metz *et al.* (1970)	63		3.2	4.7	11.6
Richards screw	Parkes (1973) quoted in Arnold *et al.* (1974)	58			18	15
Sliding nail-plate	Pugh (1955)	29			4	—
	Brown and Abrami (1964)	194			21.2	40.5
	Fielding *et al.* (1974)	256			10	17
Muscle-pedicle bone graft	Meyers *et al.* (1973)	150	5	7.3	11	8
Knowles pins	Arnold *et al.* (1974)	505	1.3	0.5	15	12
B.M.R.C.	Barnes *et al.* (1976)	1503	7.4		28	20

the displaced fractures 15% had non-union and 12% had segmental collapse.

Thus multiple pins are probably to be preferred in frail, elderly patients with an undisplaced fracture, especially if local anaesthesia is to be used.

Screw fixation

Garden (1964) introduced a new concept in the fixation of subcapital fractures by the crossed screw technique (Fig. 2.20). Screws are ideal in undisplaced subcapital fractures but are also effective in grades III and IV (Barnes *et al.*, 1976). This method gives a 70% union rate.

Technique: Once the fracture has been reduced the position of the screws is determined by two guide wires. A horizontal wire is inserted through the anterior aspect of the greater trochanter and is directed towards the inferior part of the femoral head (antero–posterior view); it should also lie in the centre of the head (lateral view). The horizontal screw is inserted using this wire as a guide.

The oblique second screw should be more posterior and skirt the calcar femorale; its tip approaching the mid-point of the articular margin of the head. The second guide wire is inserted using a special locating device applied to the lateral femoral cortex. The position of the wire is checked radiologically and the screw inserted, lying close to the posterior surface of the horizontal screw. Thus the anterior or upper screw corresponds to the direction of the lateral group of trabeculae and the posterior screw (or oblique) coincides with the line of the medial trabecular group. Usually a 3 inch anterior and 4.5 inch posterior screws are required.

Garden (1964) reported on this method in 100 patients with grades III and IV fractures. Imperfect positioning of the screws in 7 patients led to an early breakdown and non-union.

It can be concluded that crossed screws are easy to insert and provide better fixation than parallel nails or screws. They give good control of axial rotation of the femoral head and good control of lateral rotation of the distal fragment. The only criticism is that the stability against varus displacement may depend on the integrity of the shell of cortical bone in the trochanteric region and once this crumbles fixation may be lost.

Triangle pinning

Smyth *et al.* (1964) have advocated triangular pinning (Fig. 2.21) for

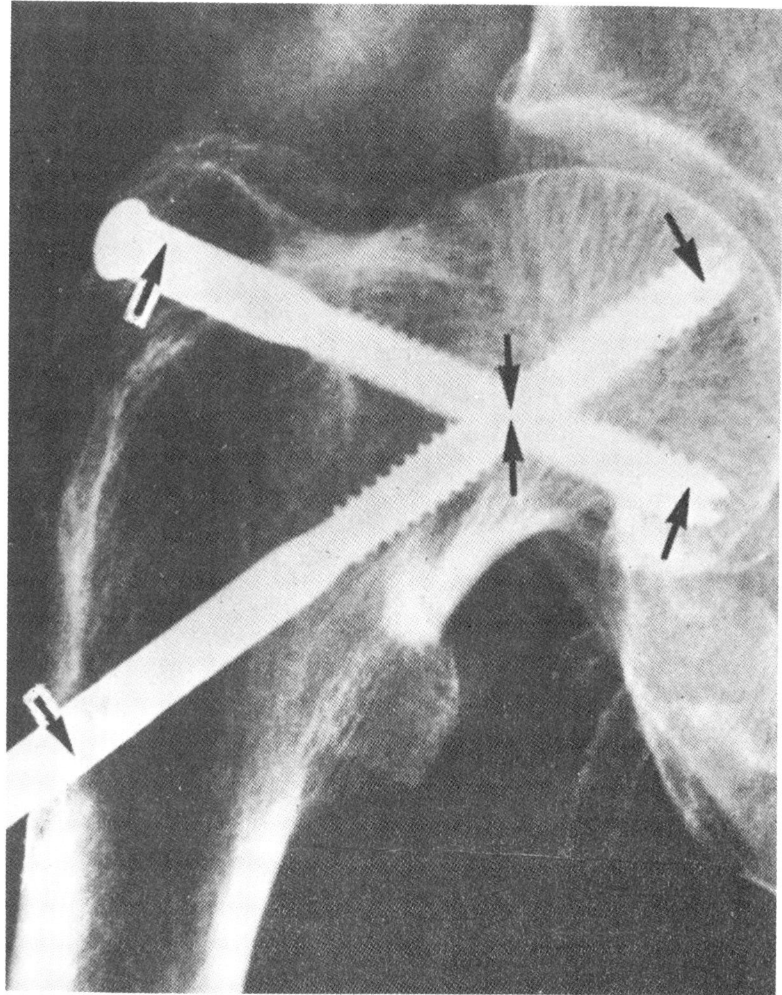

FIG. 2.20 Crossed screw technique, arrows denote key fixation points and weight transmission areas (Garden, 1964).

The single low angle screw exerts a forward and upward pressure within the femoral head, but, when combined with a horizontally disposed screw crossing it anteriorly, the direction of pressure in the capital fragment is reversed. This pressure, now exerted in a backward and downward direction, is balanced by the upward and forward thrust imparted to the femoral head by the horizontal screw. A state of equilibrium is restored. Overall postero–medial displacement of this double lever system is resisted by the calcar femorale. The posterior screw obtains a rigid fixation in the lateral cortex where it shares a common fulcrum with the horizontal screw. The latter also meets resistance where it passes through the cortex of the greater trochanter and where it lies against the posterior screw.

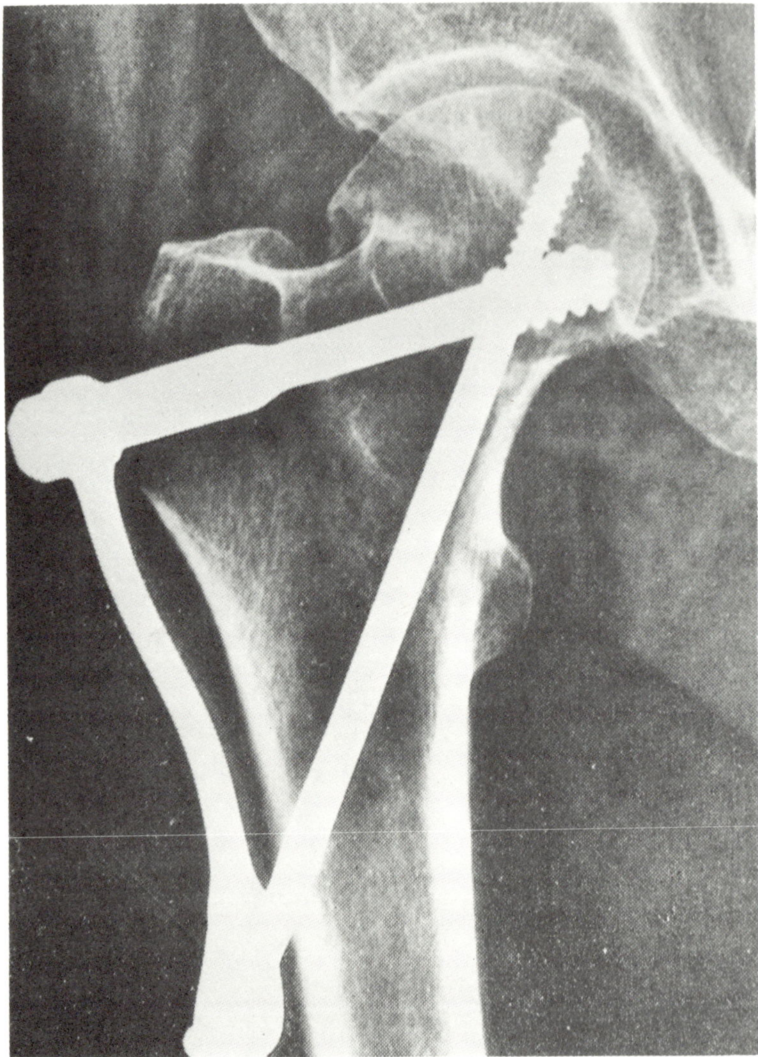

FIG. 2.21 Triangular pinning technique of Smyth *et al.* (1964, 1974).

subcapital fractures; this method gave a 70% union rate in the large series reported by Barnes *et al.* (1976).

Technique: Once the fracture is reduced a guide wire is passed through the greater trochanter close to its anterior border and directed along the neck to the inferior part of the femoral head. The wire must lie centrally in the neck and at 90° or more to the shaft.

A self-tapping screw is passed over the wire and thus directed into the femoral head. Once this has been completed a bracket is aligned in the long axis of the femoral shaft and temporarily held by a guide wire. The bracket is fixed to the upper screw by a nut, which is tightened. The lower and second screw is now inserted into the bracket, its direction being dictated by the cannulation in the inferior end of the bracket, and by the internal architecture of the reduced femoral neck. The length of both screws should be such that they extend to the periphery of the head. The strongest fixation is obtained when the whole of the threaded portions of both screws lies within the capital fragment.

Muscle–pedicle–bone graft

Meyers *et al.* (1973) have reported the technique of treating a sub-capital fracture with a fibular graft or by a muscle–pedicle–bone graft using the quadratus femoris muscle and its bone at the femoral attachment. A rectangular graft is marked out on the inter-trochanteric crest and transferred through a T-shaped incision in the posterior capsule (Fig. 2.22). However, the fracture must be stabilized with pins or screws; and one or two screws are also used to secure the graft to the posterior aspect of the femoral head and neck. This procedure is said to aid in the revascularization of the femoral head and thus prevent

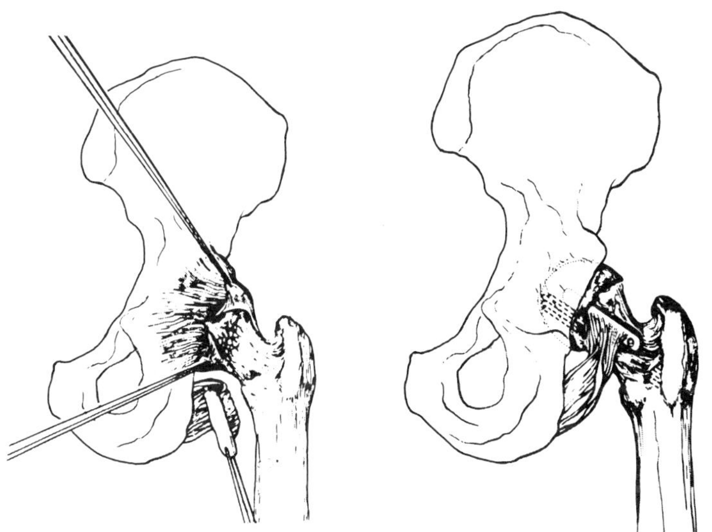

FIG. 2.22 The capsule has been incised posteriorly and the quadratus femoris muscle–pedicle–bone graft is fixed to the fracture area along the femoral neck.

non-union. However, this method has not gained wide acceptance as yet and is more complex surgically than the cross-screw or sliding nail methods.

Sliding or telescoping nail-plate

Brown and Abrami (1964) reviewed 195 patients treated with a sliding nail-plate fixation device. In 68.5% of patients there was union, 10.3% showed doubtful union, and 21.2% non-union; also 28% showed late superior segmental collapse. The Tulloch-Brown sliding nail gave 70% union in displaced fractures (Barnes *et al.*, 1976), and in this series 24% showed late segmental collapse, compared to 27.5% with crossed or triangular screw techniques and 28% with a trifin nail.

Fig. 2.23 shows two of the many varieties of sliding nail. The principle of the sliding nail is to allow firm impaction at the time of surgery and to allow for the continued impaction should reabsorption occur at the fracture site. This device can be used with a side plate (e.g.McLaughlin or Thornton) or, more commonly, incorporated into a fixed-angle blade-plate (Barr, 1973).

Technique: After reduction a guide wire is passed along the femoral neck in the usual manner lying centrally (lateral view) and just below

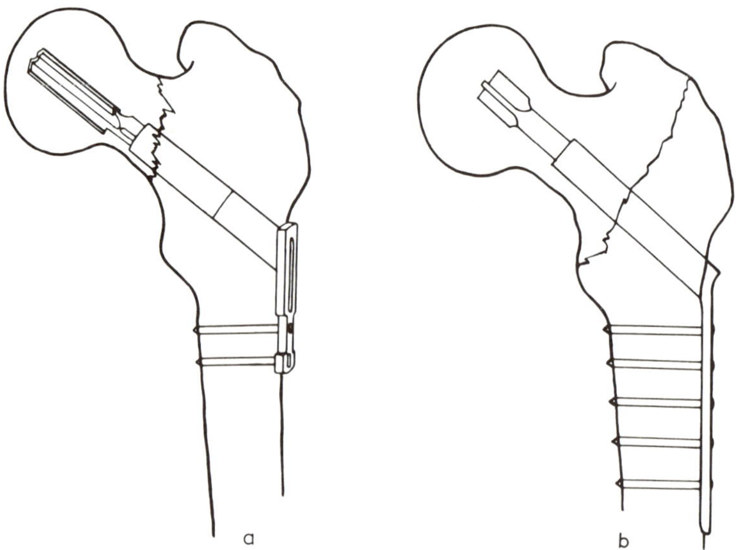

FIG. 2.23 The sliding nail can be used in both subcapital and trochanteric fractures. (*a*) Depicts the Massie nail; (*b*) shows the Ken nail.

the midline (antero–posterior view). The lateral femoral cortex is reamed using a 0.5 inch reamer and then the femoral neck is also reamed so as to produce a channel to accommodate the collar of the nail (Pugh, 1955). The nail is inserted and maintained in its shortest position. The plates are clamped to the femoral shaft. Using the driver the nail is driven to its acceptable position close to the articular margins. The plate is then secured to the shaft with screws. The tip of the nail must engage into firm bone; this requires it to be placed centrally and deeply in the femoral head, otherwise it will work loose with subsequent disimpaction of fragments.

Fielding *et al.* (1974) reviewed 256 fractures treated by a Pugh sliding nail, 90% had union and only 17% had avascular necrosis. The average telescoping was 11 mm.

Pin and plate, and other methods

Most of these methods will be described in the next section. Many centres dissatisfied with the simple trifin nail, its failure to provide adequate fixation and its inability to control rotation of the femoral head, have used either a pin and plate or a fixed-angle nail-plate, with additional screw fixation (Fig. 2.24) for both subcapital and trochanteric fractures. However, collapse of the femoral head may be associated with

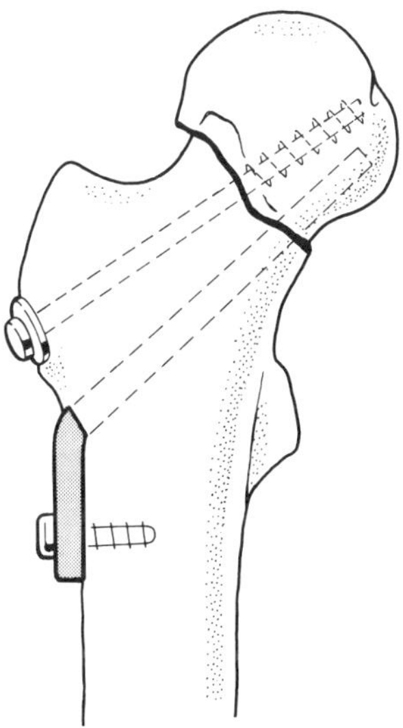

FIG. 2.24 Cancellous screw providing compression while the fixed-angle nail-plate provides support in the lower part of the femoral neck and at the lateral cortex.

pin protrusion and for this reason the sliding nail is to be preferred for subcapital fractures.

Compression hip screw

This device is gaining more widespread popularity. The procedure is outlined in Fig. 2.25. Careful reaming of the femoral neck is required for both the hip-screw shaft and the barrel of the plate. Once the hip-screw and barrel guide have been inserted the plate is slipped over the barrel guide and the latter removed. If the plate does not fit the contour of the femoral shaft it can be adjusted with bending irons. However, not more than 5° of bending is recommended. Once the plate is clamped to the femur the screw connection is firmly tightened to give compression at the fracture site in the femoral neck.

COMPLICATIONS OF SUBCAPITAL FRACTURE

In the British Medical Research Council Report (Barnes *et al.*, 1976) of 1503 subcapital fractures the mortality rate in the first month after surgery was 7.4% for women and 13.3% for men. However, there was a variation according to age; the mortality in women under 65 years being only 1.6%, but over 85 years being 20.7%. No deaths were recorded within the first month for men under 65 years, but the mortality rate was 37% in men over 84 years. The physical state of the

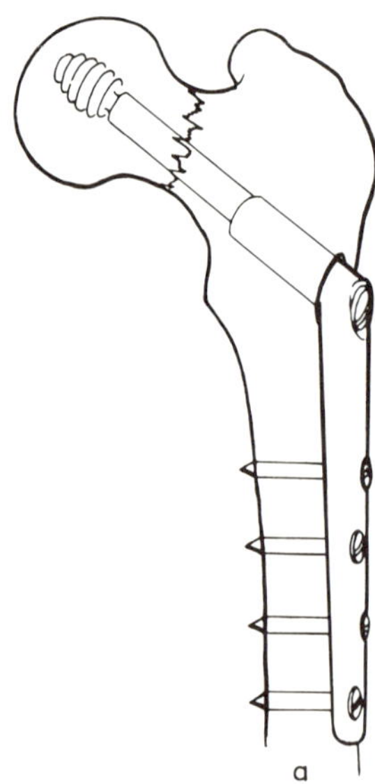

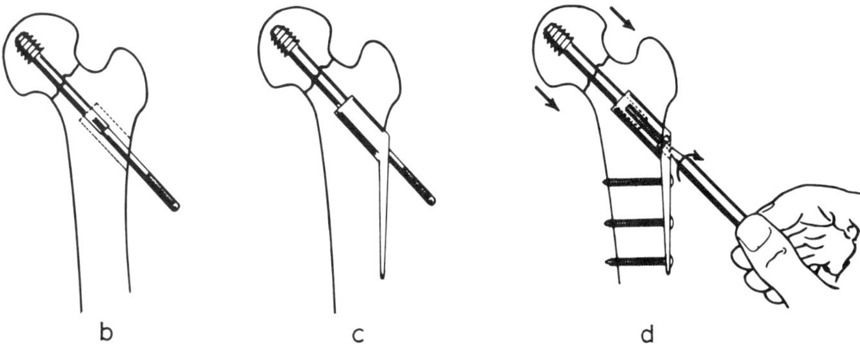

FIG. 2.25 (*a*) Compression hip screw with nail plate. (*b*) A K-wire is inserted at 45° to the femoral shaft about 2 cm below the greater trochanter, this serves as a guide for the screw. The depth setting on a calibrated reamer is set and the neck reamed for the screw. The channel is also enlarged inferiorly for the barrel of the plate. The correct screw length is determined, a screw 0.5 inch shorter should be chosen than the actual measurement (e.g. a 4 inch reamer hole uses a 3.5 inch screw). When fully inserted the end of the screw should be inside the cortex. The K-wire is removed. Then the barrel guide is inserted and turned into the end of the screw. (*c*) This provides a centring method for sliding the barrel of the plate over the shaft of the hip screw. The plate is slipped over the barrel guide and this guide removed. (*d*) The plate is clamped to the femur and screwed into place. Finally the compression screw is turned to give impaction of the fracture (adapted from Richard's Manual).

patient was found to have a profound effect on the mortality rate; one in five patients who were not fully active at the time of femoral neck fracture died within four months of the operation. The death rate was greater when the blood urea was raised, but had no direct relationship to initial anemia or to a delay of up to three days before surgery.

In the same series, the rate of non-union was 28.5% in men and 27.5% in women. It was also observed that the rate and speed of union declined with advancing age. Approximately 60% of displaced subcapital fractures united by one year in the under 65 years group, but only half that number showed union in the same period in those over 84 years. Late segmental collapse due to avascular necrosis was more common in displaced fractures in women under 75 years than in those over this age. Although the patient's weight had no obvious effect on union, late segmental collapse was more common in overweight females.

Stage I fractures almost all united and there were too few fractures in grade II for statistical analysis. In stage III fractures women had a non-union rate of 26% compared with 20% in men. In stage IV fractures 30% showed non-union in women compared with 18% in men. These figures apply after one year. By three years 31% of grade III and 35% of grade IV fractures were un-united in women compared with 28% and 26% respectively for men. An interesting feature of this report (Barnes *et al.*, 1976) was that a delay before surgery of up to one week did not affect union, nor did it lead to an increase in late segmental collapse. These figures contradict the earlier reports of Brown and Abrami (1964) who showed an 80% bony union when surgery was carried out within 24 hours of injury, compared with a 50% union when treatment was delayed.

Frangakis (1966) found a rate of avascular necrosis in 44.7% of a series of 179 patients with subcapital fractures. Avascular necrosis occurred in 38.3% of patients with established union, but in 68.7% of those with non-union. Barnes (1967) has stated that there is no agreement on the incidence of this complication apart from the observation that it is more common in grade IV injuries and when the fracture line is truly subcapital instead of basal. On radiographic evidence alone, 33% of all displaced subcapital fractures develop avascular necrosis, either partial or total; Linton (1944) reported 39% Banks (1962) 33% and Fielding *et al.* (1962) 24%. However, when the diagnosis is based on histological evidence a much higher incidence of avascular necrosis is found after subcapital fracture. Sevitt (1964) observed total or partial collapse of the femoral head in 84% of specimens removed, while Catto (1965) reported a 66% incidence in 47 femoral heads examined.

Barnes *et al.* (1976) found an incidence of late segmental collapse of 24% in women and 15% in men. A nail or screw placed high and anterior in the femoral head was associated with a considerable failure rate but the degree of penetration of the capital fragment by the fixation device had no uniform relationship to the incidence of segmental collapse. A high subcapital fracture (close to the femoral head) was associated with an increased incidence of non-union, whereas collapse of the femoral head was more common in the middle range fractures of the neck.

Finally the quality of reduction markedly affected both early and late results. When a severe varus deformity was found on check X-rays the non-union rate was 50%, compared to 25% with a satisfactory reduction. When anterior or posterior angulation of the femoral head on the neck exceeded 20° in the lateral view, there was almost a 50%

non-union rate. A very marked valgus angulation also increased the failure rate.

In conclusion almost one-third of subcapital fractures may show non-union and almost one-quarter develop avascular changes in the femoral head leading to segmental collapse. Although it appears that impacted fractures have an excellent prognosis, displaced fractures need accurate reduction and adequate fixation to offer the best chance of preserving the bony architecture of the upper femur. Unfortunately many factors are beyond the surgeon's control; these include the level of the fracture in the femoral neck, the immediate damage to the capital vessels and the age and general medical condition of the patient (Muckle, 1976). However, the quality of reduction is one of the most important factors in influencing the rate of union and avascular necrosis.

INTERNAL FIXATION OF TROCHANTERIC FRACTURES

The following section deals with fractures of the trochanteric region

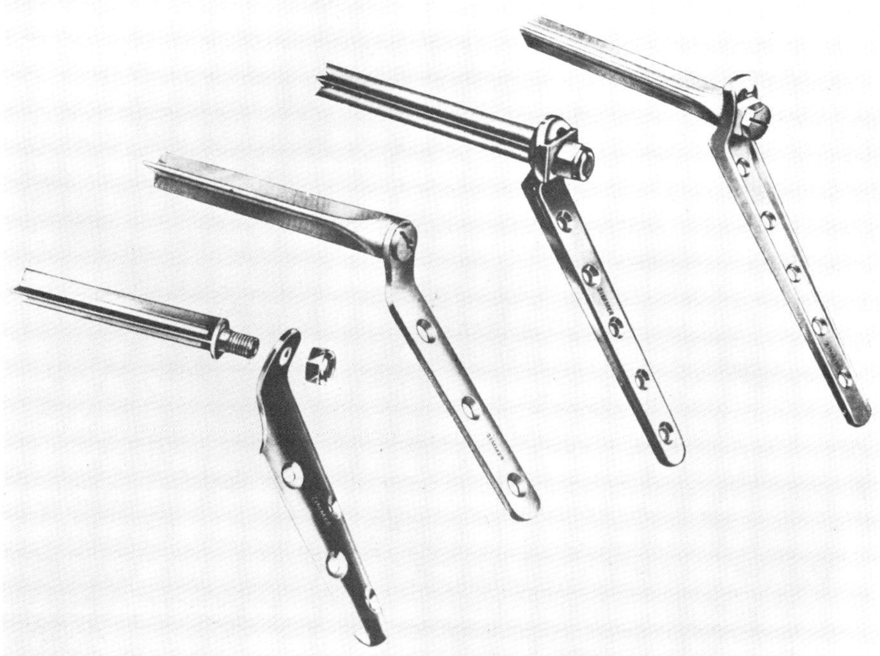

FIG. 2.26 A selection of pins and plates for fixation of trochanteric fractures (left to right) McKee, Liverpool, Northampton, and McLaughlin.

which are held with either a pin and plate or some modification such as the fixed-angle nail-plate.

Pin and plate

Fig. 2.26 shows a variety of such devices used in trochanteric fractures.

Technique: The fracture is reduced under X-ray control, but if difficulty is encountered the fragments can be palpated during surgery and further adjustments made. A lateral incision is used, and the fragments can be locked in position with bone-holding forceps. Guide wires are passed as described under subcapital fractures. Once satisfactory the pin is inserted after drilling the lateral cortex. Should this area of bone fracture then it must be reduced and fixed with oblique screws. When the nail is properly seated the plate is attached with a washer and nut but not tightly fixed. The plate should be flush with the femoral shaft and have a minimum of three holes and preferably

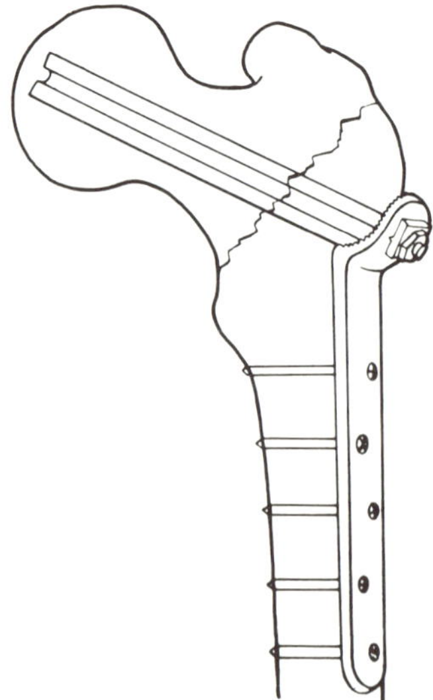

FIG. 2.27 The correct insertion of a pin and plate with the pin central in the neck and the screws at a right-angle to the plate and just penetrating the opposite cortex. A five holed-plate is preferred to a three-holed plate; a seven holed-plate can be used with low fractures of the trochanteric region. The tip of the nail should reach well into the head, if short a stress fracture will result in the femoral neck. The plate should be fixed before final impaction, otherwise a blow along the nail may be transmitted to the trochanter causing a fracture. Occasionally the iliopsoas wraps around the neck to make reduction impossible, then the muscle is divided.

five to seven, depending on the level and extent of the fracture (Fig. 2.27). The drill holes should be exactly opposite each other in the femoral cortices or the screws will not bite. Thus the drill must be held rigidly at a right-angle to the plate. The screws should not penetrate for more than a few millimetres through the far cortex. The nut connecting the pin to the plate should be firm before the screws are finally secured; if not, the plate may be lifted off the shaft when the nut is finally tightened. If a washer is used it must correspond to the nut,

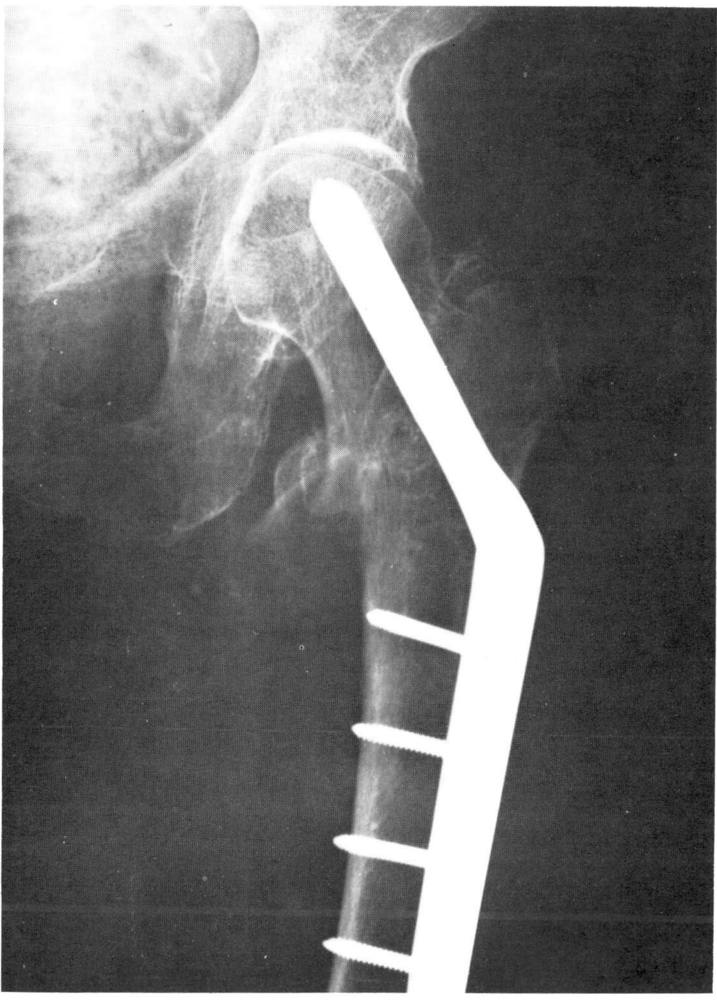

FIG. 2.28 The Jewett fixed-angle nail-plate (with overlay plate, if necessary).

a failure in correct apposition between nut, washer and pin leads to weakness at this point and eventual loosening.

Fixed-angle nail-plate

Dissatisfaction with the stability of the junction of pin and plate, and nut loosening, has led to the popularity of the above device (Fig. 2.28) (Jewett, 1956). The Jewett nail plate can be modified in several ways, and although it requires a little more expertise in both selection and insertion than a pin and plate its use is generally to be preferred to the latter.

Technique: A lateral approach is used after reduction. The guide wire is accurately positioned along the femoral neck, if necessary using a special angled insertion device (Fig. 2.29). The acute angle between shaft and wire is measured using a metal protractor and the corresponding nail-plate selected. The pin length is deducted from the guide wire. The lateral cortex is prepared with a cannulated reamer. An important point is that when the nail is being driven into the neck an assistant must hold the side plate exactly parallel to the shaft. When

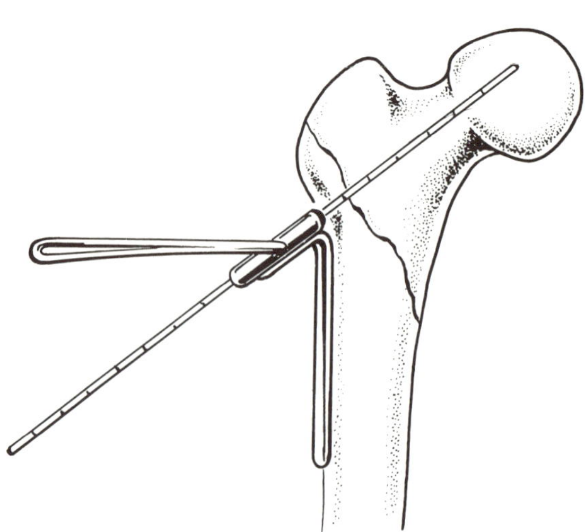

FIG. 2.29 The Jewett guide aids in correct insertion of the nail-plate. A metal protractor scored at intervals which correspond to the variations in Jewett nails can be used.

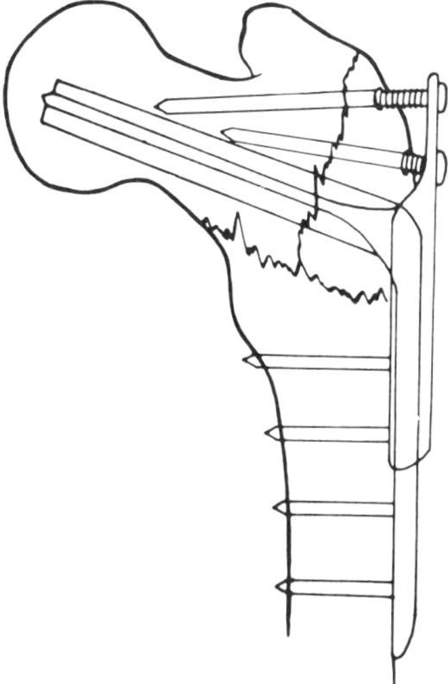

FIG. 2.30 A buttress plate gives added support to the Jewett nail when there is comminution of the trochanteric region.

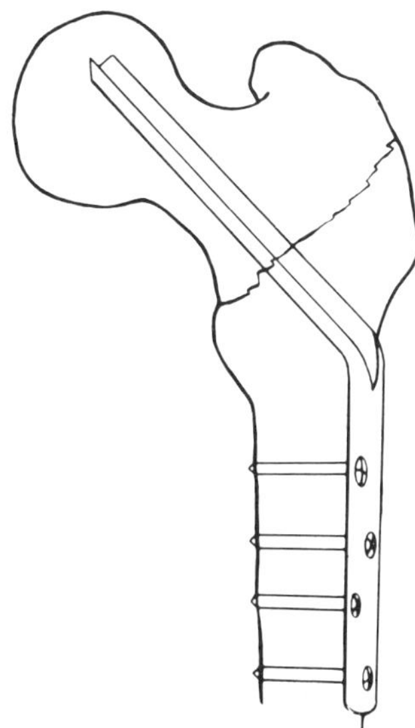

FIG. 2.31 The Neufeld nail-plate.

a Jewett nail-plate does not give adequate support a buttress plate can be added (Fig. 2.30).

Some centres use the Neufeld nail (Fig. 2.31) which allows some correction of angulation since the V part of the nail approximates to the guide wire but does not necessarily follow. Fracture of the nail-plate junction and bending of the nail (Chapter 1) have been reported (Fielding, 1973).

Comminuted, unstable inter-trochanteric fractures

Fig. 2.32 depicts the unstable inter-trochanteric fracture. Routine fixation with a nail-plate or a pin and plate results in late displacement and varus deformity. As the fragments displace, the nail may penetrate the head, bend, break or cut out of the bone. Thus the main objective is to achieve bony stability to prevent these complications.

This stability can be produced by using a medial displacement osteotomy at the level of the lesser trochanter and then firmly fixing the fragments with a nail-plate. When a Jewett plate is used the femoral neck can be tilted into valgus and before the side plate is attached, the shaft can be forcibly jammed over the remaining femoral neck and head segment; this impaction of the shaft on the neck is facilitated by cutting a slot on the lateral cortex of the shaft (Dimon, 1973; for details). A limb shortening of 0.5 to 1 inch may occur (Hughston, 1964).

Sarmiento (1973) has fully documented the use of the I-beam nail-plate fixation of these fractures. He emphasizes the importance of accurate reduction of the medial cortex of the femur as the main point of stability.

Technique: When comminution is present so that accurate closed reduction is impossible and only partially achieved by internal reduction, an oblique osteotomy in the lower fragment is required extending from below the flare of the greater trochanter, medially to a point approximately 1 cm below the apex of the fracture (Sarmiento and Williams, 1970). Once the osteotomy is completed, the resulting wedge-shaped fragment is retracted laterally to expose the medullary canal in the upper fragment (Fig. 2.32). A guide wire is driven into the upper femur parallel to the anterior cortex and at a right-angle to the plane of the fracture. When the fracture is very vertical the wire can be introduced at less than 90°. However, it is important that the distance between the guide wire entry point and the medial cortex (w–x) must equal the width of the osteotomized surface on the lower fragment (y–z). An allowance is also made for the width of the nail, thus the guide wire is correctly inserted 0.5 cm above this estimated point. X-rays confirm the position of the wire and a short, usually 6.4 cm I-beam at 135° is driven over the guide wire and into the femoral

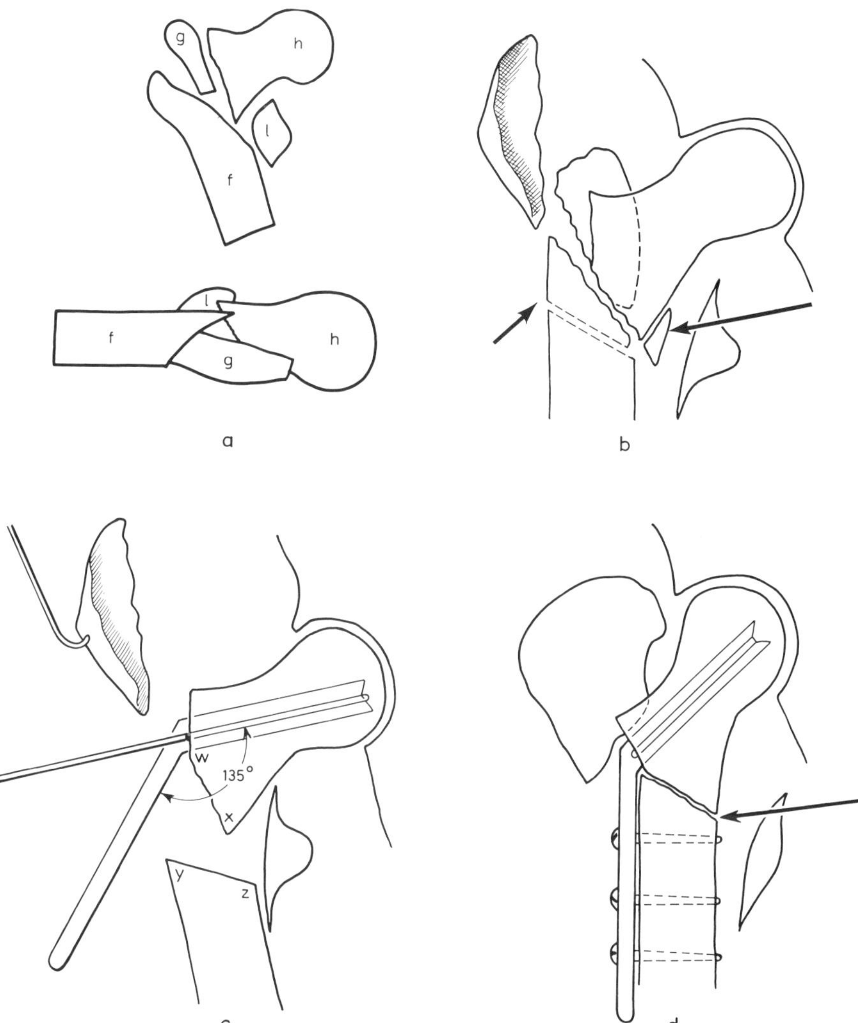

FIG. 2.32 (*a*) Unstable inter-trochanteric fracture showing the major components: (h) head; (f) shaft; (l) medial fragment and (g) posterior fragment. (*b*) oblique osteotomy below the flare of the greater trochanter (level arrowed). (*c*) fixation with guide wire and I-beam. (*d*) reduction of medial cortex (arrow) with stability. (After Sarmiento and Williams, 1970.)

head (Fig. 2.32*c*) Since the distance from the medial cortex of the upper fragment and the entry point of the nail is equal to the osteotomized surface of the lower fragment, abduction of the lower fragment brings the medial cortices into exact opposition (Fig. 2.32*d*). Any bone on the lateral aspect of the upper fragment which interferes with contact of the plate may be removed with a rongeur. Some internal rotation of the lower fragment may be required because during insertion of the nail the upper fragment is often rotated internally. The valgus position of the proximal fragment compensates for any loss in limb length.

Acrylic cement can be used to reinforce the nail-plate (Harrington, 1975), although it is best reserved for the elderly with fragile bones and when there is excessive comminution.

Subtrochanteric fractures

These have been divided into three levels (Fig. 2.33) (Fielding and Magliato, 1966). Boyd and Griffin (1949) found that they constitute almost 27% of trochanteric fractures and were the most difficult to treat. They can occur through the weakened femoral cortical bone when an excessive number of guide wires have been used during the fixation of subcapital fractures. Coxa vara, medial migration and non-union are more common in subtrochanteric fractures. Type 1 fracture usually shows 90% union, type 2 shows 66% union and type 3 shows 43% union (Fielding, 1973).

Because of the stresses applied to this area of the femur, strong plates are required. Holt and Massie fixation devices have been em-

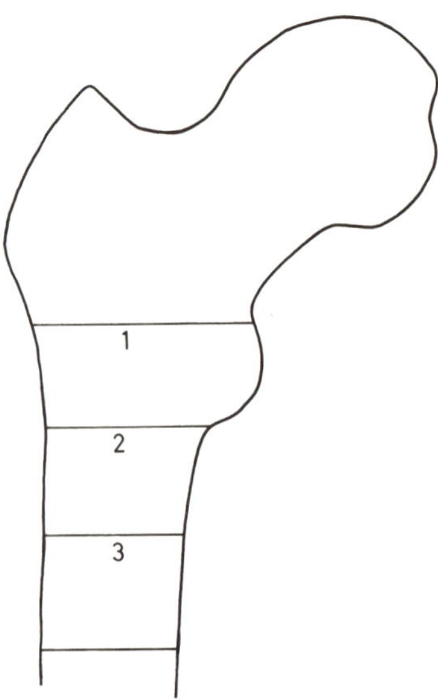

FIG. 2.33 Areas involved in subtrochanteric fractures. (After Fielding and Magliato, 1966.)

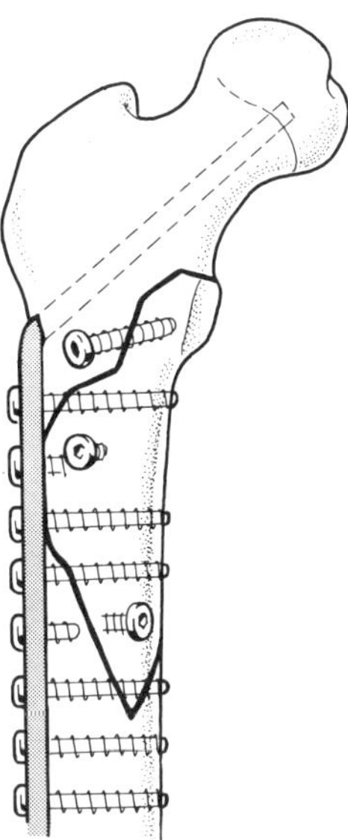

FIG. 2.34 Rigid internal fixation of the large fragment is obtained from lag screws, then the 130° blade-plate is introduced. Some of the screws on the plate are short so that they do not penetrate the fractured area. (Müller *et al.*, 1970.)

ployed and a variety of nail-plates with an extended plate, but early weight-bearing (less than 12 weeks) can be the cause of appliance failure and non-union. Additional bone grafting may be required especially when comminution is present and there is danger of poor fixation. The pertrochanteric plate (Müller *et al.*, 1970) with interfragmental compression is probably the treatment of choice (Fig. 2.34). This technique may be supplemented with a bone graft. After surgery the patient is non-weight bearing for 6–10 weeks.

When there is comminution of the lateral cortex of the upper fragment, the strong adductor pull may force the lower fragment medially and cause penetration of the pin through the head. Several types of buttress plates have been used (Fig. 2.30) to offset this strong adducting force; in addition, medial displacement of the lower fragment can be carried out before fixation. Fielding (1973) has advocated an intramedullary rod with nail fixation (Zickel nail) in low subtrochanteric fractures.

AO-fixation techniques

The recent interest in compression techniques of internal fixation has not escaped femoral neck fractures (Müller *et al.*, 1970). When the

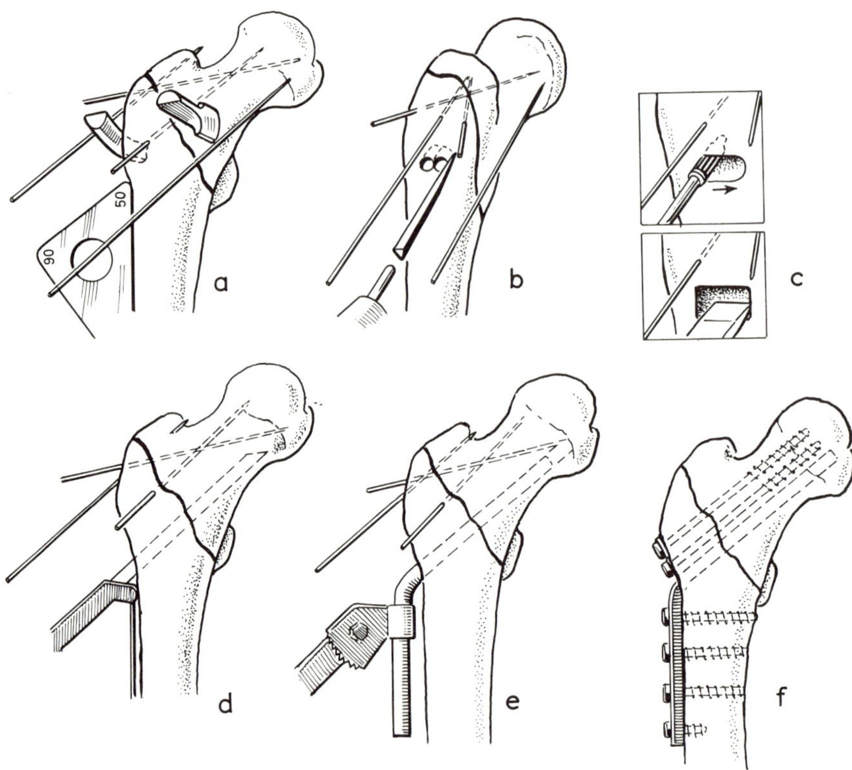

FIG. 2.35 Special features of the angled blade-plate. The channel for the blade of the plate is cut by a special seating chisel which has an identical profile to the blade of the plate. (*a*) The lower K-wire lies along the front of the neck while a second is inserted at 50° (using the triangular positioning plate). (*b*) An area 2.5 cm below the prominence of the greater trochanter is drilled with a 4.5 mm drill. (*c*) The holes are enlarged and the oblique part of the lateral cortex cut with a fine chisel, this area is used to seat the shoulder of the plate. Since the shaft of the blade-plate must lie flat on the femoral shaft, it is necessary that the flap of the chisel guide lies parallel with the femoral shaft while the seating chisel is hammered in. (*d*) The seating chisel with its chisel guide parallel to the K-wire in the greater trochanter is inserted. (*e*) The chisel is removed and the angled blade-plate driven home. (*f*) Further fixation is provided by two cancellous lag screws which apply compression between fragments. (After Müller *et al.*, 1970.)

lateral cortex of the femur is intact most fractures can be stabilized with a 130° pertrochanteric plate, and the technique is depicted in Fig. 2.35. When there is weakness of the lateral cortex a condylar plate with bone cement, if necessary, can be used; cancellous bone screws can be employed for interfragmentary compression.

These techniques are becoming increasingly popular and are to be recommended, especially in low fractures of the trochanteric region.

The results of internal fixation are routinely gratifying in trochanteric fractures and the treatment of choice is the fixed-angle blade-plate, although accurate apposition between bony fragments and the establishment of stability at the fracture site (by a displacement osteotomy if necessary) is required to prevent the fixation appliance from cutting out of the bone on weight-bearing. The commonest error is to fix the limb in external rotation or varus with an associated shortening which may require a raise on the shoe when above 3 cm.

COMPLICATIONS OF TROCHANTERIC FRACTURES

A mortality rate of 21.7% has been recorded after fixation of trochanteric fractures, the average age in the series being 73.2 years (Sweet, 1967). However, Horn and Wang (1964) reported a series of 170 inter-trochanteric fractures with an average age of 69.6 years and a mortality rate of 5.3%. All their patients were treated non-operatively with Russell traction. Evans (1949) calculated a 33.7% mortality among 1194 patients treated by 13 authors.

Non-union is not a feature of trochanteric fractures, Boyd and Griffin (1949) reporting only 4 cases of non-union in 209 patients reviewed. Avascular necrosis is also rare after this type of femoral neck fracture: Mann (1973) reported 1 case in 239 fractures reviewed and added another 5 cases to the literature. He suggests that the internal fixation device could interfere with the vascularity of the head especially the lateral epiphyseal vessels when the nail or screw is placed high in the superior and posterior quadrants.

Boyd and Griffin (1949) reported a coxa vara deformity of 10% and a medial migration of the fragments in 5% of 209 trochanteric fractures treated by a nail-plate. Subtrochanteric fractures were described as the most difficult of all trochanteric fractures to stabilize. Watson *et al.* (1964) reported a 19% non-union in these fractures treated by a Jewett nail-plate or a Kuntscher nail with supplementary fixation. Fielding (1973) found that 12 out of 46 subtrochanteric fractures treated with nail-plates showed non-union due to nail breakage occurring at the nail-plate junction or through the plate portion at a screw hole, usually at the level of the fracture site. Eight of the un-united subtrochanteric fractures healed after bone grafting and further internal fixation.

REFERENCES

ARNOLD, W.D., LYDEN, J.P. and MINKOFF, J. (1974). *J. Bone Jt. Surg.* **56A**, 254.
BANKS, H.H. (1962). *J. Bone Jt. Surg.* **44A**, 931.
BARNES, R. (1967). *J. Bone Jt. Surg.* **49B**, 607.
BARNES, R, BROWN, J.T, GARDEN, R.S. and NICOLL, E.A. (1976). *J. Bone Jt. Surg.* **58B**, 2.
BARR, J.S. (1973). *Clin. Orth. & Rel. Res.* **92**, 63.
BÖHLER, L. Quoted in STUCK, W.G. (1949). S. *Afr. med. J.* **42**, 1021.
BOYD, H.B. and GEORGE, I.L. (1947). *J. Bone Jt. Surg.* **29**, 13.
BOYD, H.B. and GRIFFIN, L.L. (1949). *Arch. Surg.* **58**, 853.
BOYD, H.B. and SALVATORE, J.E. (1964). *J. Bone Jt. Surg.* **46A**, 1066.
BROWN, J.T. and ABRAMI, G. (1964). *J. Bone Jt. Surg.* **46B**, 648.
CATTO, M. (1965). *J. Bone Jt. Surg.* **47B**, 749.
DEYERLE, W.M. (1965). *Clin. Orthop.* **39**, 135.
DIMON, J.H. (1973). *Clin. Orth. & Rel. Res.* **92**, 100.
EVANS, E.M. (1949). *J. Bone Jt. Surg.* **31B**, 190.
FIELDING, J.W. WILSON, J.H. (jun) and ZICKEL, R.E. (1962). *J. Bone Jt. Surg.* **44A**, 965.
FIELDING, J.W. and MAGLIATO, J. (1966). *Surgery Gynec. Obstet.* **122**, 155.
FIELDING, J.W. (1973). *Clin. Orth. & Rel. Res.* **92**, 86.
FIELDING, J.W., WILSON, S.A. and RATZAR, S. (1974). *J. Bone Jt. Surg.* **56A**, 1464.
FLYNN, M. (1974). *Injury* **5**, 309.
FRANGAKIS, E.K. (1966). *J. Bone Jt. Surg.* **48B**, 17.
GARCIA, A., NEER, C.S. and AMBROSE, G.B. (1961). *J. Trauma*, **1**, 128.
GARDEN, R.S. (1961). *J. Bone Jt. Surg.* **43B**, 647.
GARDEN, R.S. (1964). *J. Bone Jt. Surg.* **46B**, 630.
GARDEN, R.S. (1971). *J. Bone Jt. Surg.* **53B**, 183.
HARRINGTON, K.O. (1975). *J. Bone Jt. Surg.* **57A**, 744.
HORN, J.S. and WANG, Y.C. (1964). *Br. J. Surg.* **51**, 574.
HOROWITZ, B.G. (1966). *Surg. Gynec. Obstet. with Int. Abst. Surg.* **123**, 565.
HUGHSTON, J.C. (1964). *J. Bone Jt. Surg.* **46A**, 1145.
JEWETT, E.L. (1956). *Am. J. Surg.* **91**, 621.
LINTON, P. (1944). *Acta Chirug. Scand.* 86 suppl.
LINTON, P. (1949). *J. Bone Jt. Surg.* **31B**, 184.
MAKIN, M. (1965). *J. Bone Jt. Surg.* **47B**, 198.
MANN, R.J. (1973). *Clin. Orth. & Rel. Res.* **92**, 108.
MASSIE, W.K. (1962). *Clin. Orthop.* **22**, 180.
METZ, C.W., SELLERS, T.D., FEAGIN, J.A., LEVINE, M.I., ONKEY, R.G., DYER, J.W. and EBERHARD, E.J. (1970). *J. Bone Jt. Surg.* **52A**, 113.
MEYERS, M.H., HARVEY, J.P. and MOORE, T.M. (1973). *J. Bone Jt. Surg.* **55A**, 257.
MÜLLER, M.E., ALLGÖWER, M. and WILLENEGGER, H. (1970). *Manual of Internal Fixation.* Springer-Verlag, Berlin.
MUCKLE, D.S. (1976). *Injury* **8**, 98.
PAUWELS, F. (1935). *Z. Orth. Chir.* **63**: suppl.
PUGH, W.L. (1955). *J. Bone Jt. Surg.* **37A**, 1085.
SARMIENTO, A. (1973). *Clin. Orth. & Rel. Res.* **92**, 77.

SARMIENTO, A., WILLIAMS, E.M. (1970). *J. Bone Jt. Surg.* **52A**, 1309.
SEAL, P.V. (1972). *J. Bone Jt. Surg.* **54B**, 200.
SEVITT, S. (1964). *J. Bone Jt. Surg.* **46B**, 270.
SMYTH, E.M.J., ELLIS, T.S., MANIFOLD, M.C. and DEWERY, P.R. (1964). *J. Bone Jt. Surg.* **46B**, 664.
SMYTH, E.M.J. and SHAH, V.M. (1974). *Injury* **5**, 197.
SMITH-PETERSEN, M.N. (1937). *Surg. Gynec. Obstet.* **64**, 287.
STRANGE, F.G.ST.C. (1969). *J. Bone Jt. Surg.* **51B**, 574.
SWEET, M.B.E. (1967). *J. Bone Jt. Surg.* **49B**, 199.
WATSON, K., CAMPBELL, R.D. (jun). and WADE, P.A. (1964). *J. Trauma*, **4**, 457.
WILSON, P.D. (1938). *Experience in the Management of Fractures and Dislocations.* Lippincott Co., London & Philadelphia.

Chapter Three

FRACTURES OF THE FEMORAL NECK: PART 2

D. S. Muckle

Prosthetic replacement of the femoral head ~ Treatment of avascular necrosis of the femoral head ~ Impacted fractures ~ Stress fractures ~ Fractures of the greater and lesser trochanter ~ Fractures of the femoral neck with a stiff hip ~ Post-irradiation fractures ~ Fractures of the femur in Paget's disease of bone ~ Fractures through metastases ~ Fractures through primary bone tumours ~ Fractures of the femoral head ~ Infection after hip operations ~ Physiotherapy and rehabilitation

PROSTHETIC REPLACEMENT OF THE FEMORAL HEAD

In 1920 Hey Groves used an ivory hip prosthesis to treat femoral neck fractures. An acrylic-type prosthesis was popularized by the Judet brothers in 1948. In 1954 Thompson introduced a vitallium prosthesis, although in 1939 Moore and Bohlman had used a similar prosthesis to replace the proximal femur in a patient with a giant cell tumour. In the 1950s the total hip arthroplasty, as exemplified by the McKee-Farrar and Charnley prostheses, was under development.

The use of the endoprosthesis after a femoral neck fracture has certain advantages, namely early weight-bearing, the avoidance of avascular necrosis and non-union; while hospital stay can be reduced by approximately 30% compared to internal fixation (Gossling and Hardy, 1969).

However, the contra-indications to the use of a prosthesis include acetabular disease (either from injury, osteoarthrosis, infection or some degenerative disorder), a non-ambulatory patient, and the presence of local or generalized infection, including sacral sores, skin ulceration, bladder infection and incontinence.

Prosthetic replacement is usually used as a primary procedure in displaced subcapital fractures in elderly patients (over 70 years) especially if the capital fragment cannot be reduced or if internal fixation is delayed. Although it was commonly taught that a delay in internal fixation of over three days was prejudicial to the femoral head, Barnes *et al.* (1976) showed that a delay of up to 7 days could be tolerated and was not associated with an increased incidence of non-union or of late collapse of the femoral head.

Other factors should be taken into account. Frail, elderly patients, when there is a history of epileptiform seizures or spasmodic contractions of the muscles (such as Parkinsonism where movement of the fracture may cause non-union), are candidates for prosthetic replacement. Such replacement of the femoral head is obligatory in undiagnosed fractures showing non-union, or when the nail or pin has slipped or fractured, when the femoral head has developed avascular necrosis and segmental collapse and when there are neoplastic deposits in the femoral head. Other indications include a fracture–dislocation of the hip, especially if the fracture involves the superior weight-bearing surface of the head; a fracture and complete dislocation of the femoral head; and in post-irradiation fractures in the femoral neck where avascular necrosis is a real possibility.

Types of prosthesis

Fig. 3.1 shows the two most commonly used prostheses, the Austin Moore and the Thompson (1954). The latter is often used with bone cement and its smaller size makes it easier to insert through an antero-lateral incision.

However, the pure lateral incision is not recommended for this form of hip arthroplasty since access is limited and it is not unknown for the femoral shaft to be damaged either during reaming of the medullary cavity or during insertion of the prosthesis, especially the bulky Moore's prosthesis.

The posterior approach gives a bountiful view of the acetabulum and allows easy insertion of the prosthesis and has been the most commonly used approach. However, the sciatic nerve or its peroneal branch are at risk; while an inadequate repair of the capsule and external rotators can lead to a posterior dislocation. The series of 243 patients reported by Chan and Hoskinson (1975) confirmed the findings of the author, namely that the rate of infection and frequency of dislocation were

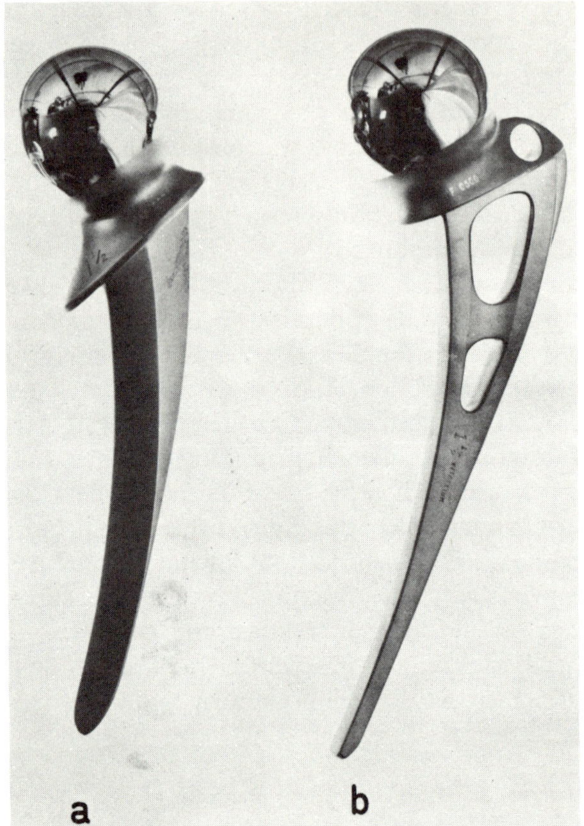

FIG. 3.1 (*a*) The Thompson prosthesis; (*b*) The Austin Moore prosthesis.

much greater when a posterior approach was used compared to an anterior (antero-lateral) approach. In the former approach the infection rate was 18.5% and the number of dislocations were 19 compared to 6.5% and 1 dislocation with the latter method.

The antero-lateral approach, basically a Smith-Petersen approach, is the method of choice. Since the capsule is divided anteriorly, the prosthesis is more stable with the hip in the position of flexion and medial rotation (whereas with the posterior approach, the hip is more stable in a position of extension and lateral rotation).

Technique of insertion of prosthesis

The hip is dislocated and the head removed with a cork-screw remover; sometimes the head is so friable that it has to be removed with bone nibblers. However, it is best to retain the femoral head if possible as an accurate assessment of size allows for a correct selection of prosthesis. The neck is shaped for correct angulation by aligning the prosthesis on the outer aspect and making two small saw marks on each cortex of the neck. The medullary canal is cleared of cancellous tissue; a rasp, flexible reamer or large curette is used. The latter is to be preferred when there is marked osteoporosis because the rasp or reamer can easily penetrate the femoral cortex. A notch is cut in the medullary canal of the neck, the direction of this notch will be reflected in the final position of the prosthesis, thus care must be taken at this stage.

The trial prosthesis is inserted and any minor modifications to the angulation of the femoral neck carried out using either a small saw or bone nibblers; however, enough calcar must remain to support the medial aspect of the prosthesis. Once the prosthesis fits snuggly a trial reduction is made. A swab can be placed in the acetabulum so that the prosthesis can be dislocated with ease. If the limb will not reduce more bone is removed from the femoral neck. It is often surprising how little needs removing to allow reduction, often 5–10 mm will suffice. A failure to insert the stem into the shaft is often due to incorrect reaming especially in the region of the greater trochanter where the cancellous bone can press against the hump of the prosthesis. The isthmus may be very narrow in small, elderly women and this area of bone may require gentle expansion with a K-nail reamer. Once the prosthesis is in close approximation to the shaft and neck it can be tapped gently into position. Cement may be used and should completely surround the stem. Care must be taken on reducing the prosthesis into the acetabulum since a rotatory strain can fracture the shaft.

TOTAL HIP ARTHROPLASTY

In the relatively young patients (65 years and less, approximately) a total hip arthroplasty can be advantageously employed (Charnley, 1964), especially if the acetabulum is damaged or diseased. In all patients who have wearing of the articular cartilage of the acetabulum after simple prosthetic replacement, usually denoted by hip pain or prosthetic migration into the acetabular bone, a total hip arthroplasty can be substituted.

Pseudarthrosis

As a final procedure, especially in the presence of severe or deep-seated infection, a Girdlestone pseudarthrosis can be carried out with removal of the prosthesis (or fixation device) and the diseased tissues.

COMPLICATIONS OF PROSTHETIC REPLACEMENT

Glass (1965) in a review of 259 Moore arthroplasties found a mortality of 13.4% and an infection rate of 10%. Fracture of the femur during insertion of the prosthesis occurred 5 times and dislocation of the hip 14 times. In a late review of 78 patients he found that 10 had had their prosthesis removed because of sepsis or recurrent dislocation. Chan and Hoskinson (1975) in their review of 243 Thompson arthroplasties found a mortality rate of 14.4% at six weeks, an infection rate of 13.2% (including 2.1% of patients having a deep infection) and a dislocation rate of 8.2%. In relatively fit elderly patients there is little difference in the complication rate after internal fixation or prosthetic replacement. However, in unfit elderly patients the mortality rate can be almost three times greater after prosthetic replacement, Raine (1973) reported a 33% mortality after the insertion of a prosthesis compared to 12% after internal fixation.

Dislocation can occur in almost 10% of all prosthetic replacements being especially common after a posterior approach. Chan and Hoskinson (1975) in their comparison of dislocation rates (0.9% anterior; 14% posterior) suggested an inherent instability in the posterior approach when the Thompson prosthesis was used. The design of this prosthesis with its curved varus stem facilitates insertion through an anterior incision and Thompson himself preferred the Smith-Petersen approach (Thompson, 1954). They also noted that 75% of dislocations occurred in the posterior group during the first two weeks of surgery while the patient was confined to bed, and the supine position conferred no advantage. Indeed observations on the standard nursing procedure in turning patients emphasized the difficulty in maintaining hips in the stable position of extension and lateral rotation after the posterior approach.

The seeming stability at the time of reduction and the use of traction conferred no benefit in reducing the incidence of dislocation, and although an incorrect version of the prosthesis was not a great factor in leading to dislocation, any minor degree of malposition associated with excessive residual neck length, was prejudical to joint stability (Fig. 3.2) (Chan and Hoskinson, 1975).

Infection is a serious complication and may not be associated in the elderly with a rise in temperature; it is discussed later.

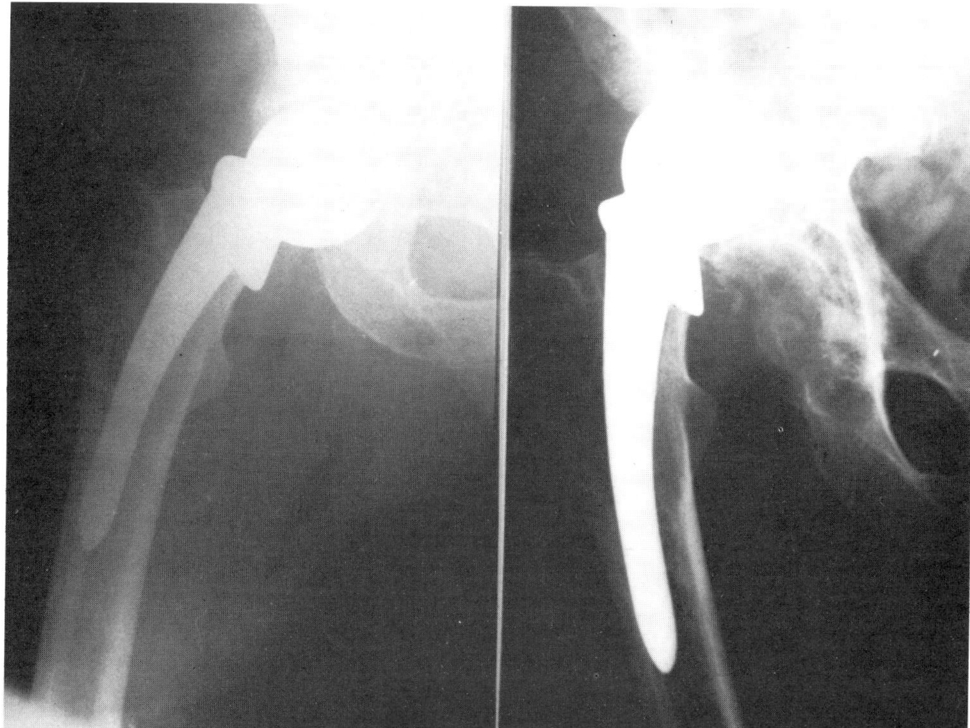

FIG. 3.2 Inadequate resection of the femoral neck endages the stability of the Thompson's prosthesis. A radiograph taken twelve days after operation showing dislocation of the prosthesis (J. Hoskinson, personal communication).

Other late complications include loosening of the prosthesis, proximal migration, distal migration, heterotopic ossification, metal fatigue and pain (Coventry, 1964). The X-ray changes associated with loosening are absorption of the femoral neck, deepening of the acetabulum, acetabular sclerosis, a radio-lucent zone in the femoral shaft, and motion of the prosthesis with traction and rotation.

In conclusion it can be said that prosthetic replacement of the femoral head should not be undertaken lightly because of the associated mortality in the unfit elderly, while in the younger patient the preservation of the femoral head by internal fixation is desirable.

TREATMENT OF AVASCULAR NECROSIS OF THE FEMORAL HEAD

The treatment of an avascular femoral head depends upon the age of the patient. In younger subjects especially when the acetabulum is diseased or injured (as for example following a dislocated hip or a failed pinning operation) the most advantageous operation is a total hip arthoplasty. In older or more frail subjects a Thompson or Moore's arthroplasty will suffice.

About one-third of displaced subcapital fractures will undergo ischaemic necrosis (Fielding *et al.*, 1962) and unless the patient is followed at three monthly intervals over the first year and six monthly intervals the following year, then the true incidence of failed pinning operations will not be realized. Not all patients who develop segmental necrosis will require replacement of the femoral head; some patients manage surprisingly well with little or no pain, while in others the patient's mobility may be hindered by concurrent disease, such as hemiplegia or Parkinson's disease. Complete necrosis of the femoral head after a pin or pin and plate operation usually means removing the metallic implant and substituting a Thompson's or a Moore's prosthesis, or a total hip replacement. This second operation is required in about 10% of all subcapital fractures treated by internal fixation (usually grade III fractures), although the incidence rises to about 20% when grade IV fractures are included.

IMPACTED FRACTURES

Fractures of the femoral neck are considered to be impacted (Fig. 3.3) when they do not displace during movements of the hip; however, most observers regard these fractures as only the initial stage (I) in subcapital fractures, and doubt whether a separate terminology is needed.

The criteria of impaction are (a) absence of deformity at the affected hip; (b) ability to rotate and flex the hip; (c) painless passive movement and (d) radiographic evidence showing close apposition of fragments.

Two methods of treatment are proposed: conservative treatment (Crawford, 1965) is said to give a high rate of union and a low incidence of avascular necrosis; and surgery (Banks, 1962; Garden, 1964). Proponents of the latter method point out that impacted fractures often displace spontaneously in recumbency or early weight-bearing.

Bentley (1968) reviewed 70 patients with impacted femoral neck fractures, and compared the two methods; 47 patients having conservative treatment and 23 internal fixation. In the group treated conservatively 88% had fracture union and the average period to

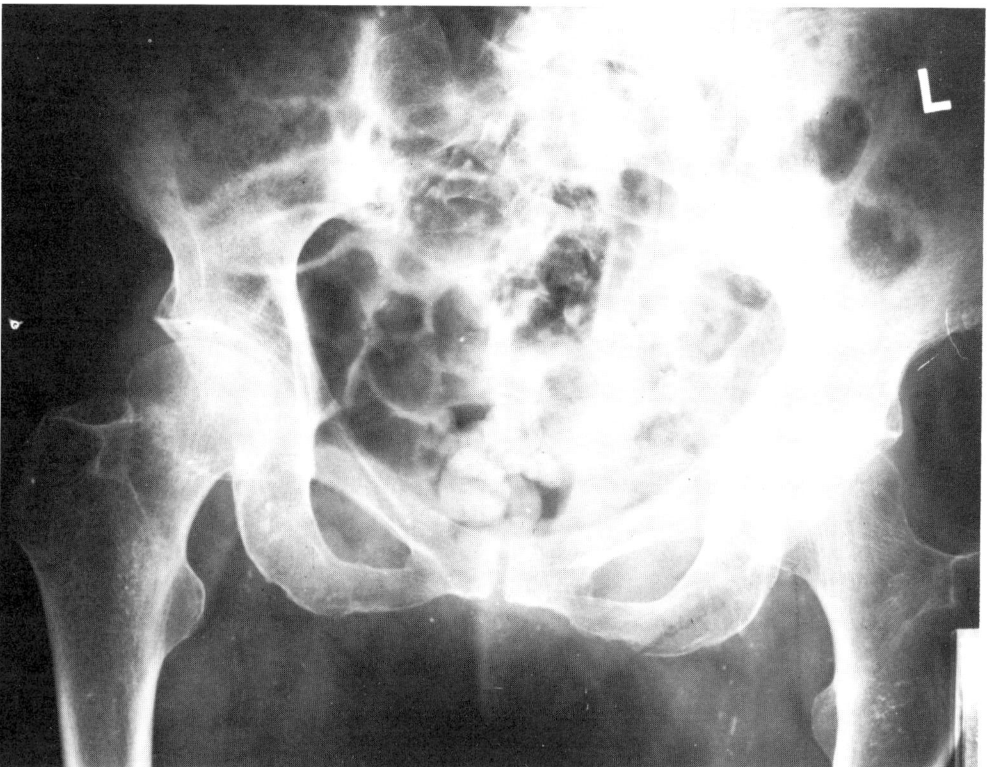

FIG. 3.3 An impacted fracture in the neck of the right femur.

weight-bearing was 8.5 weeks. In the 12% of cases when displacement occurred, the average period to fragment separation was 3 weeks. This complication required internal fixation or arthroplasty. However, after internal fixation patients were able to mobilize within a few days, and 96% had good or excellent results. The overall incidence of avascular necrosis was 15%, being similar in both groups.

Thus internal fixation is the method of choice, preference being given to multiple pins or screw fixation techniques.

STRESS FRACTURES

Devas (1965) reported 25 cases of stress fractures in the femoral neck. He described two distinct radiological types: compression fractures, and transverse fractures. Clinically it is impossible to distinguish between the two types, although the compression fracture is more common in youth and transverse in the aged.

Compression fractures usually present as a haze of internal callus in the inferior part of the femoral neck, with the subsequent appearance of a crack or the area becomes sclerosed. This type of stress fracture has little tendency to displace and usually responds to a limitation of athletic activity.

The earliest sign of a transverse stress fracture is a minute crack in the upper surface of the femoral neck. If the hip is not correctly positioned in the antero–posterior radiograph the crack may be hidden by the outline of the greater trochanter. Once displacement begins, the fracture becomes obvious on the upper cortex. Ultimately the fragments become opened but not widely displaced, with little callus. Since transverse fractures have a tendency for separation, they require internal fixation with pins or screws. Nails should not be used since they tend to cause segmental necrosis (Devas, 1965).

In the early diagnosis of stress fractures tomograms can be used, but are often not necessary since the fracture is usually visible on ordinary X-rays. This fracture can be seen at any age including the young and athletic. The patient presents with a limp and hip pain. Both hips can be affected at once. Osteoporosis, osteomalacia and steroid therapy may be associated with a stress fracture and often there is no history of injury (Jeffery, 1962).

FRACTURES OF THE GREATER AND LESSER TROCHANTER

A direct blow over the greater trochanter may cause an isolated fracture but complete separation and displacement of the trochanter usually occurs from muscle violence—the abductor and lateral rotator muscles avulsing the bony fragment which comes to lie above the neck of the femur. Surgery is seldom needed. A hip spica can be employed with the limb in abduction, or the bone fragments can be wired together. Often the fractures unites with bed rest and gentle mobilization non-weight bearing on crutches.

Avulsion of the epiphysis of the lesser trochanter is sometimes caused by a powerful contraction of the iliopsoas, as in rugger when the player attempts to stop suddenly. Operative intervention is not required. Three to four weeks of restricted movements with an initial period of resting the limb on a pillow, with flexion at the hip, will suffice.

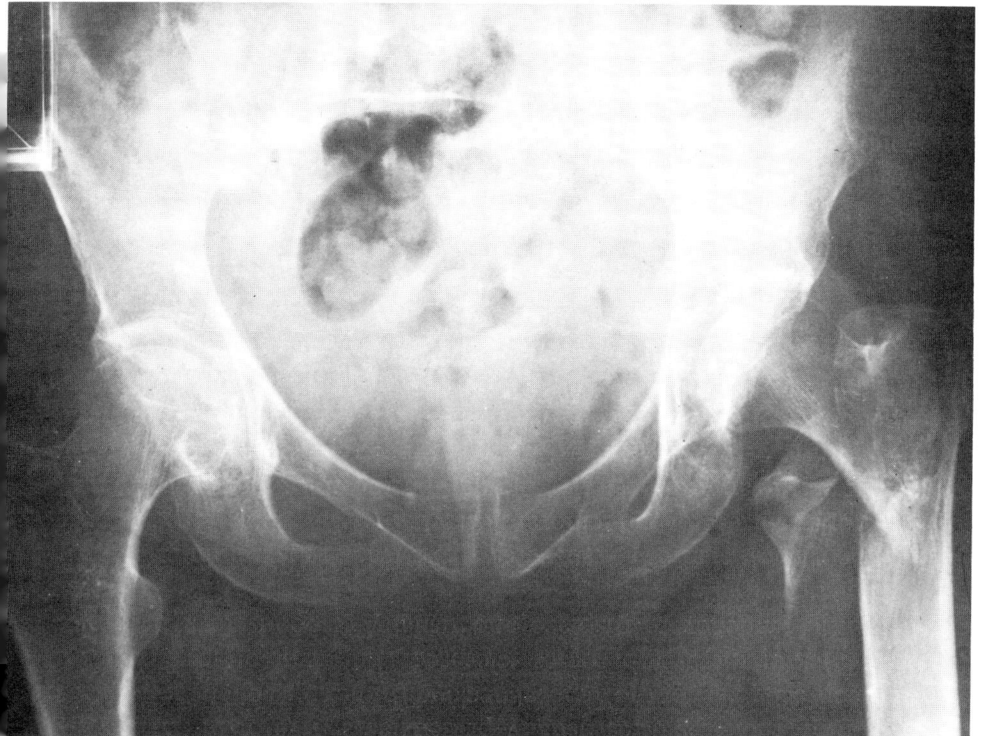

FIG. 3.4 Displacement of the lesser trochanter in a trochanteric fracture.

Horn and Wang (1964) have described adult fractures of the lesser trochanter due to varus impaction or compression during a fall which generally fractures the femoral neck or greater trochanter (Fig. 3.4). Kumar (1972-73) has studied fractures of the lesser trochanter associated with femoral neck fractures. In a series of 18 patients he found that, although internal fixation of the major fracture (femoral neck) was satisfactory clinically, these patients had a weakness of the iliopsoas due to the associated lesser trochanteric fracture. This weakness was indicated by an inability to flex the hip or sit with the knees at the same level. There were also problems in walking due to an inability to stand upright and some inco-ordination of knee and hip movements. He also noted some initial swelling and tenderness in the groin, and late effects were permanent psoas shortening and weakness. He concluded that the associated fracture of the lesser trochanter could be a disabling factor in femoral neck injuries.

FRACTURES OF THE FEMORAL NECK WITH A STIFF HIP

The association of a fractured femoral neck with a stiff (and/or painful) hip poses complications in surgical management because attempts at procuring hip mobility produces movement at the fracture site and mobilization becomes hindered by hip pain. Usually the stiffness is due to osteoarthrosis or rheumatoid arthritis, but may follow a hip arthrodesis (Morris, 1966).

If the fracture is at the subcapital level, it is best to proceed at once to a total hip replacement, if the patient's general condition allows. An alternative in a frail subject with minimal acetabular disease is to use a Thompson's or Moore's prosthesis. However, basal and trochanteric fractures may require a modified total hip arthroplasty using a long-neck or long-stem femoral component.

Low lying and comminuted fractures of the trochanteric region often require either a period of bed rest (up to twelve weeks) to allow healing or fixation with a pin and plate and, if necessary, lag screws to allow consolidation. A total hip arthroplasty can be carried out later when the fracture has united, but reaming of the medullary canal can pose problems.

Occasionally the femoral neck can be built up with cement for a few centimetres to allow the use of a Thompson prosthesis, for example in basal fractures with little acetabular disease in the elderly.

POST-IRRADIATION FRACTURES

White *et al.* (1969) have reported femoral neck fractures occurring in women who have had irradiation of the genital tract. In 16 patients reported, 5 had been bilateral, giving a total of 21 fractures in all. Irradiation fractures must be differentiated from fractures through metastases. 7 were treated by bed rest, 2 by nailing, 2 by an Austin Moore prosthesis, 3 by osteotomy, and 5 by pseudarthrosis (Girdlestone). The 2 fractures that had been nailed had united. Studies had shown that the irradiation in the region of the obturator vessels and the iliac vessels was often greater than that received by the cervix. Angiography had shown extensive arterial damage, and this may be an aetiological factor.

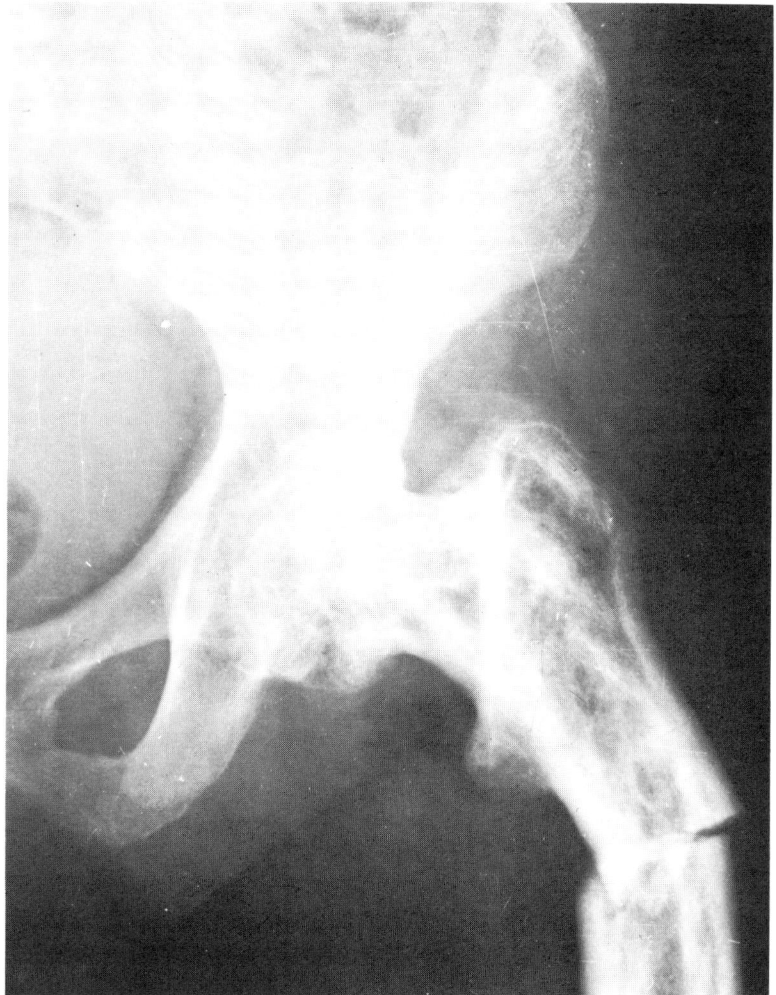

FIG. 3.5(*a*) Fracture in the subtrochanteric region in Paget's disease,

FRACTURES OF THE FEMUR IN PAGET'S DISEASE OF BONE

Grundy (1970) reviewed 63 fractures of the femur in Paget's disease (Fig. 3.5). 11 femoral neck fractures in this series failed to unite; it was suggested that neither fixation nor prolonged conservative treatment had any advantage over the other. Subtrochanteric fractures required

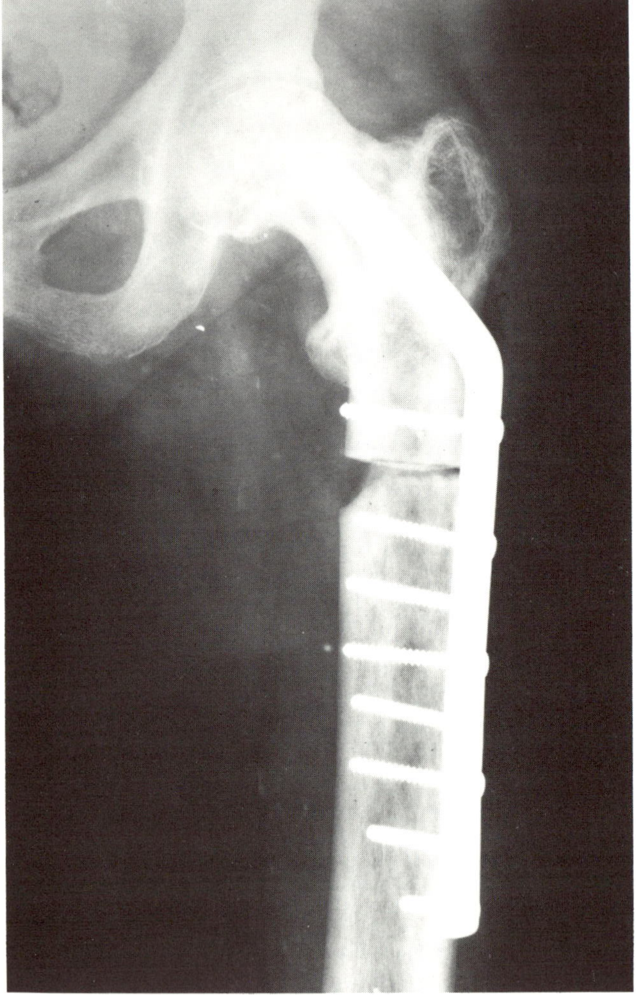

FIG. 3.5(*b*) Treated by fixed-angle nail-plate.

intramedullary fixation although shaft fractures were best treated by conservative methods. Sarcomatous change at the fracture site was not observed in this series.

Fractures of the femoral neck have also been reported in low calcium and magnesium convulsions following parathyroidectomy (Davies and Friedman, 1966).

FRACTURES THROUGH METASTASES

Although all fractures through the femoral neck are pathological in one sense, the true neoplastic fracture deserves special mention. One-sixth of all neoplastic fractures are found in the proximal fourth of the femur (Clain, 1965). Conservative treatment leads to union in only 5%. The period of survival after fracture is 8 months on average, and since the condition is often bilateral it is desirable to maintain adequate fixation. Poigenfurst *et al.* (1968) reviewed 110 operations, 44 being treated by internal fixation, 46 by resection of the head and a pseudarthrosis and 20 by prosthetic replacement. In 52 patients the fracture was in the femoral neck and in 58 in the inter-trochanteric region. 55 patients had mammary carcinoma, 5 had renal carcinoma, 5 had carcinoma of the lung and 4 had thyroid carcinoma. There were various other tumours including multiple myeloma, leukaemias, and sarcomas. Of all the methods employed, prosthetic replacement proved the most advantageous, giving good fixation and stability thus allowing early mobilization. However, patients with diffuse metastatic disease of the ilium were not suitable for prosthetic replacement and resection of the femoral head was employed. This is a less traumatic procedure and was useful in the palliative treatment of patients in poor general condition. Internal fixation with pins and plate led to complications such as the pin penetrating the acetabulum, or collapse of the femoral neck into the extreme varus.

Bone cement can be used to buttress pins or the prosthesis when there is widespread trochanteric involvement. There is a danger of refracture below the stem of the normal length prosthesis and a long-stemmed prosthesis with cement is advocated. The cement not only fills the defect caused by the neoplasm, but its hyperthermic effect may destroy local bone deposits. Radiotherapy can be given to the upper femur before or after surgery.

FRACTURES THROUGH PRIMARY BONE TUMOURS

Primary bone tumours may be found in the region of the femoral neck and may cause pathological fractures. Treatment may include excision, curettage, bone grafting (including the use of a fibular graft), internal fixation or prosthetic replacement and radiotherapy, according to the nature of the lesion. Solitary enchondroma, solitary bone cyst, giant cell tumours, chondrosarcoma, osteogenic sarcoma, benign osteoblastomas, Ewings sarcoma, multiple myeloma are all reported in the femoral neck (Lichenstein, 1972). Fibrous dysplasia can cause excessive bending of the femoral neck and the 'Shepherd's crook' deformity, which may progress despite internal fixation (see also Chapter 5).

FRACTURES OF THE FEMORAL HEAD

The femoral head may be fractured alone or in combination with a femoral neck fracture or a dislocated hip (Chapter 7). If the fragment is attached to a strip of perisoteum it can be reduced into a satisfactory position by rotatory manipulation of the hip; however, a completely detached fragment requires surgical removal because it causes pain and locking in the joint.

Osteochondritis dissecans may be occasionally found in the hip causing similar symptoms, and loose bodies occur in osteoarthrosis, and other forms of degenerative joint disease.

INFECTION AFTER HIP OPERATIONS

Table 3.1 gives the infection rate after prosthetic replacement. The routine use of antibiotics as a pre-operative loading dose or during surgery has not gained wide acceptance, although a continuous infusion of antibiotics during surgery has been shown to give a satisfactory inhibitory level in bone (Kolczun *et al.*, 1974). Usually antibiotics are given only if superficial or deep seated infection is suspected, although

TABLE 3.1 Complications after primary prosthetic replacement (for references see Arnold *et al.*, 1974)

AUTHOR	CASES	MORBIDITY (%)	MORTALITY (%)	INFECTION (%)
Garcia *et al.* (1961)	100	58	18	6
Stein and Costen (1962)	85	18.8	11.8	2.4
Hinchey and Day (1964)	294		3.7	4.1
Smith *et al.* (1972)	211		6.1	
Arnold *et al.* (1973)	160	24	11.3	16

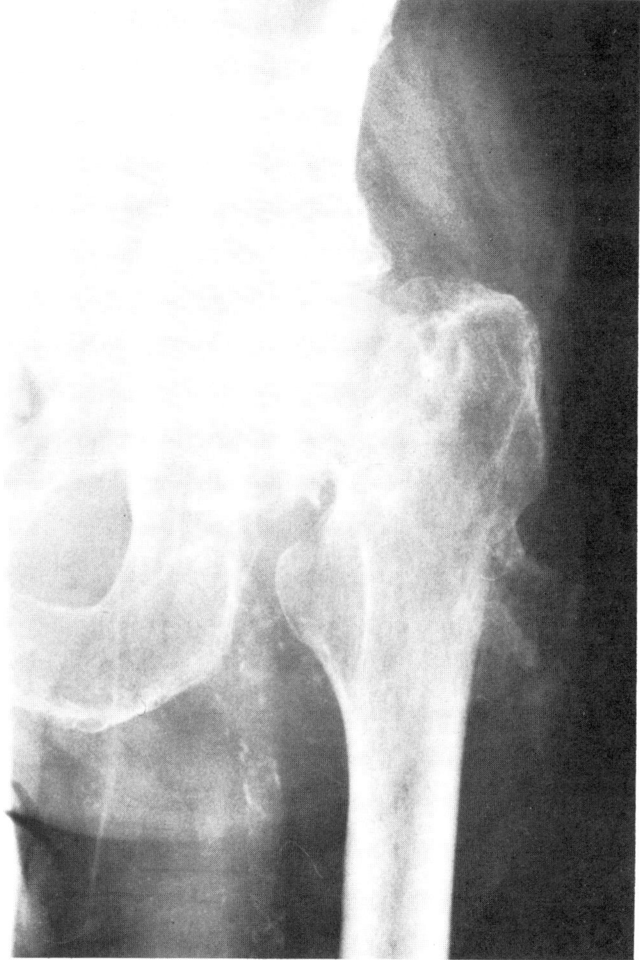

FIG. 3.6 The nail has been removed because of infection. There is collapse of the femoral head, cystic changes in the trochanteric region and heterotopic bone. The proven presence of infection makes the further use of a metallic implant hazardous, and a pseudarthrosis was performed.

the latter may not be preceded by signs of superficial infection. A large haematoma may mimic an infection and by tracking down the lateral compartment of the leg (beneath tensor) simulate a deep vein thrombosis. Deep seated pain, a raised ESR and radiological changes (Chapter 1) can confirm the diagnoses of deep infections, although the elderly may not show a rise in temperature and only a small rise in pulse rate and white cell count. The infection can loosen the prosthesis or cause collapse of the fracture site or medial migration of the prosthesis. In these circumstances the metallic device is removed (Fig. 3.6), and antibiotics given for 2–3 months. Devitalized tissue is excised and the wound coapted with nylon sutures (long and deeply placed) with drainage and antibiotic lavage, if necessary.

When an implant becomes surrounded by infective material within a few weeks of surgery, the difficult decision has to be made regarding removal of the implant and the subsequent problems of non-union. In this situation the infected area is incised and drained and all dead tissue removed. The wound can be packed with a dressing impregnated with an antiseptic or antibiotic. After several days (usually 5–7) a secondary suture can be performed. Antibiotics are given during this period according to sensitivity. Once fracture union is thought to have occurred the implant is removed along with all dead bone and sequestra. If non-union is found or the infection is impossible to control in the early stages due to the presence of the implant then it is probably better to proceed to a pseudarthrosis with removal of the femoral head, neck and all devitalized fragments and foreign materials.

Patients with concurrent infection (chest, sacral ulcers, skin sores, urinary tract infections) or who are incontinent may require a broad-spectrum antibiotic such as ampicillin supplemented by benzyl penicillin or flucloxacillin. Under these circumstances, other possible antibiotics are sulphonamides, tetracyclines and co-trimoxazole.

The common causal organisms in wound infections are: *Staphylococcus aureus*; *Staphylococcus albus*; *Haemophilus influenzae*; *Streptococcus pyogenes*; *Streptococcus faecalis*; Gram-negative bacteria; *E. coli*, *Proteus*; *Ps. aeruginosa*; *Kl. aerogenes*; *Salmonella*.

Approximately 90% of all infections are due to *Staphylococcus aureus*, *Staphylococcus albus* and the Gram-negative organisms. In acute infections with abscess formation it may be assumed that the infecting organism is *Staphylococcus aureus* and appropriate antibiotic therapy commenced. However, before the drugs are given a swab should be taken from the wound, and, if necessary blood culture, sputum and urine specimens sent for bacteriology. Anaemia should be corrected, and a blood sugar estimation taken to exclude latent diabetes. Old people do not always have the raised ESR and leucocytosis in the presence of infection that younger people show. Aspiration of the hip joint may be helpful when a low grade infection is suspected.

The most reasonable choice of antibiotic rests between cloxacillin (flucloxacillin) plus, ampicillin or benyzl penicillin; cephalosporins or fusidic acid. Acute infections require 2–3 weeks of therapy if the infection is superficial but 2–3 months if the infection is much deeper and involves bone. As mentioned under chronic infections, the metallic implant may have to be removed along with dead bone in refractory cases.

When the infection does not resolve promptly the cause of the antibiotic failure may be:

(1) Wrong antibiotic
(2) Inadequate dosage
(3) Wrong route
(4) Inadequate duration
(5) Development of resistance
(6) Antibiotic antagonism
(7) Wrong organism (lab. report)
(8) Underlying pathology (e.g. necrotic bone)
(9) General ill-health (anaemia, steroids etc.)
(10) Poor surgical drainage
(11) Presence of foreign body (e.g. metallic implant).

PHYSIOTHERAPY AND REHABILITATION

Physiotherapists are concerned with the maintenance of function during the acute episode, such as a femoral neck fracture, not only by maintaining joint range and muscle power but also by ensuring effective early mobilization and short-term rehabilitation. The role of the occupational therapist has to be envisaged in much longer terms with an emphasis given to the functional assessment of the patient's capabilities, exploitation of their residual skills and the institution of planned retraining to compensate for permanent disability.

The integration of the patient into social, domestic and occupational networks is the ultimate aim of the surgeon, although many patients by their infirmity will never return to a normal life or even to a life-style they had adopted prior to the accident. However, the object of physiotherapy (especially early mobilization after surgery) is to prevent complications such as deep vein thrombosis, chest infection and sacral ulceration; while later enhancing muscle recovery and locomotor skills such as walking. The physiotherapy regimen needs direction from the medical staff as to the type of therapy employed, its duration and timing after surgery. Each patient will require individual consideration depending upon such factors as the type of accident, the locomotor ability of the patient prior to the accident, the general condition of the patient (including cardio-respiratory function and weight) and the nature and success of the surgical procedure. Ancillary forms of physiotherapy such as heat, cold, ultrasonics and electrotherapy, can be used after femoral neck fractures. Remedial exercises are important.

Within 24 h of any hip operation the physiotherapist can carry out passive movements of the limb concerned, and if these movements are gently performed then no additional bleeding or trauma will ensue. Such passive exercises maintain proprioceptive sense in the muscles and joints as well as joint mobility. The physiotherapist should encourage deep breathing exercises and gentle leg movements to combat the dangers of broncho-pneumonia and deep vein thrombosis. Within 2–3 days the patients can sit out of bed and begin a series of assisted movements, that is the patient actively collaborates with the therapist by contracting the muscles while the therapist assists the movement. After prosthetic replacement the patient may have to remain recumbent for 10 days, especially if a posterior approach has been used. The lateral approach allows the patient to sit out of bed much earlier (2–3 days).

As the patient progresses free movement is achieved when the patient moves the limb without help from the therapist. During this stage muscle tone, power and bulk improve, especially in the flexors of the hip and extensors of the knee. Resisted exercises are employed prior to full mobilization. Isometric exercises are performed when the joint is immobilized (e.g. in a plaster cast), isotonic exercises are used to build up muscle power by applying predetermined weights and instructing the patient to perform a number of resisted movements.

Full mobilization is encouraged by 2 weeks since several series have shown that this regimen did not increase the incidence of failure of fixation or non-union; indeed a greater number of cases developed superior segmental collapse when weight-bearing was deferred for 12 weeks (Abrami and Stevens, 1964; Graham, 1968). Mobilization exercises are often preceded by the application of heat or ice-packs, or they may be performed in water (hydrotherapy) or in suspension apparatus, or using a gymnasium apparatus (wall bars, parallel bars). Patients with femoral neck fractures, after successful fixation, can be mobilized within 7–14 days; walking frames are ideal for this purpose. Some centres have even suggested a more rapid return to partial weight-bearing within 72 h of surgery. However, the onset of discomfort or pain in the hip may herald complications such as angulation or refracture and there is little point in rushing the period of early mobilization if the future of the femoral head or hip joint may be jeopardized. Frankel *et al.* (1971) have shown that after internal fixation and biotelemetric studies, the load on the tip of the nail is of similar magnitude whether the patient was kept in bed and nursed by turning; assisted in transfer to a wheelchair; or allowed to walk with a walking frame. A hip spica was shown to limit the loading on the head, but upward bending movements of the nail may occur. The ideal, after all hip operations, is to promote an early return to walking while safeguarding the fracture and cartilage from further damage.

As recovery proceeds, the specific exercise designed to aid future normal life are commenced, e.g. walking exercises, getting out of bed, standing while dressing, etc. This is an area for collaboration between physiotherapist and occupational therapist. With planned physiotherapy and rehabilitation, many patients with femoral neck fractures may be fully mobile and independent in 4–6 weeks.

REFERENCES

ABRAMI, G. and STEVENS, J. (1964). *J. Bone Jt. Surg.* **46B**, 204.
BANKS, H.H. (1962). *J. Bone Jt. Surg.* **44A**, 931.
BARNES, R., BROWN, J.T., GARDEN, R.S. and NICOLL, E.A. (1976). *J. Bone Jt. Surg.* **58B**, 2.
BENTLEY, G. (1968). *J. Bone Jt. Surg.* **50B**, 551.
CHAN, R.N-W. and HOSKINSON, J. (1975). *J. Bone Jt. Surg.* **57B**, 437.
CHARNLEY, J. (1964). *J. Bone Jt. Surg.* **46B**, 518.
CLAIN, A. (1965). *Br. J. Cancer*, **19**, 15.
COVENTRY, M.B. (1964). *J. Bone Jt. Surg.* **46A**, 200.
CRAWFORD, H.B. (1965). *J. Bone Jt. Surg.* **47A**, 830.
DAVIES, D.R. and FRIEDMAN, M. (1966). *J. Bone Jt. Surg.* **48B**, 117.
DEVAS, M.B. (1965). *J. Bone Jt. Surg.* **47B**, 728.
FIELDING, J.W., WILSON, J.H. (Jr.) and ZICKEL, R.E. (1962). *J. Bone Jt. Surg.* **44A**, 965.
FRANKEL, V.H., BURSTEIN, A.H., BROWN, R.H. and LYGRE, L. (1971). *J. Bone Jt. Surg.* **53A**, 1023.
GARCIA, A., NEER, C.S. and AMBROSE, G.B. (1961). *J. Trauma*, **1**, 128.
GARDEN, R.S. (1964). *J. Bone Jt. Surg.* **46B**, 630.
GLASS, K.D. (1965). *J. Bone Jt. Surg.* **47B**, 598.
GOSSLING, H.R. and HARDY, J.H. (1969). *J. Trauma.* **9**, 423.
GRAHAM, J. (1968). *J. Bone Jt. Surg.* **50B**, 562.
GRUNDY, M. (1970). *J. Bone Jt. Surg.* **52B**, 252.

HORN, J.S. and WANG, Y.C. (1964). *Br. J. Surg.* **51**, 574.
JEFFERY, C.C. (1962). *J. Bone Jt. Surg.* **44B**, 543.
KOLCZUN, M.C., NELSOM, C.L., MCHENRY, M.C., GAVAN, T.L. and PINOVICH, D. (1974). *J. Bone Jt. Surg.* **56A**, 305.
KUMAR, V. (1972–73). *Injury* **4**, 327.
LICHENSTEIN, L. (1972). *Bone Tumours.* 4th Edn., Mosby, St. Louis.
MOORE, A.T. and BOHLMAN, H.R. (1943). *J. Bone Jt. Surg.* **25A**, 688.
MORRIS, J.B. (1966). *J. Bone Jt. Surg.* **48B**, 260.
POIGENFURST, J., MARCOVE, R.C. and MILLER, T.R. (1968). *J. Bone Jt. Surg.* **50B**, 743.
RAINE, G.E.T. (1973). *Injury* **5**, 25.
THOMPSON, F.R. (1954). *J. Bone Jt. Surg.* **36A**, 489.
WHITE, J., PROTHEROE, K., GLENNIE, J. and JACKSON, W. (1969). *J. Bone Jt. Surg.* **51B**, 569.

Chapter Four

METABOLIC ASPECTS

R. Smith

INTRODUCTION

The great majority of fractures of the femoral neck occur in elderly people, and the main cause is a reduction in the normal amount of mineralized bone. This reduction may be due to osteoporosis, where there is less bone than there ought to be (but it is of normal composition), or to osteomalacia, where the amount of bone tissue is normal but poorly mineralized. Osteoporosis is the commonest known cause of femoral neck fracture but osteomalacia accounts for a significant number of cases, and is probably more frequent than we suspect. Some patients may have both conditions.

Discussion of these two abnormalities of bone will occupy most of this chapter, and rarer causes of femoral neck fracture will be dealt with briefly. The main emphasis will be on diagnosis and management and on those points which cause practical difficulty. Recent work will be summarized. Good accounts of osteoporosis will be found in Nordin (1973) and Morgan (1973); aspects of other metabolic disorders of bone are well dealt with in *Clinics in Endocrinology and Metabolism* (1972).

OSTEOPOROSIS

In osteoporosis there is a reduced volume of bone tissue relative to the volume of anatomical bone (Nordin, 1971) (Fig. 4.1(*b*).). In practice the term implies a general loss of skeletal tissue in which trabecular bone is generally more affected than cortical bone.

It should come as no surprise that the femoral neck fractures when there is least bone in it; the possible ways in which this reduction in bone mass comes about require brief consideration, so that we can better understand its cause, management and treatment. Much of the work done on the relationship between osteoporosis and femoral neck fracture has been admirably reviewed by Morgan (1973).

CAUSES

Osteoporosis may conveniently be regarded as primary or secondary (Nordin, 1973). In the primary disorder, where the cause is unknown, the commonest form is associated with bone loss with increasing age after the menopause (post-menopausal osteoporosis) and in old age (so-called senile osteoporosis). There is every reason to think that in this primary group we are dealing with the lower range of a population of normal distribution (as far as the skeleton is concerned), in which age related bone loss is excessive. In secondary osteoporosis the loss of bone, (presumably superimposed on the normal changes in the skeleton with age) is due to some additional factor not present in the rest of the population; such as thyrotoxicosis, steatorrhoea, hypogonadism, or treatment with corticosteroids.

The reason for the normal loss of bone with age has been widely debated (Morgan, 1973). It seems clear that with advancing age the two active processes of formation and resorption of bone become dissociated, so that bone loss, which is mainly endosteal, exceeds bone formation, which is mainly subperiosteal. Bone loss occurs more rapidly and begins earlier in women than in men, and in women is clearly related to the menopause. The overall skeletal loss between youth and old age is about 15%, and women aged 70—80 years old may have lost up to 30% of their early adult bone mass. This loss does not occur equally from all parts of the skeleton. Trabecular bone rather than cortical is lost, and rearrangements of architecture occur, with loss of the less important trabeculae (Nordin, 1973. Fig. 1.20). The rate of bone loss probably slows in old age; if it continued at a linear rate, the vertebrae of all old people would ultimately collapse at the age of 80 (Nordin, 1973).

In women post-menopausal bone loss has long been considered to be due to the decline in ovarian hormones, which normally antagonize

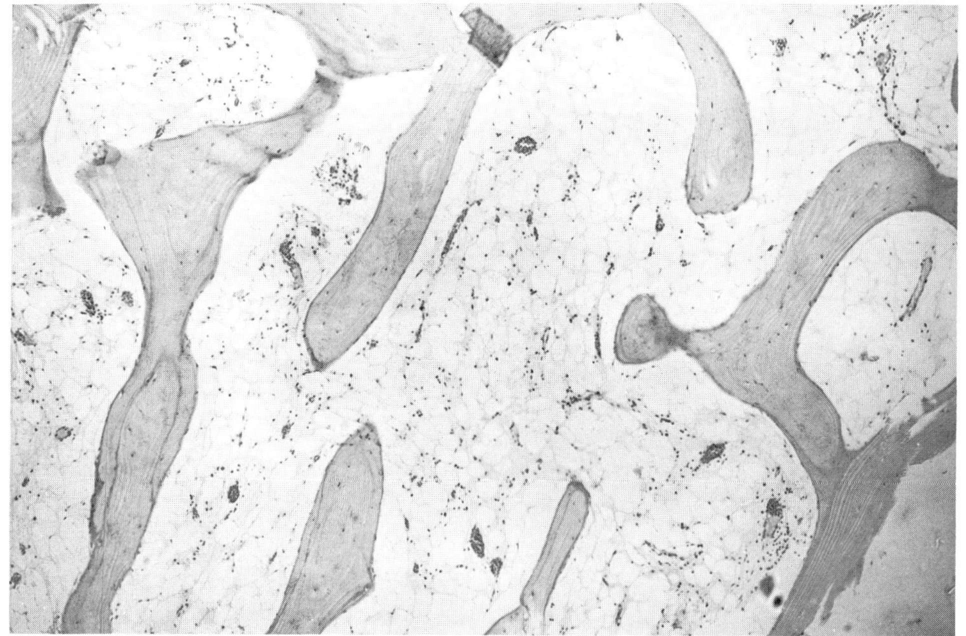

FIG. 4.1(*a*)

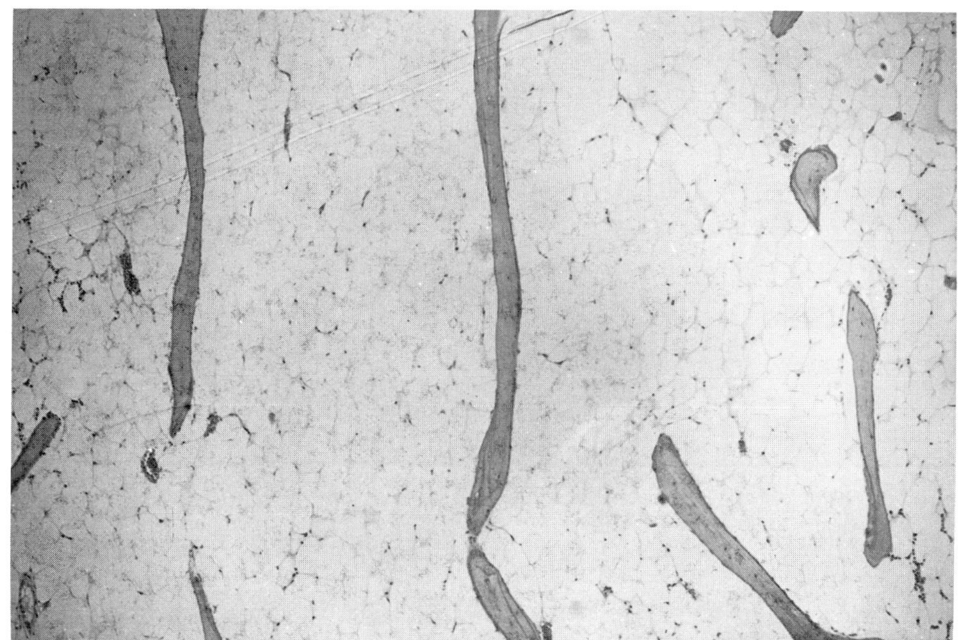

FIG. 4.1(*b*)

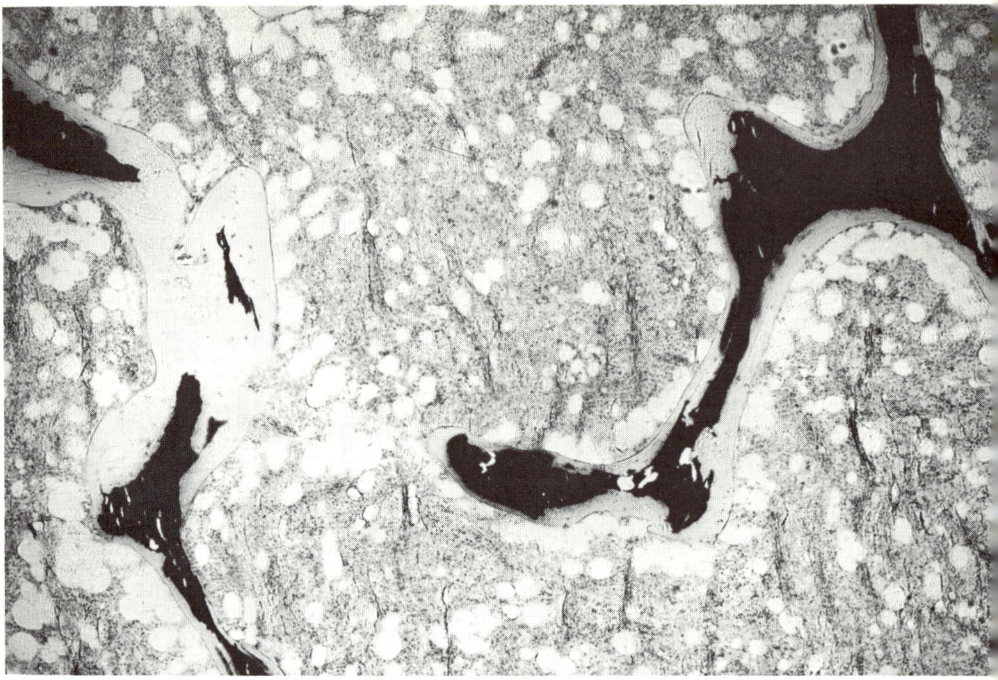

FIG. 4.1(*c*)

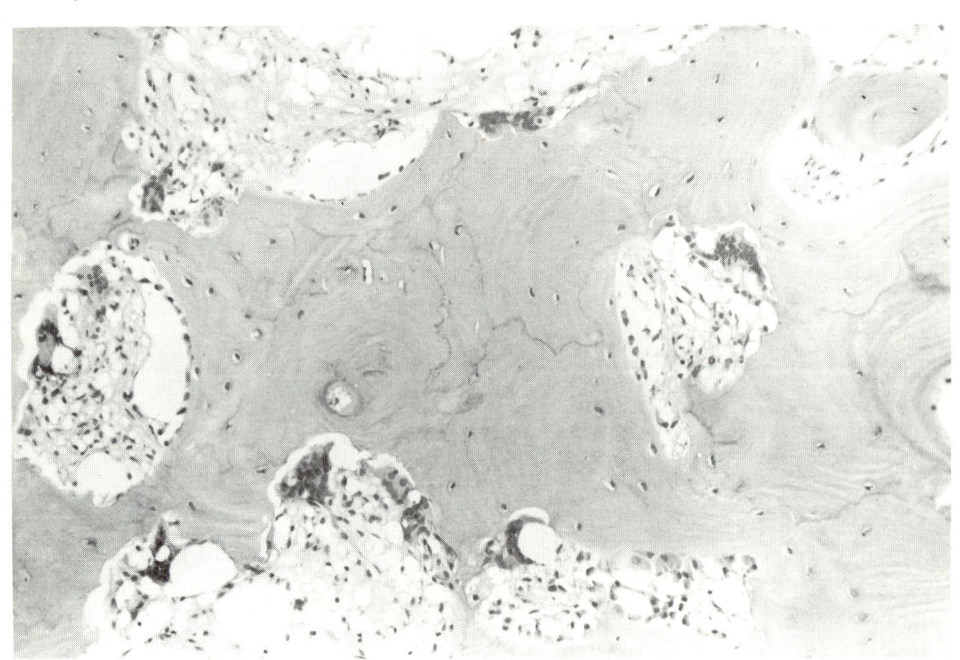

FIG. 4.1(*d*)

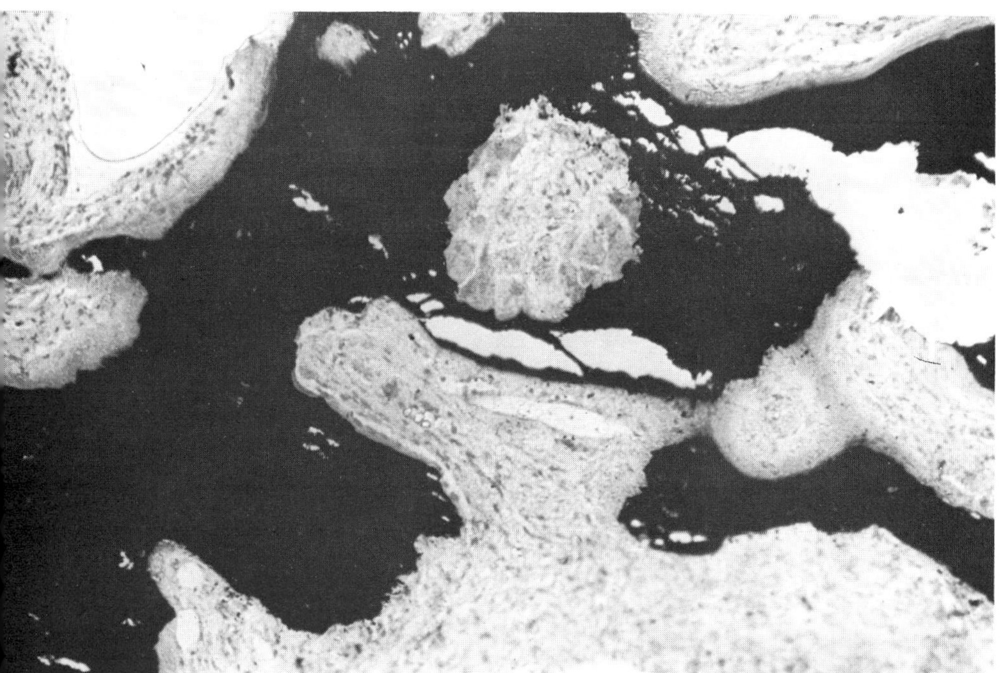

FIG. 4.1 (*e*)

FIG. 4.1 The appearance of trabecular bone in iliac crest biopsies from subjects with (*a*) normal bone; (*b*) osteoporosis; (*c*) osteomalacia; (*d*) Paget's disease; and (*e*) osteitis fibrosa (parathyroid bone disease) is shown. (*b*) Osteoporosis: the number of trabeculae are less than normal and individual trabeculae are thinner than normal. There is little cellular activity. (*c*) Osteomalacia: the amount of bone tissue is normal but mineralization is defective. A thick layer of osteoid (unmineralized bone matrix) covers the bone surfaces. Mineralized bone is shown in black. (*d*) Paget's disease: there is disorderly formation of bone with cement lines. Multinucleate osteoclasts and osteoblasts are increased, and the marrow shows an increase in fibrous tissue. (*e*) Osteitis fibrosa: the main features are excessive osteoclastic bone resorption with increased fibrous tissue. × 90 (*a–c*); × 200 (*d,e*).

the bone resorbing action of parathyroid hormone. Oophorectomy in women before the age of 45 significantly increases the incidence of osteoporosis (Aitken *et al.*, 1973). After the menopause the fasting urine and plasma calcium increase slightly, suggesting an increase in resorption of bone, particularly at night. Normally nocturnal calcium loss is balanced by calcium absorption from food during the day. In post-menopausal patients it seems that nocturnal calcium loss is higher than the possible day time absorption.

It has been implied (Nordin, 1971) that the cause of senile osteoporosis is different from that of post-menopausal osteoporosis. After about the age of 70, bone loss continues in women, and develops in men; it might be argued that the decline in sex hormones is the cause in both sexes. Since however the 24 h urine calcium tends to fall in this older age group and there is a pronounced decrease in intestinal calcium absorption, this malabsorption may be the most likely explanation of the senile form of osteoporosis.

By the age of 70–80, the female is a hundred times more prone to a femoral neck fracture than she was in her youth. Three important factors contribute to her orthopaedic downfall; a reduction in bone mass; more frequent falls; and in some patients increased weight. The first of these is the most important, but its effect is not predictable since fractures do not necessarily occur where the reduction in bone mass is most marked. Although there is a strong presumption that the increasing rate of femoral neck fracture with age is due to osteoporosis in the fracture region, absolute proof of this is difficult to obtain.

An important factor, which must account for a large part of the variation between individuals, sexes and races is the amount of bone present in the skeleton in early adult life. Thus for a given rate of resorption (or imbalance between resorption and formation) those persons with the greatest initial bone mass (with thickest bones and densest skeletons) will resist structural failure the longest.

DIAGNOSIS

The diagnosis of osteoporosis as the cause of a fractured femoral neck in an elderly patient is likely to be right, since it is the most common one; but alternatives should always be considered, especially since some may be capable of being treated.

Where the fracture is due to osteoporosis, the patient is likely to be elderly and female, and may have had an early menopause or hysterectomy. There may be a history of intermittent backache or of previous fractures. Quite considerable loss of trunk height may have gone unnoticed, although clothes may no longer fit. Examination will often show a kyphosis, and transverse abdominal crease, in addition to the local sign of fracture.

The X-ray diagnosis of borderline osteoporosis is not easy; however, fractures usually occur only when the osteoporosis is advanced. Generalized rarefaction of the bones is difficult to be certain about on a routine film and difficult to interpret and obvious structural changes are often more useful in diagnosis. Thus the vertebral bodies may show irregular wedge-shaped collapse (Fig. 4.2) or asymmetrically biconcave end plates; the width of the metacarpal cortex may be reduced, (the metacarpal cortical/total area ratio is inversely related to the rate of proximal femoral fracture), and a corresponding change may be seen in the larger limb bones. It has been emphasized by Nordin (1973) that osteoporosis may affect some bones more than others; and that, for instance, vertebral collapse, producing the crush fracture syndrome, may be independent of the changes in the rest of the skeleton. Nevertheless osteoporosis is often generalized. In the femoral neck, osteoporosis produces loss of trabeculae with alteration in their pattern and a thin calcar femorale.

The plasma calcium, phosphate and alkaline phosphatase are normal, as usually are the urine calcium and phosphate. An exception is the rapid osteoporotic bone resorption in immobilized young subjects, when the urine calcium may be greatly increased. The normal range of daily urine calcium excretion is approximately 100–400 mg in males and lower in females (Morgan and Robertson, 1974).

Histology of the undecalcified bone taken at an operation or at iliac crest biopsy (Fig. 4.1*b*) will probably show thin scanty trabeculae with little cellular activity and no excess of osteoid. Nordin (1973) states that the amount of trabecular bone in the iliac crest may be normal for the age of the patient in patients with femoral neck fracture, but severely reduced in patients with crush fractures of the vertebral bodies. This may only apply to those patients in whom femoral neck fracture is associated with osteomalacia. In general the state of the trabecular bone of the iliac crest indicates its condition in the rest of the skeleton. Borderline osteoporosis is also difficult to diagnose by histology. Correct interpretation requires knowledge of a considerable

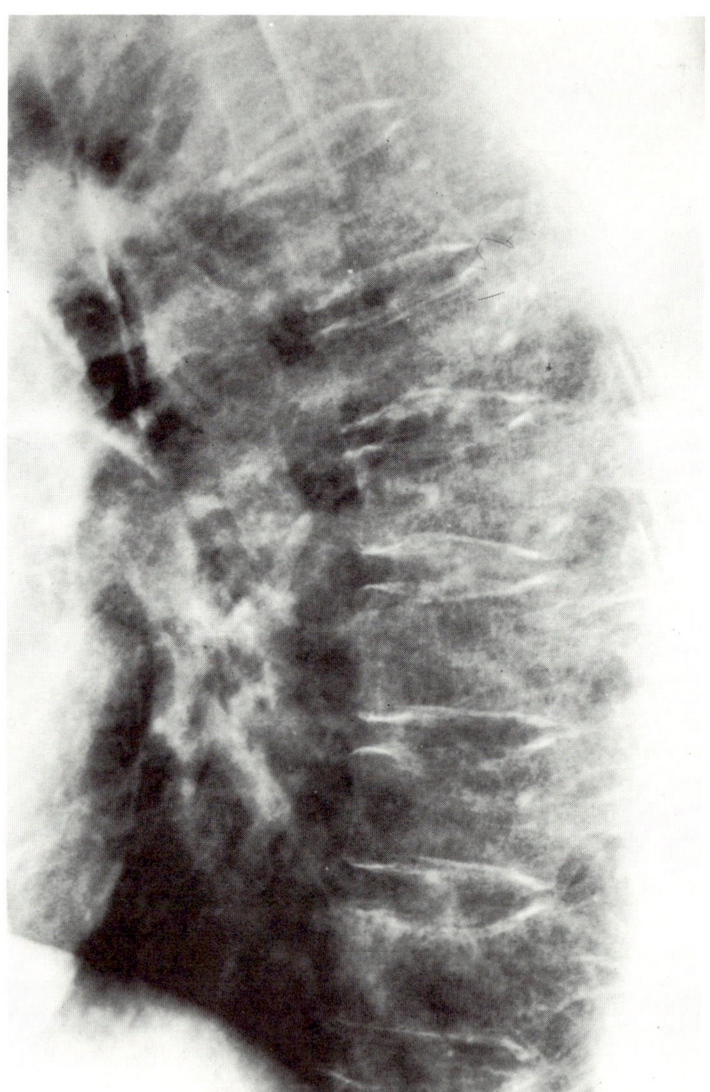

FIG. 4.2 Appearance of the spine in a woman of 61 years with severe osteoporosis who had a hysterectomy and oophorectomy at the age of 34. Note the irregular wedge-shaped collapse of the vertebral bodies and generalized rarefaction.

range of normal biopsies. Practically, the histological diagnosis of marked osteoporosis presents no difficulty, and in milder cases histology is useful to exclude other causes of fracture.

DIFFERENTIAL DIAGNOSIS

Possible causes of secondary osteoporosis such as immobilization and disuse, thyrotoxicosis, hypogonadism and Cushing's syndrome should be considered; neoplastic conditions, such as secondary carcinoma, myeloma or leukaemia are important; and metabolic disorders such as osteomalacia, Paget's disease and parathyroid bone disease must be excluded (see later).

Localized or generalized immobilization rapidly produces osteoporosis, the cause of which is still debated. However, it is well known clinically that a limb which has been immobilized may readily fracture.

Thyroid hormone increases bone matrix turnover and breakdown, and may cause osteoporosis. In the elderly, thyrotoxicosis may not be clinically obvious, but suspicion may be aroused by unexplained loss of weight, atrial fibrillation without obvious cause, agitation and fatiguability; it is important to look for thyroid enlargement (which may be slight or retrosternal) and if doubt exists to ask for tests of thyroid function. Rarely hypercalcaemia may occur, and both urine calcium and hydroxyproline (derived from collagen) may be increased.

Cushing's syndrome due to spontaneous adrenal cortical overactivity is rare, but iatrogenic disorder due to prolonged steroid therapy is more common. Both may cause severe osteoporosis. Clues to the diagnosis may be a 'moonface', hirsutes, striae, central obesity, hypertension, easy bruising and hyperglycaemia. In Cushing's syndrome, fractures are said to heal with excess callus. In the spontaneous disorder the most useful biochemical estimation is the night-time plasma cortisol.

In the male, hypogonadism as a cause of osteoporosis should not be missed. The patient is usually tall, with disproportionately long legs compared with the trunk and with absent secondary sex characteristics. The voice is high pitched, the hairline low and the face smooth, wrinkled and hairless. In partial and complete pituitary failure, osteoporosis may also be severe; sexual development, growth and skeletal maturation are much delayed.

Osteogenesis imperfecta may be considered clinically as a cause of secondary osteoporosis; in this condition, where the bone matrix is not properly formed, fractures often occur in childhood. They usually become less frequent in adult life. However age-related bone loss presumably occurs in these patients and in mild cases fractures may occur after the menopause for the first time. Osteogenesis imperfecta is suggested by bluish sclerae and a positive family history. It should be recalled that the sclerae may normally be bluer at the extremes of life.

The exclusion of neoplastic disease is important in femoral neck fracture. Neoplasm is suggested where the clinical situation is wrong for idiopathic osteoporosis, although both occur commonly together. For example, fracture of the femoral neck in a man around 50 without sufficient trauma might suggest myeloma rather than osteoporosis as a cause. Such a fracture might be the first indication of myeloma, or might occur in a patient who is generally unwell, possibly with recent infections (of the lungs or skin, for instance). Alternatively, myeloma can be an undiagnosed cause of rapid loss of height, suggesting progressive osteoporosis. Investigations show an anaemia, with abnormal plasma cells, with rouleaux formation and a very high ESR, and abnormal plasma proteins, with a dense 'M' band on electrophoresis. The urine may show Bence Jones protein. X-rays of the rest of the skeleton may show numerous areas of rarefaction particularly in the skull. Further specialized investigation will establish which type of myeloma is present.

Secondary deposits, from a primary carcinoma elsewhere (which may include kidney [Fig. 4.3], lung, breast and prostate) may cause femoral neck fractures. For this reason, clinical examination should be as full as possible, to exclude obvious primary lesions.

It is important to consider all these possibilities in a patient with a fractured femoral neck, particularly in an inappropriate age group, since it is amongst the minority that some remedial cause may be found. Further possible causes are considered by Dent and Watson (1966). It should be remembered that malabsorption may cause osteoporosis as well as osteomalacia (see below).

TREATMENT OF OSTEOPOROSIS

By the time osteoporotic femoral neck fracture has occurred, bone loss is considerable, and medical treatment can at the best only slow down further loss of bone. Since the two main causes of osteoporosis appear to be the decline in sex hormones with increasing years, and immobilization, these provide the main clues for treatment.

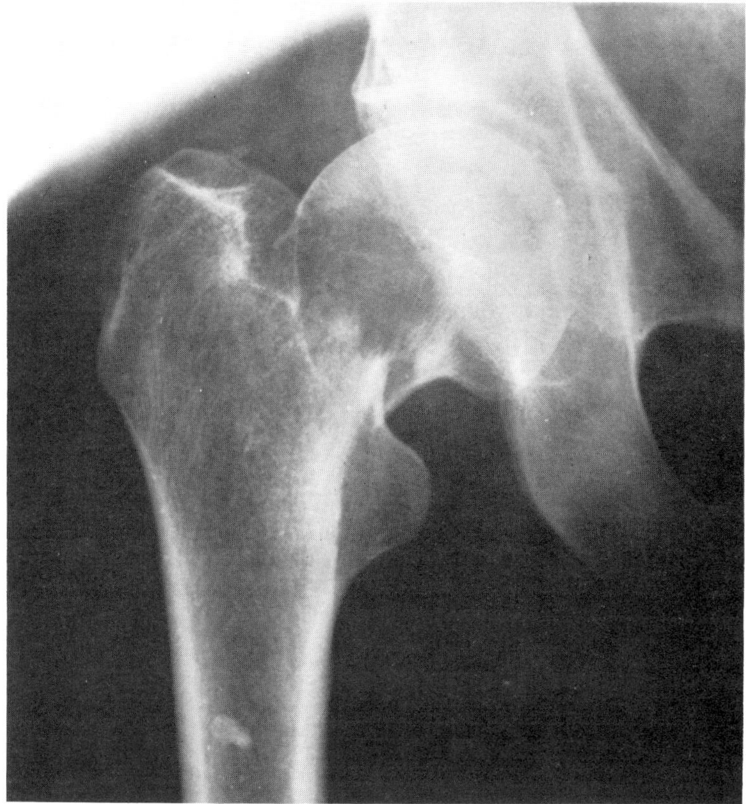

FIG. 4.3 Pathological fracture in the femoral neck of a man of 54, due to a secondary deposit from a hypernephroma. The plasma values were calcium 2.9 mmol l^{-1} (11.6 mg per 100 ml) phosphorus 0.9 mmol l^{-1} (2.9 mg per 100 ml) and alkaline phosphatase 21 King Armstrong units per 100 ml. They resembled those of osteitis fibrosa but were due to the neoplasm.

The question of the use of oestrogens in post-menopausal osteoporosis is a vexed one. Oestrogens appear to protect against parathyroid-induced bone resorption and reduce the fasting plasma calcium in post-menopausal women. It is presumed that they do not antagonize the stimulating action of parathyroid hormone on calcium absorption from the gut or renal tubule. Since all females lose bone mass after the menopause, although at a variable rate, universal post-menopausal hormone replacement to prevent subsequent osteoporosis might seem advisable (Henneman, 1972). In practice, this is not possible. It is usual to restrict such treatment either to those who are particularly at risk—young women after a total hysterectomy and oophorectomy, or those who develop symptoms due to progressive osteoporosis at a comparatively early age. The easiest regime is stilboestrol 1–3 mg daily for periods of 3–4 weeks, interrupted by a week, and continued in cycles. Ethinyl oestradiol 50 μg daily can be used in the same way.

The avoidance of immobility is most important. The continuing formation of bone depends on the stresses and strains through it; physical exercise is important to build up skeletal mass in youth and to prevent its too rapid decline in later life. There are practical difficulties; thus after a femoral neck fracture, mobility may be difficult to maintain and pain may prevent it. Likewise the pain of vertebral collapse may prevent mobility, and external forms of spinal support will relieve symptoms but may make the bones more osteoporotic. Many of these fractures are discovered on X-rays taken for other reasons.

In most patients with osteoporosis additional oral calcium should be given, either in the form of additional calcium (often as effervescent calcium 'Sandoz'), or by increasing the calcium intake in the diet, or both. Calcium was initially given because of the idea, subsequently modified, that calcium deficiency contributed to senile osteoporosis. However, its use may be logical for two reasons. Firstly, there is good evidence that bone resorption usually occurs at night after the day's oral calcium has been absorbed, and that this resorption increases after the menopause; secondly, there is also evidence that there may be a group of elderly patients with osteoporosis in whom absorption of calcium is very poor. Evening supplements of calcium may therefore be advisable (Belchetz *et al.*, 1973). The administration of vitamin D or its derivatives in relatively large doses to overcome the impaired calcium absorption (Peacock *et al.*, 1974) is more controversial.

Of other possible treatments, there is no good evidence that anabolic steroids can increase the mass of bone matrix collagen, although they may increase the protein of muscle. It has not yet been convincingly proved that calcitonin (which reduces bone resorption), diphosphonates (which appear to prevent experimental animal osteoporosis) or fluoride (which appears to stimulate new bone matrix formation) are of therapeutic value in human osteoporosis, and the usefulness of calcium infusions has not yet been confirmed (Dudl *et al.*, 1973). For further discussions, see *Seminars in Drug Treatment* (1972).

Finally, on the rare occasions where osteoporosis is due to a clear underlying cause, such as hypogonadism, Cushing's syndrome or thyrotoxicosis, it is obviously important to treat this.

OSTEOMALACIA

Osteomalacia is the most important treatable cause of fractured femoral neck, and a recognized cause of subtrochanteric fracture (Chalmers, 1970); it should always be considered because it is easy to treat. With rare exceptions, osteomalacia in adult life (and rickets in childhood) is due to a deficiency of vitamin D or to a disturbance of its metabolism. In recent years there have been rapid physiological and clinical advances of which the reader should be aware.

The only practical distinction between rickets and osteomalacia is one of age, and the terms are often used interchangeably. Rickets occurs when bone growth is still going on; whereas the term 'osteomalacia' is applied to the bone disease in adults. Clearly there are situations, as in adolcsccncc, when the features of both may be present.

It is now recognized (Kodicek, 1974) that vitamin D undergoes important conversions in the body before it produces its biological effects. Vitamin D comes from food (such as oily fishes and dairy products) and from u. v. irradiation of its precursors in the skin; it is first converted to 25-hydroxycholecalciferol (25-HCC) by the liver, and 25-HCC together with native D forms the main storage form of the vitamin. Measurement of 25-HCC levels in plasma appears to give a very good indication of the vitamin D status of the patient. The second conversion occurs in the kidney to produce the active metabolite 1,25-dihydroxycholecalciferol (1,25-DHCC), the so-called kidney hormone. This is active in very small (µg) amounts, and has known effects on intestine and bone, and possibly other tissues such as kidney and muscle.

In the last few years osteomalacia has been recognized as an increasing nutritional problem in this country particularly amongst immigrants, in the elderly (both indigenous and immigrant), and sometimes also amongst adolescents. Further, with the increasing care of patients with renal glomerular failure (in whom the production of 1,25-DHCC may be defective), and the prolongation of life with haemodialysis, osteomalacia due to renal disease is a growing problem. The reported incidence of osteomalacia in patients with fractured femoral necks is very variable, because of the different biochemical, histological and radiological criteria often used for its diagnosis.

The reasons for the recent increase in osteomalacia are multiple, and may in part be due to increasing awareness of the diagnosis.

However, dietary surveys and measurement of 25-HCC levels in the plasma have established that the average person in Great Britain receives little vitamin D, either through sunlight or food. The amount will clearly differ with the time of the year. In normal persons the amount of 25-HCC in the plasma is more in the summer than in the winter, (McLaughlin *et al.*, 1974); in Asian immigrants there appears to be spontaneous cure of vitamin D deficiency in the summer (Gupta *et al.*, 1974); and in the elderly the histological incidence of osteomalacia in patients with femoral neck fracture is said to be seasonal (Aaron *et al.*, 1974*a*).

CAUSES

Within the general statement that osteomalacia (rickets) is due to a deficiency of vitamin D, or a disturbance of its metabolism, there are three main causes, namely, vitamin D deficiency (so-called nutritional rickets); malabsorption; and renal disease.

Vitamin D deficiency is probably now (for the first time since the Victorian era) the commonest cause of osteomalacia, especially in the elderly.

Malabsorption is most often due to gluten sensitive enteropathy (or coeliac disease) in which there is atrophy of the small intestinal mucosa. Partial gastrectomy is a less common cause.

Osteomalacia due to renal disease may be due to renal tubular disorders (particularly X-linked hypophosphataemia) or to renal glomerular disease. It is important to draw a distinction between these two types, and not just to consider renal rickets as one disease, since the cause, clinical presentation, treatment and prognosis in renal tubular rickets is entirely different from that due to renal glomerular failure.

Less common causes of osteomalacia which are nevertheless of clinical importance include the prolonged use of anticonvulsants, osteomalacia associated with non-endocrine tumours, and the rare but extremely severe inherited form known as vitamin D-dependent rickets.

DIAGNOSIS

The diagnosis of osteomalacia should be suspected on the historical and clinical features, and confirmed by biochemistry, radiology and, if necessary, bone biopsy. In the fully developed disorder, the symptoms are quite characteristic, comprising bone pain and tenderness, often proximal muscle weakness and sometimes deformity, together with the symptoms of the underlying disorder and sometimes those of hypocalcaemia.

The musculo-skeletal symptoms are most important. The bones may be spontaneously painful as well as tender; all bones are affected, but tenderness of the ribs is probably most characteristic. The tenderness may be so severe that the patients may wake themselves up when turning over in bed at night. Normal activities may be limited by pain, and pain may be locally increased in the area of pseudo-fractures.

Weakness of the proximal muscles does not always occur, but when present is of considerable diagnostic significance. A false diagnosis of muscular dystrophy in a young patient is not unknown, and some patients with osteomalacia may be unable to walk (Leeming, 1973) because of progressive weakness of the proximal muscles together with a variable degree of bone pain. An early symptom of the weakness is a waddling gait; later there is difficulty in getting out of low chairs and out of bed, and inability to go upstairs except on all-fours. Complaint may be made of stiffness as well as of weakness. Since the proximal muscles of the pelvis and trunk are most used in daily life, weakness is first noticed in these, but weakness of the shoulder girdle muscles may also be noticed, with inability for instance, to reach objects from a high shelf.

Deformity in osteomalacia may be due to past or present disease. There may be evidence of previous rickets in childhood; in the chronic forms of rickets, such as vitamin D resistant rickets, and in vitamin D-dependent rickets, dwarfism, bowing of the long bones and disproportion between the upper and lower segments of the body may occur. A patient who develops osteomalacia for the first time in adult life may lose trunk height. In the elderly person with recent osteomalacia, general deformity may be absent.

To these cardinal features of bone pain, proximal muscle weakness and deformity should be added those of the underlying disorder and sometimes those of hypocalcaemia. It is important to consider the patient as a whole and to look for symptoms of general illness; thus a woman may have had unrecognized coeliac disease all her life but the features of dwarfism, or late onset of periods, or iron deficiency anaemia resistant to iron, or of intermittent diarrhoea with bulky stools may suggest it. Similarly a history of repeated 'cystitis', of nocturia or

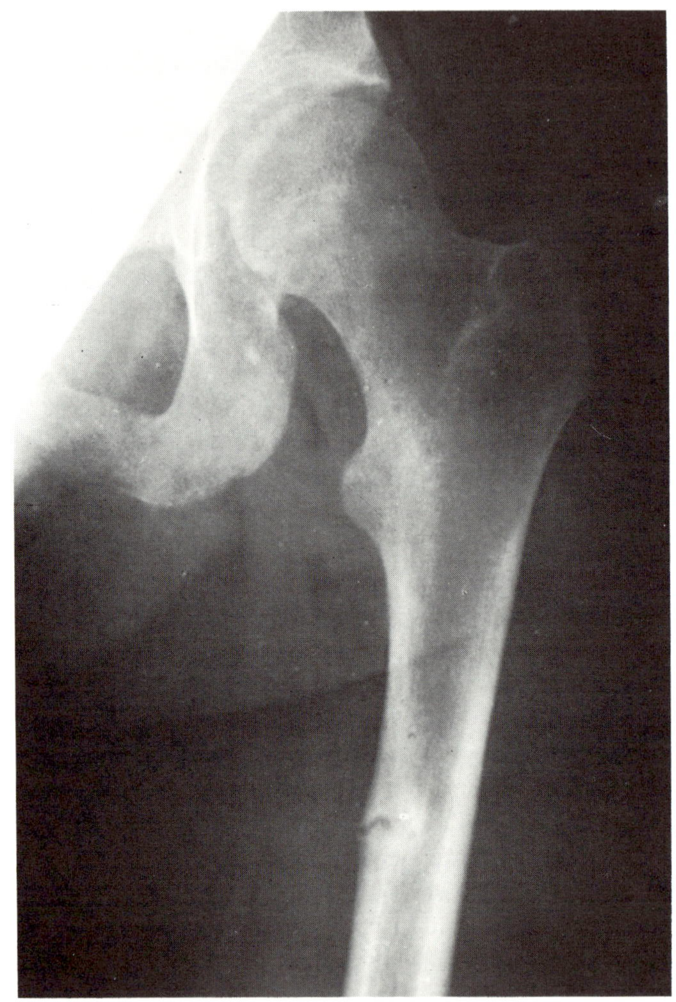

FIG. 4.4 Loozer zone in a woman of 20 with osteomalacia. Two years history of difficulty in walking, with a waddling gait, and tenderness of the ribs, without the correct diagnosis. The plasma phosphate was 0.5 mmol l^{-1} (1.7 mg per 100 ml).

thirst, of anaemia or of pigmentation may suggest unsuspected renal failure. Not all patients with osteomalacia have hypocalcaemia; occasionally this may provide the leading symptom of tetany, with tingling and carpopedal spasm which may go unrecognized.

Examination will confirm the features. Obvious abnormalities such as dwarfism or anaemia must not be missed. Bone tenderness and proximal muscle weakness should be looked for, and latent tetany most easily detected by Chvostek's sign.

Exact confirmation of the diagnosis of osteomalacia depends on radiology, biochemistry and often bone biopsy. In the elderly patient with a fractured femoral neck, one has to choose those investigations which will most simply and rapidly give the diagnosis, since if such a patient has osteomalacia it is likely to be 'nutritional' in origin, rather than due to some more obscure cause, and will respond well to relatively small doses of vitamin D.

The radiological hall mark of osteomalacia is the Loozer zone, a ribbon-like area of decalcification which extends partly across the border or shaft of a bone (Fig. 4.4). There is little evidence for the idea that this occurs where arteries cross bone surfaces and they may be found in nearly all parts of the skeleton. However, they tend to occur on the concave side of long bones, such as the femur, in the pelvic bones, in the ribs and around the scapulae; Loozer zones are seen only in a proportion of patients with osteomalacia, but if present they are diagnostic. Other radiological features of osteomalacia due to softening of the bones include deformity of the rib cage, with crowding and bending of the ribs and sometimes a triradiate appearance of the pelvis.

The vertebrae may show a regular biconcave appearance, sometimes with end-plates which are denser than the body of the vertebrae (an appearance sometimes called 'rugger jersey spine', Fig. 4.5) said to be most common in patients with osteomalacia due to renal failure. Further, in most types of osteomalacia with hypocalcaemia there are the X-ray changes of secondary hyperparathyroidism with subperiosteal erosion of bone. This erosion is most commonly seen in the phalanges, but may also occur around the pubic symphysis, the sacroiliac joints and the femoral necks. The X-ray appearances of osteomalacia may differ with the cause, which may be diagnostically useful.

The main biochemical investigation is measurement of the plasma calcium, phosphate and alkaline phosphatase. The plasma calcium is often reduced but hypocalcaemia is not necessary for the diagnosis.

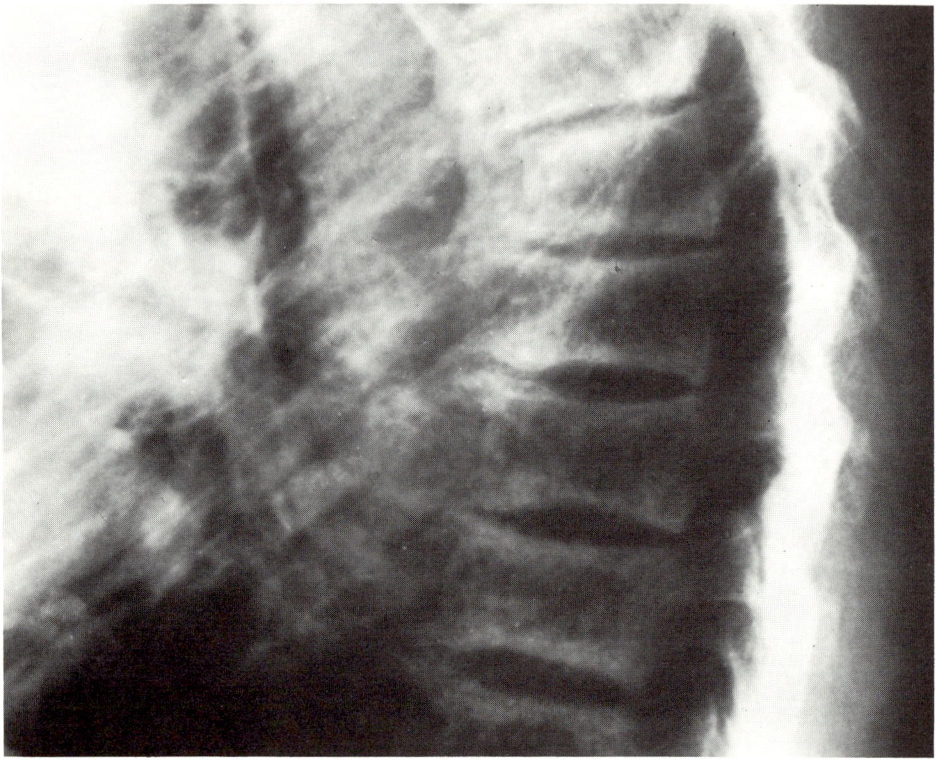

FIG. 4.5 Appearance of the spine of a woman of 70 with severe osteomalacia. The density of the end plates in comparison to the body of the vertebra gives a 'rugger jersey' appearance.

Due correction should be made if the plasma albumin is low, and appropriate formulae are available (Berry *et al.*, 1973). The plasma inorganic phosphate is important, but sometimes it is not measured or the result is ignored; it is almost always low in osteomalacia, except where there is renal glomerular failure. Secondary parathyroid overactivity (stimulated by hypocalcaemia) will accentuate the hypophosphataemia, whereas it will tend to return the plasma calcium to normal. The plasma alkaline phosphatase, which reflects osteoblastic activity, may be quite normal, although it is usually increased, especially in the later stages of osteomalacia. One should remember that it is higher in adolescents than in adults and may increasingly be expressed in milli-international units per litre (rather than the more familiar King Armstrong units per 100 ml). A very low 24 h urinary calcium, in the range of 5–30 mg supports the diagnosis of osteomalacia.

Further results which may suggest its cause include a raised blood urea due to renal failure; a low plasma CO_2 and an increased chloride due to renal tubular acidosis; and glycosuria and proteinuria due to renal tubular disorder.

Rarely osteomalacia may be present despite normal X-rays and biochemistry. Bone histology is then necessary to establish or to exclude the diagnosis. Bone can be obtained at operation on the fractured femur or by transilliac trephine biopsy. It is necessary to examine undecalcified bone. Osteomalacia (Fig. 4.1*c*) is diagnosed by an increase in the amount of osteoid (unmineralized bone matrix) which is present as lamellae of doubly refractile collagen on the bone surfaces. Typically, there is an increase in both the fraction of bone surfaces covered with osteoid, and the thickness of the osteoid itself. In the borderlinc casc the criteria to be used are disputed. Where the clinical picture is still suspicious but the diagnosis is in doubt, a therapeutic trial of vitamin D (see under Treatment) may cause a striking improvement and establish the diagnosis.

DIFFERENTIAL DIAGNOSIS

In a patient with bone pain and tenderness and proximal muscle weakness, osteomalacia must always be considered. Delays in diagnosis for years are not uncommon. When the diagnosis is not thought of, it is usual for these patients to be dealt with initially in departments of physical medicine or rheumatology, because of the complaints of generalized pain and 'stiffness'; rheumatoid arthritis may be diagnosed (in the absence of arthritis) or the common condition of polymyalgia rheumatica may be considered. Where the proximal muscle weakness and progressive inability to walk are prominent features, muscular dystrophy may be suggested. In all of these the plasma alkaline phosphatase is normal, and in polymyalgia, which occurs in the elderly with stiffness and pain in the proximal muscles and general malaise, the ESR is considerably increased and response to steroids is dramatic.

Osteomalacia may be confused with other metabolic bone diseases. Distinction from osteoporosis is not difficult. The features of Paget's disease do not resemble those of osteomalacia, but the raised plasma alkaline phosphatase is a feature of both and confusion may be possible (Fig. 4.6). Hyperparathyroidism with bone disease may initially be difficult to distinguish because its clinical features of bone pain, deformity and muscle weakness may closely resemble those of osteo-

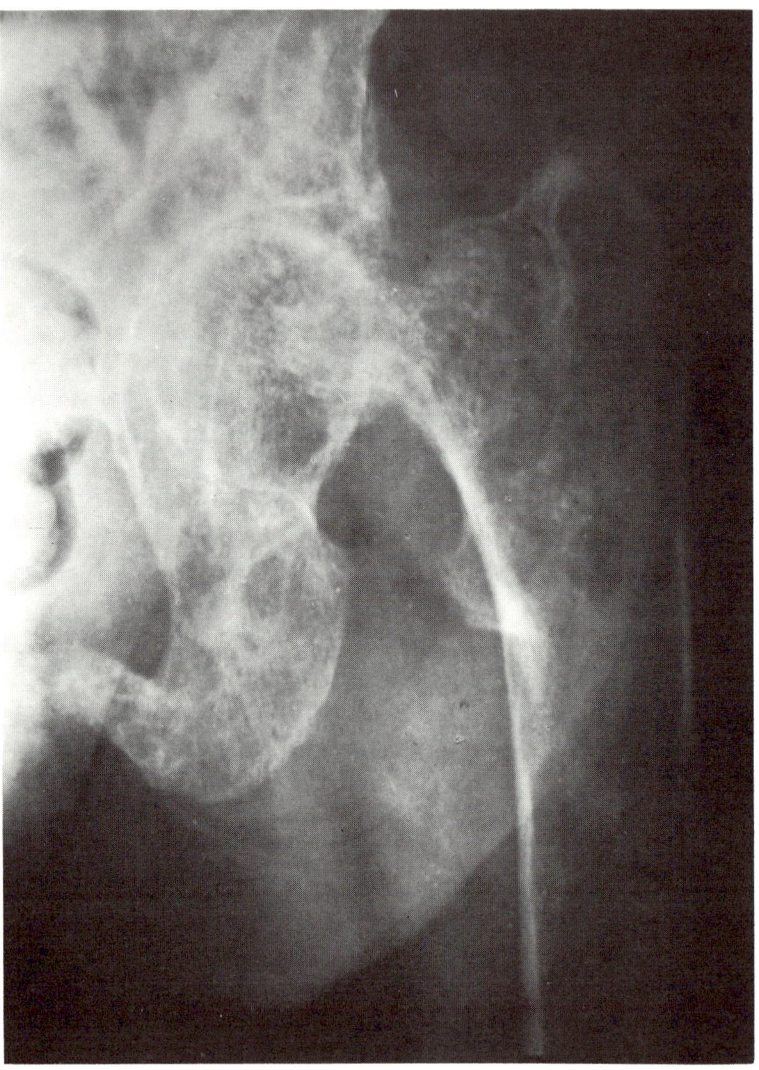

FIG. 4.6 The pelvis and upper part of the left femur in the same patient, with a pathological fracture of the femoral neck. An erroneous diagnosis of Paget's disease had been made. She had been unable to walk for several years. Osteomalacia was proved by histology, and the plasma values were calcium 2.4 mmol l^{-1} (9.6 mg), phosphorus 0.7 mmol l^{-1} (2.3 mg per 100 ml) and alkaline phosphatase 80 King Armstrong units per 100 ml. The osteomalacia was probably due ot a poor intake of vitamin D and prolonged treatment with anticonvulsants for epilepsy.

malacia, as do the X-ray and biochemistry, and the conditions may co-exist. However in osteomalacia the plasma calcium is not raised as it is in primary hyperparathyroidism.

TREATMENT

The intake of vitamin D is generally low, and much osteomalacia, especially in the elderly, could be prevented by appropriate dietary supplements. It is not easy to encourage old people to have more exposure to ultraviolet light, even if this were practicable. The oral requirements should be satisfied by Caps A and D B.P.C., 2 daily, which will provide 900 i.u. and this should be an appropriate outpatient maintenance dose. Advice should also be given to eat some of those foods which contain vitamin D–particularly the oily fishes, and less importantly, dairy products.

In established osteomalacia it is usual to start off treatment with much higher doses of vitamin D to heal the bones quickly, to improve mobility and to replenish the stores of vitamin D. Calciferol 50 000 i.u. (1.25 mg) daily may be given by mouth for an arbitrary period of, for instance, 1–2 weeks, followed by a smaller maintenance dose. This high dose should not be continued indefinitely, or as an outpatient, or where facilities for frequent accurate estimations of the plasma calcium are not available. In some patients prolonged treatment may be required and elderly patients may have an increased requirement for the vitamin D; but if vitamin D resistance is encountered in the presence of proven osteomalacia, this may be due to renal glomerular failure or to coeliac disease; or rarely to one of the uncommon forms of inherited rickets. These will require specialist advice.

OTHER METABOLIC CONDITIONS

Rarely femoral neck fracture is associated with other metabolic bone diseases. Two of these deserve brief mention.

PAGET'S DISEASE

This disorder is common (Leeming, 1973) but most patients have no symptoms. Although its cause is obscure, the histological and biochemical features are well known. There is excessive and disorderly resorption and formation of bone (Fig. 4.1*d*); early in the course of the disorder resorption may predominate, but later there is excessive bone formation as well. The new bone is structurally weak and fractures may occur.

The diagnosis of Paget's disease is based on the clinical, radiological and biochemical findings; rarely is biopsy necessary. The affected bone is characteristically larger than normal, warm and deformed and may be painful. There are many X-ray appearances, but the most common are an area of resorption or rarefaction with a clear cut edge, or an enlarged and deformed bone with a disturbance of the trabecular pattern. Paget's disease may occur in any bone.

In long-standing Paget's disease, numerous small partial fractures–microfractures–may occur, particularly well seen on the convex outer border of the bowed femur (Fig. 4.7). These differ from the wide and less numerous Loozer zones of osteomalacia, which may occur on the concave border of long bones. Paget's disease should always be considered as a cause of unusual appearance of bone, if only because of its frequency.

The outstanding biochemical abnormality in Paget's disease is an increase in the plasma alkaline phosphatase, which may be very considerable. The plasma calcium and phosphate are normal, unless the patient is immobilized, in which case both the plasma and urine calcium may increase, or in the rare situations where there is co-existent osteomalacia or hyperparathyroidism. Another indication of the very rapid turnover in this condition is an increase in the urinary total hydroxyproline, derived from bone collagen. In adults the normal daily excretion is less than 50 mg.

It is now possible to suppress the excessive and disorderly bone activity in Paget's disease with agents such as the calcitonins or phosphonates, but they should probably not be given when a fracture is present. Their exact mode of action is not known but they act at cellular level; complications are few although the phosphonates may produce excess osteoid tissue. Resistance to calcitonin may develop after 3 months but does not depend on the level of antibodies.

Hyperparathyroidism (osteitis fibrosa)

The majority of patients with hyperparathyroidism have no clinical bone disease. In those who have (approximately 20%), the main pathological changes are a mixture of excessive osteoclastic bone

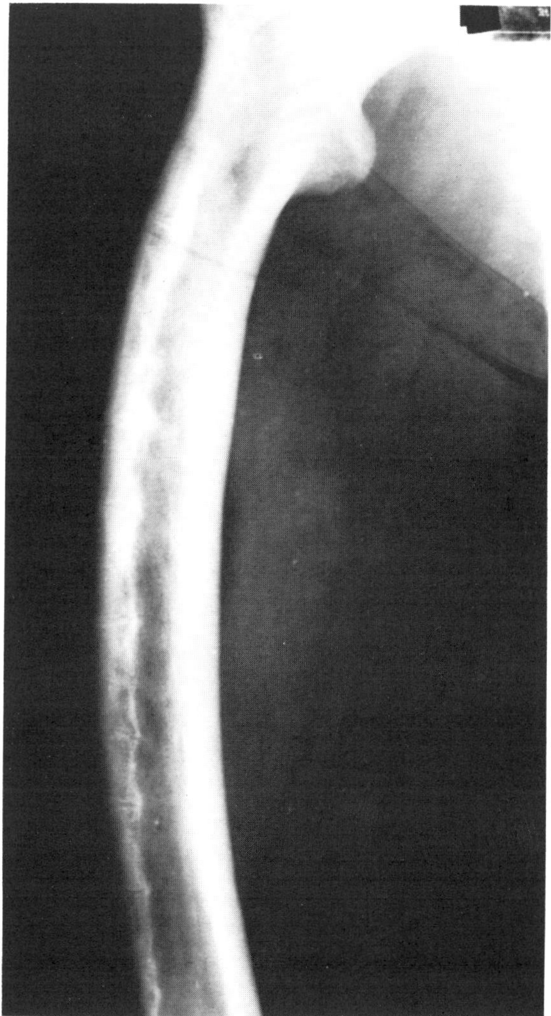

FIG. 4.7 The appearance of microfractures on the convex border of a thickened and deformed femur in a man of 70 with Paget's disease.

resorption and fibrosis of the marrow (Fig. 4.1*e*), sometimes with the formation of cyst-like areas–hence the term osteitis fibrosa cystica. The bone disease may sometimes be limited to a 'cyst' in a bone such as the pelvis or femur; more often it is generalized.

Generalized bone disease due to hyperparathyroidism can lead to bone pain, deformity (with loss of height), fractures and muscle weakness. The weakness may be generalized and due to the hypercalcaemia (although other causes have been suggested). Hypercalcaemia may also cause other important symptoms, including thirst, nocturia (due to inability of the kidney to resorb water), anorexia, nausea, vomiting and constipation. Depression is also common; and also unexplained difficulty in walking with stiffness and joint pain.

The biochemistry is characteristic, with an elevated plasma calcium and low plasma phosphate. The plasma alkaline phosphatase is increased only in that minority of hyperparathyroid patients who have bone disease. The diagnosis is virtually excluded by a normal plasma calcium but the plasma phosphate is not invariably low; the urine calcium is often, but not always, increased above normal (upper limit in males not more than 400 mg a day); clearly these are important points of distinction from osteomalacia.

In generalized osteitis fibrosa, the radiological hallmark is subperiosteal bone resorption, particularly of the phalanges, when it is best seen on the radial borders of the phalanges of the fingers; it is said to occur most often in those fingers which are used most (such as the right hand in right-handed people). There is erosion and sometimes loss of the terminal phalanges. In primary hyperparathyroidism with bone disease such erosions may be the only feature; if the excessive parathyroid activity is secondary to hypocalcaemia due to osteomalacia, the feature of this disorder may also be present.

In those patients with generalized parathyroid bone disease the diagnosis can be confirmed by bone biopsy, but this is hardly necessary where the characteristic X-rays are present. A difficulty may arise in a patient with a fractured femoral neck who has hypercalcaemia but no evidence of bone disease. Although the hypercalcaemia may be due to hyperparathyroidism it should be recalled that the commonest cause of hypercalcaemia in the elderly is neoplasm. Persistent hypercalcaemia always requires further investigation.

PRACTICAL POINTS IN DIAGNOSIS

In practice, patients do not present with diagnoses but with complaints, and the problem is to find the likely cause. How do we decide on the likely cause of femoral neck fracture? Since most of these occur in the elderly and in females, occurrence in the young or in men without due trauma suggests an unusual diagnosis, such as neoplasm, myeloma, osteitis fibrosa or renal osteodystrophy. In the elderly female osteoporo-

TABLE 4.1 Metabolic causes of femoral neck fractures.

DIAGNOSIS	TYPE OF PATIENT	HISTORY	PHYSICAL SIGNS	X-RAY	BIO-CHEMISTRY	BONE BIOPSY	DIFFEREN-TIAL DIAGNOSIS
Osteoporosis	Elderly female	Loss of height; back pain. Sometimes early or artificial menopause	Loss of height. Kyphosis. Abdominal crease	Thin cortices. Wedge shaped vertebral bodies. Loss of trabeculae. Rarefaction	Normal	Few thin trabeculae	Myeloma. Metastases. Osteomalacia
Osteomalacia	Any age; common in elderly and immigrant	Proximal muscle weakness. Generalized bone pain and tenderness. Loss of height; Unable to walk	Waddling gait. Myopathy. Tender ribs. Sometimes Chvostek positive. Signs of underlying disorder	Loozer zones. Triradiate pelvis. Deformed chest. Symmetrically biconcave vertebrae	Ca ↓ or N. P ↓. P, ase ↑ or N. Urine Ca low	Normal amount of bone. Excess osteoid	'Arthritis' 'Fibrositis'. Polymyalgia rheumatica. Muscular dystrophy
Pagets disease	Elderly either sex. May start in 30s	Deformity; often localized to one long bone. Bone pain	Deformed thick bowed bone. Warm	Rarefaction early; later thick cortex; abnormal trabeculae large bone sometimes microfractures	CaN PN P, ase ↑ Urine hydroxy proline increased	Disorganized bone. Excess osteoclastic resorption osteoblasts formation. Fibrosis marrow. Cement lines	Metastases in bone. Sarcoma Osteomalacia
Osteitis fibrosa	Any age or sex. Commonest in post menopausal females	Bone pain. Deformity. Difficulty in walking. Symptoms of hypercalcaemia	Tender bones. Deformity. Corneal calcification	Subperiosteal resorption of phalanges. Resorption elsewhere. Localized cysts in bones	Ca ↑ P ↓ P, ase ↑ in primary HPT. If secondary to Ca ↓, biochem. of underlying disorder	Excessive osteoclastic bone resorption. Marrow fibrosis	Osteomalacia. Neoplasm with 2° deposits. Other causes of hypercal caemia

N, Normal; ↑, increased; ↓, decreased; P'ase, Plasma alkaline phosphatase; Normal biochemical values in plasma. Calcium 2.12–2.65 mmol l^{-1}(9.0–10.6 mg per 100 ml); Inorganic phosphate 0.80–1.45 mmol l^{-1}(2.8–4.8 mg per 100 ml); Alkaline phosphatase 35–80 i.u. l^{-1} (3–12 King Armstrong units per 100 ml).

sis is most likely, and if the X-rays and biochemistry support this, no further investigation is necessary.

Since X-rays are often more familiar and more notice is taken of them than of biochemistry, the initial differential diagnosis is often based on radiology. An X-ray of the femoral neck usually includes one of the pelvis, and if a Loozer zone or triradiate deformity is seen strongly suggesting osteomalacia, this should then be confirmed biochemically. An X-ray showing resorption, for instance of the femoral neck or localized 'cystic' lesions, should be followed by one of the hands, to check for subperiosteal erosions, and by plasma biochemistry. If hypercalcaemia with an increased alkaline phosphatase is present the diagnosis of primary hyperparathyroidism is virtually established. If the plasma calcium is low or normal in the presence of radiological parathyroid bone disease, the hyperparathyroidism is presumably secondary to a low plasma calcium; and the commonest causes are malabsorption and renal glomerular disease. The plasma urea (and electrolytes) should also be requested.

The X-ray may suggest Paget's disease. Since in this disorder the affected bone is typically larger than its normal counterpart, with a coarse trabecular structure, confusion only rarely arises. Paget's disease may produce almost any radiological appearance; and if microfractures are confused with Loozer zones, osteomalacia may be suggested. Since only the alkaline phosphatase is increased in Paget's disease, and the plasma calcium and phosphate are normal, these estimations will clarify the picture. Although the correct diagnosis can often be made by X-ray, biochemistry is also essential since the situation may be complex and bone biopsy may be necessary. The accompanying Table 4.1 emphasises these points.

RECENT AND FUTURE WORK

Recent work in metabolic bone disease has concentrated on two points which are of particular importance to orthopaedic surgeons. These are the cause and possible prevention of postmenopausal and senile osteoporosis, and the increasing incidence of osteomalacia.

Osteoporosis is by far the commonest metabolic bone disease and the commonest cause of femoral neck fracture. It is also the least remediable. The demonstration of the protective effect of oestrogens against parathyroid hormone-induced bone resorption provides a logical basis for hormonal treatment of osteoporosis, although its application may be difficult. If senile osteoporosis has a different cause, it may be that treatment to overcome the poor intestinal absorption of calcium in this disorder is correct. Since relatively large doses of vitamin D or its metabolites are required, it is clear that there is not merely a simple deficiency of vitamin D.

The high incidence of osteomalacia in femoral neck fracture has been demonstrated by the Leeds group (Aaron *et al.*, 1974*b*), by O'Driscoll (1973) and by Jenkins *et al.*, (1973). Its exact incidence is debated (Hodkinson, 1974). Although the argument is largely histological and statistical it is clinically important since the treatment of osteomalacia with vitamin D is so simple and effective.

Thus Aaron *et al.* (1974*a*) suggested that their 125 patients could be divided into three groups; those with normal bone histology for age (50 patients) (which included some with 'osteoporosis') and a fracture rate higher than young persons; those with probable osteomalacia, (at most 46 patients), 10 of whom also had osteoporosis, with a high fracture risk; and those with severe osteoporosis alone (29 patients) with possible predisposing causes, including corticosteroid therapy, in 10.

Aaron *et al.*, (1974*a*) also showed that in the same patients the incidence of histological osteomalacia in femoral neck fractures was seasonal (40–50% in the spring and 10–20% in the autumn). This correlates well with the seasonal variation of 25-HCC in healthy people (McLaughlin *et al.*, 1974) and the spontaneous cure of the osteomalacia of Asian immigrants in the summer (Gupta *et al.*, 1974). The data of the Leeds group have however been challenged by Hodkinson (1974).

REFERENCES

AARON, J.E., GALLAGHER, J.C. and NORDIN, B.E.C. (1974*a*). *Lancet* **ii**, 84.

AARON, J.E., GALLAGHER, J.C., ANDERSON, J., STASAIK, L., LONGTON, E.B., NORDIN, B.E.C. and NICHOLSON, M. (1974*b*). *Lancet* **i**, 229.

AITKEN, J.M., HART, D.M., ANDERSON, J.B., LINDSAY, R., SMITH, D.A. and SPIERS, C.F. (1973). *Br. med. J.* **2**, 325.

BELCHETZ, P.E., LLOYD, M. H., JOHNS, R.G.S. and COHEN, R.D. (1973). *Br. med. J.* **2**, 510.

BERRY, E.M., GUPTA, M.M., TURNER, S.J. and BURNS, R.R. (1973). *Br. med. J.* **4**, 640.

CHALMERS, J. (1970). *J. Bone Jt. Surg.* **52B**, 509.

Clinics in Endocrinology and Metabolism (1972) Vol. 1. (Ed. MacIntyre I.) W.B. Saunders Co., London.

DENT, C.E. and WATSON, L. (1966). Osteoporosis. *Postgrad. Med. J.* **42**, 581. (supplement).

DUDL, R.J., ENSINCK, J.W., BAYLINK, D., CHESNUT, C.H., SHERRARD, D., NELP,

W.B. and PALMIERI, G.N.A. (1973). *Amer. J. Med.* **55**, 631.

GUPTA, M.M., ROUND, J.M. and STAMP, T.C.B. (1974). *Lancet* **i**, 856.

HENNEMAN, P.H. (1972). *Seminars in Drug Treatment* **2**, 15.

HODKINSON, H.M. (1974). *Lancet* **ii**, 1008.

JENKINS, D.H.R., ROBERTS, J.G., WEBSTER, D. and WILLIAMS, E.O. (1973). *J. Bone Jt. Surg.* **55**B, 575.

KODICEK, E. (1974). *Lancet* **i**, 325.

LEEMING, J.T. (1973). *Br. med. J.* **4**, 472.

MCLAUGHLIN, M., RAGGATT, P.R., FAIRNEY, A., BROWN, D.J., LESTER, E. and WILLS, M.R. (1974). *Lancet* **i**, 536.

MORGAN, B. (1973). *Osteomalacia, Renal Osteodystrophy and Osteoporosis.* Charles C. Thomas, Springfield, Illinois.

MORGAN, D.B. and ROBERTSON, W.G. (1974). *Clin. Orth.* **101**, 254.

NORDIN, B.E.C. (1971). *Br. med. J.* **1**, 571.

NORDIN, B.E.C. (1973). *Metabolic Bone and Stone Disease.* Churchill Livingstone, Edinburgh and London.

O'DRISCOLL, M. (1973). *J. Bone Jt. Surg.* **55B**, 882.

PEACOCK, M., GALLAGHER, J.C. and NORDIN, B.E.C. (1974). *Lancet* **i**, 385.

Seminars in Drug Treatment (1972). **2**, No. 1. Drug Treatment of Bone. (Eds. Di Palma, J. R. and Calesnick, B.) Grune and Stratton.

Chapter Five

AVASCULAR NECROSIS AND PATHOLOGICAL FRACTURES

C. G. Woods

AVASCULAR NECROSIS

As we have seen in Chapter 1, the blood supply of the mature femoral head arrives via the medullary cavity of the neck and by vessels passing through the joint capsule and the ligamentum teres. Complete fracture through any part of the femoral neck will interrupt the flow into the head through the medullary vessels. Displaced fractures proximal to the capsular reflexion compress or sever the transcapsular blood vessels, and these structures may also be damaged during attempts to realign the proximal fragment. Vessels entering the fovea are sometimes damaged by misdirected nails.

Displaced intracapsular fracture almost inevitably disrupts the superior retinacular vessels, and the possibility for survival of the femoral head (Fig. 5.1) after such an injury depends upon the integrity of the inferior metaphyseal and medial epiphyseal vessels and the extent of the distribution of their branches within the head.

Injection studies (Trueta and Harrison, 1953; Sevitt and Thompson, 1965) show that the blood supply is essentially territorial with overlap and that the size of the territories is widely variable (Fig. 5.2). The vessels passing through the ligamentum teres rarely ramify throughout the major part of the head and commonly terminate within a short distance of the fovea.

It should, therefore, be anticipated that a high proportion of femoral heads separated by subcapital fracture will suffer a degree of necrosis

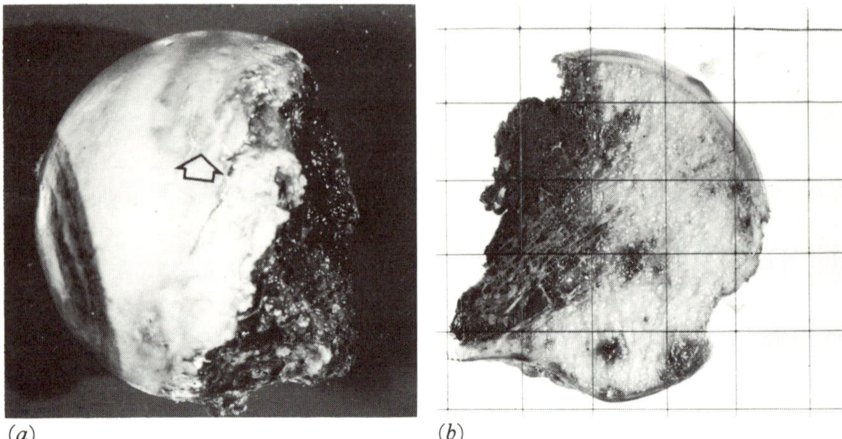

(*a*) (*b*)

FIG. 5.1 Avascular necrosis of the femoral head after subcapital fracture. (*a*) The head shows softening on its superior surface prior to segmental collapse (arrow); (*b*) a section through the femoral head shows infarction and an avascular area (J. C. Scott).

beyond that which occurs adjacent to every fracture and that in some this will involve a very large part of the head.

BONE NECROSIS, RESORPTION AND REVASCULARIZATION

Studies of femoral heads removed because of subcapital fracture and at autopsy (Sevitt, 1964; Catto, 1965*a*) have provided evidence of the incidence and extent of necrosis and of the possibilities of revascularization.

In an account of her observations, Mary Catto places due emphasis on the distinction between loss of osteocytes which occurs commonly in normal bone of elderly people and bone necrosis due to rapid devascularization. She also emphasized the time lag between fracture and the appearance of unequivocal histological evidence of necrosis of marrow and bone tissues. Regarding the latter, it is clear that the features of marrow necrosis may not appear until the fourth day or later after fracture and that trabeculae within necrotic areas may still contain osteocyte nuclei which are seemingly normal for as many as 28 days after fracture.

Bearing in mind that the specimens examined came from fractures treated in different hospitals and by several surgeons, the findings of Sevitt and Catto are in accord, indicating that about 70% of femoral heads separated by subcapital fracture will undergo partial or total necrosis soon after injury. Revascularization of the dead tissue is a less predictable event, some totally necrotic heads being unchanged at 40 weeks and others being completely revascularized in less than that time. When some of the bone remains viable, there is a greater chance of revascularization commencing but the rate at which it occurs appears to be highly variable. The process of revascularization may stop short of completion, a fact which has important consequences for the integrity of the head months or years after the fracture.

Accepting that the time scale is imprecise and that there are no sharply defined stages, the histological changes due to devascularization are as follows. 'Foamy' cells and dead haematopoietic cells are seen in the marrow from about the fourth day and small cysts may appear about the same time (Fig. 5.3).

Empty osteophyte lacunae begin to appear about the fourth day also (Fig. 5.3). The bone tissue first affected is normally close to the fracture line and cells within a zone 0.5 cm from a fracture can be expected to die (McLean and Urist, 1953), irrespective of what happens elsewhere.

In avascular areas further from the fracture site loss of osteocyte nuclei may not occur until the fourth week and should not be expected to occur within the first week.

Resorption of dead soft tissue and the repair process begin within a short time if there is viable tissue in direct contact with the devascularized area. A few neutrophil polymorphonuclear leucoctyes may migrate a short distance into the devitalized zone within 24 h to be followed by phagocytic cells, many of which become 'foamy' histiocytes. Capillary and fibroblast proliferation, which, in favourable circumstances is active from the third day, initiates the repair process. Slightly behind the advancing front of revascularization, resorption of dead bone and osteoclastic differentiation may occur or new bone may be deposited on the unmodified surfaces of necrotic trabeculae. These changes in bone structure are not invariable and some revascularized marrow may be filled by fibrous connective tissue without any evidence of differentiation of osteoblasts or osteoclasts, (Fig. 5.4). The factor determining the form of repair process is unknown.

Equally mysterious and unpredictable is the extent and rate of revascularization once the process has started. Of 36 femoral heads classified as totally necrotic by Catto (1965*b*), 8 showed evidence of revascularization, which was complete in some specimens within 42 days of fracture; whilst heads which were only partially necrotic

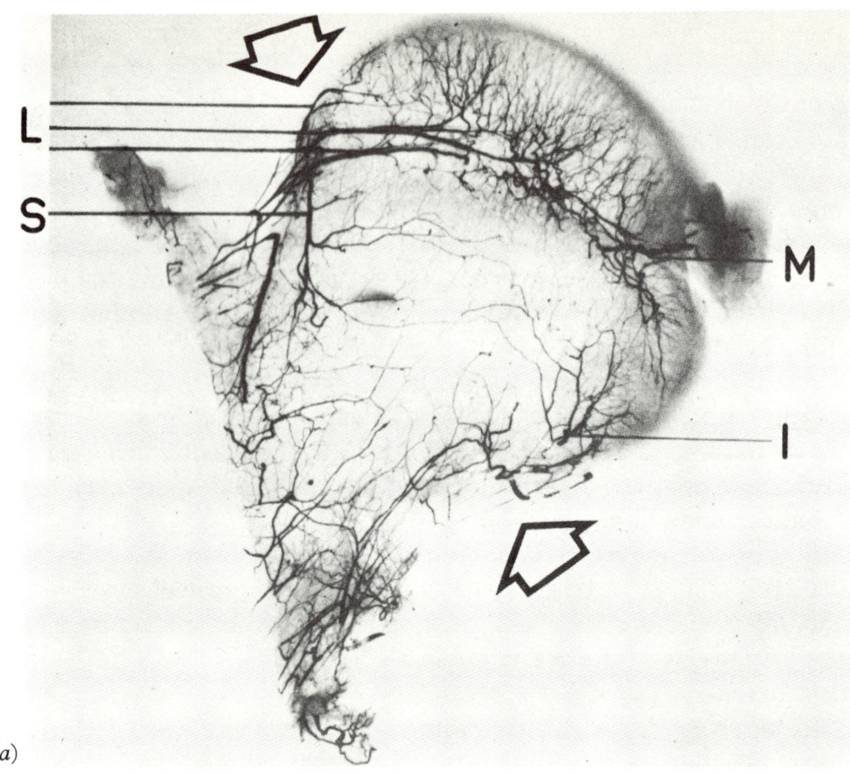

(*a*)

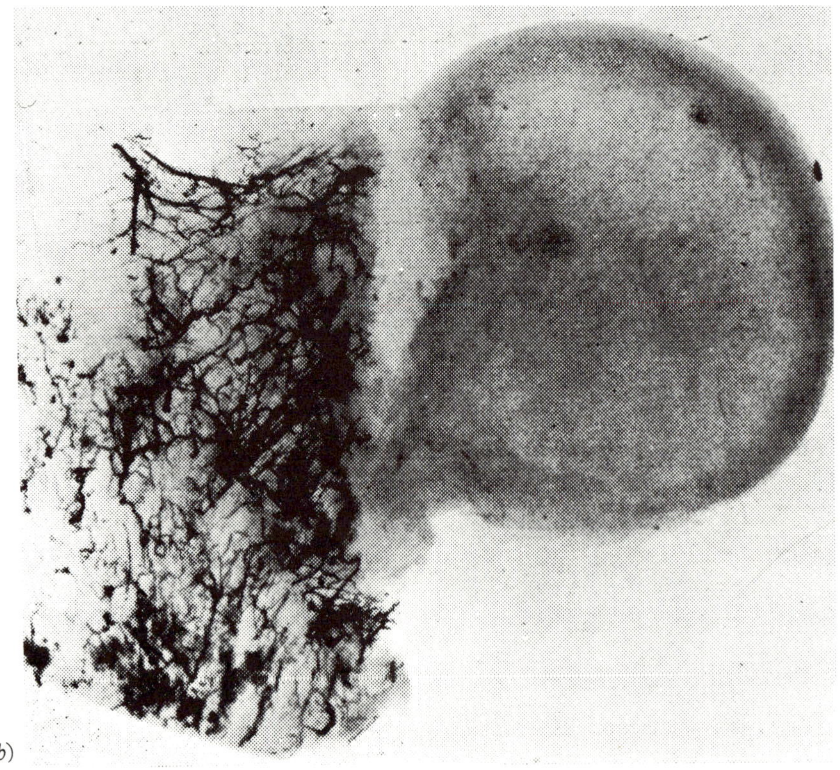

(*b*)

were not revascularized completely in the same period. The most serious consequence of avascular necrosis – late collapse of the head – is due to the persistence of an unrevascularized portion of the head for months and sometimes years. If only part of the head is devascularized, it is almost always the superior part of the bone which is affected and failure of revascularization usually leaves a conical shaped area, with the base in the subchondral plate, necrotic. This is the 'weight-bearing' area of the femoral head.

Fracture union is not generally possible when the head is completely avascular. Phemister (1949) found that non-union was four times more frequent when the capital fragment was necrotic than when it was not. The case for accurate reduction and fixation to minimize the incidence of non-union and late segmental collapse has been made on many occasions (Sherman and Phemister, 1947; Garden, 1971), but there is no method of fracture treatment which will guarantee restoration to a wholly viable state.

If it were possible to determine easily and reliably whether the capital fragment is vascularized or not shortly after fracture, it would be possible to assess the effects of different techniques of management more scientifically and have a more rational attitude to treatment than exists at the moment.

The histological changes seen in decalcified preparations stained by haematoxylin and eosin afford little help in the immediate post-fracture period and a biopsy sample might be unrepresentative even if one were to use the Feulgen reaction as a more sensitive indication of cell death (Nelson and Haynes, 1970). Radiology is of no value until revascularization is well established or porotic changes are manifest in adjacent bones.

Other methods for early detection which have been tested include: arterial assay (McGinnis *et al.*, 1958), venous assay (Harrison, 1962), oximetry (Woodhouse, 1962) Coomassie blue dye injection directly into the femoral head (Price, 1962) and radioactive phosphorous uptake

---

FIG. 5.2 (*a*) Blood supply to the femoral head (shown by lateral and medial epiphyseal vessels; and superior and inferior metaphyseal vessels. L and M stand for lateral and medial epiphyseal vessels respectively; S and I for superior and inferior metaphyseal vessels respectively. (*b*) Arteriography depicts the avascularity of the head and proliferation of new vessels on the neck below the fracture (fracture line depicted by arrows).

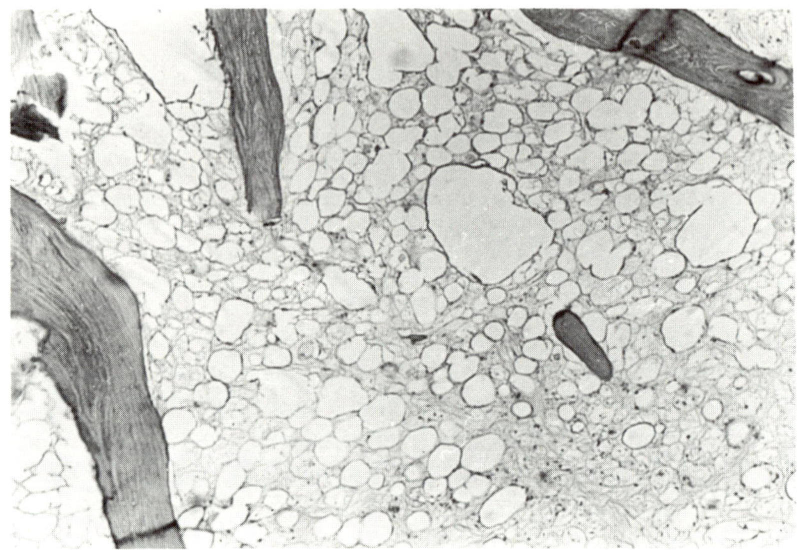

FIG. 5.3 Avascular necrosis. In the bone marrow there are large spaces, presumably due to coalescence of the contents of necrotic fat cells. The cells in the haematopoietic tissue have pyknotic nuclei. Many of the osteocyte lacunae appear empty.

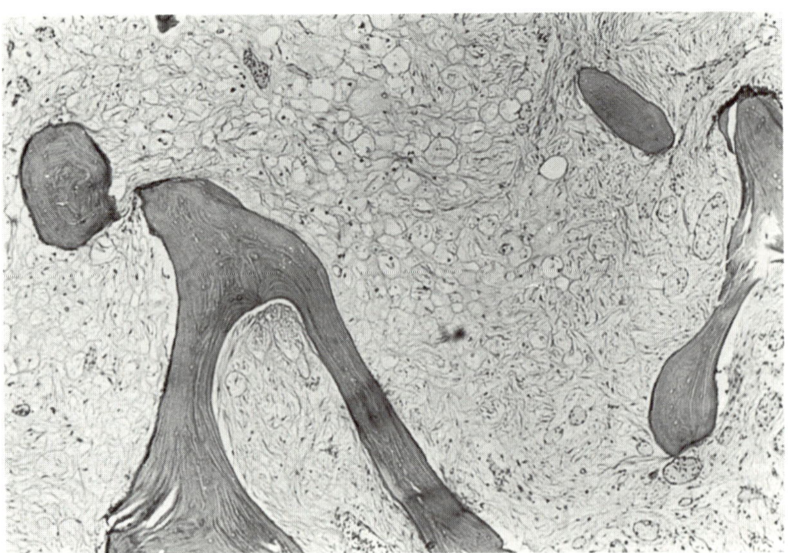

FIG. 5.4 Avascular necrosis with dense fibrosis of marrow tissue. There is no resorption of dead bone nor differentiation of new bone.

(Boyd and Calandruccio, 1963). None has been considered satisfactory and a reliable and safe technique has yet to be developed.

FEMORAL HEAD COLLAPSE

If a subcapital fracture soundly unites and the patient is permitted free mobility with weight-bearing through the affected hip joint there is a possibility that the femoral head will collapse. The reported incidence of this complication varies considerably (Green, 1960; Garden, 1961). Some of the variation can be accounted for by the length of time over which the patients are observed after fracture, for whilst it is generally agreed that most instances of this complication will have appeared within two years of the fracture, others will occur in later years.

There is abundant evidence to support the view expressed by Hodges (1954) that collapse of the head is 'late' but the causative necrosis is early. Although later displacement of a head which remained viable or was revascularized after the original fracture can cause necrosis, it is a relatively infrequent occurrence and usually occurs several months before collapse begins.

Examination of femoral heads which have begun to collapse or have fragmented reveals that the affected heads are almost invariably only partially necrotic and that it is the superior part of the bone of the head which is dead (Fig. 5.1). Usually the dead bone represents a residue which has failed to revascularize, a phenomenon previously mentioned. An interesting aspect of this frustrated repair process is that it is commonly accompanied by an excessive deposition of bone in the front edge of the repair tissue (Fig. 5.5). It is not clear why this occurs. Perhaps it is analogous to the ossification which occurs around unresorbed dead tissue or blood clot in soft tissues or perhaps it is a response to forces transmitted through the dead tissue when the patient becomes mobile.

It is important because it is often the first radiographic clue to incomplete revascularization and the possibility of collapse, and because fracture of trabeculae often occurs in the dead tissue adjacent to the sclerotic zone. Once disintegration of the bone has begun it continues fairly quickly, usually through necrotic tissue and generally close to the interface between living and dead tissue. The process leads to the separation of a saucer or conical-shaped area of bone, the rim or base of which is in the subchondral plate. Loss of structural con-

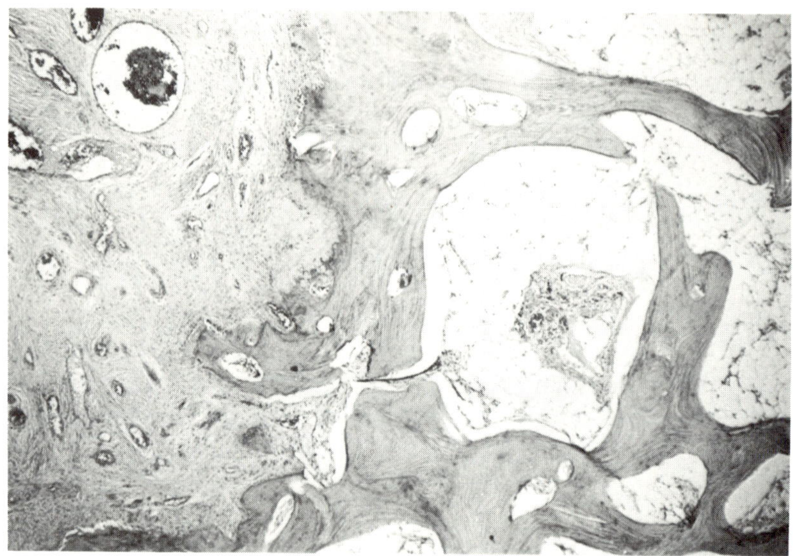

FIG. 5.5 Avascular necrosis with arrested repair. Resorption of dead bone and fibrous replacement have occurred in part of the necrotic bone. Bone has been deposited at the interface between the scar tissue and the dead marrow to form a sclerotic plate. In this femoral head separation of the necrotic fragment had occurred through the necrotic tissue.

tinuity allows the superior articular surface to collapse, at first during weight-bearing and eventually permanently. Furthermore, the articular cartilage is torn near the edge of necrotic bone which then becomes completely loose. The segment of bone and the covering cartilage may then fragment with liberation of the pieces into the synovial cavity.

If the femoral head is not removed at this stage, continued use of the joint will lead to fibrillation and erosion of the surviving cartilage (Fig. 5.6). There are occasions when the articular cartilage is damaged at the time of fracture but they are relatively infrequent. By far the greatest proportion of necrotic heads which are still complete have an intact covering of viable articular cartilage.

The proportion of united, partly necrotic femoral heads which eventually disintegrate is not known and cannot be until the existence of partial necrosis can be reliably identified. Whilst, therefore, the suggestion that weight-bearing is a crucial factor in late collapse (Sherman and Phemister, 1947) is a reasonable one, as is the principle that careful re-alignment of the fracture fragments and of the femoral head within the hip joint will reduce the incidence of late collapse

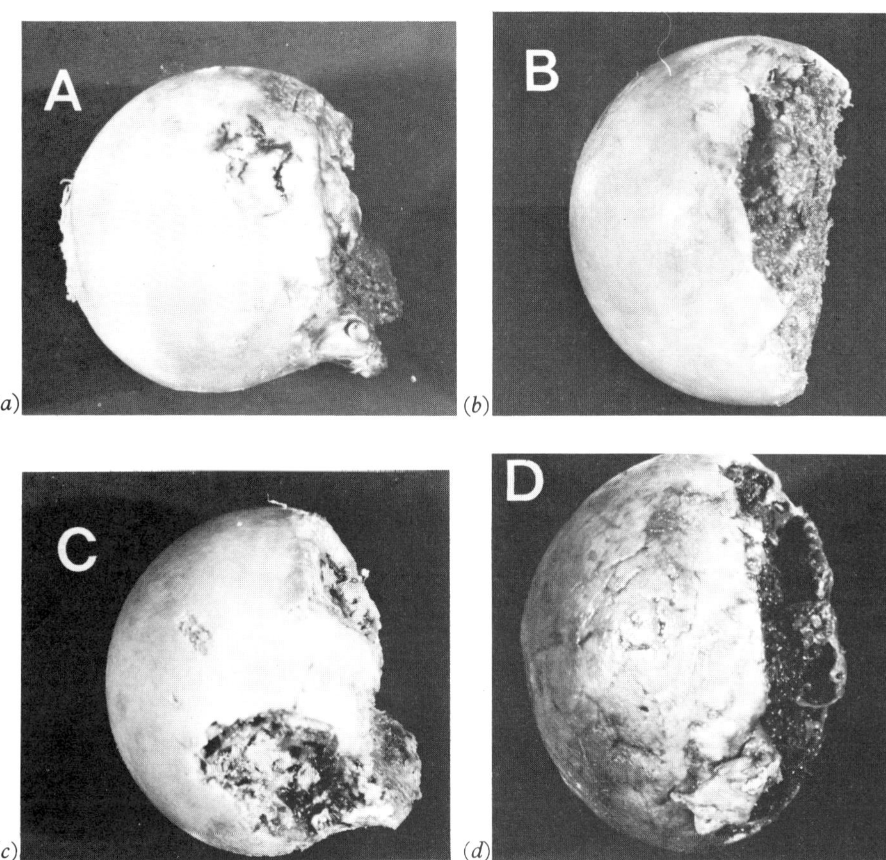

FIG. 5.6 Femoral heads removed at operation. (*a*) Two days after subcapital fracture, damage to the femoral head on its superior aspect; (*b*) femoral head removed 7 days after injury, there is some loss of the normal glistening appearance of the hyaline cartilage; (*c*) an osteochondral fragment has been detached from the inferior aspect of the head; (*d*) 4 weeks after injury, the femoral head shows degeneration in the cartilage and early collapse of the head.

(Garden, 1971), objective evidence in support of these ideas is still required.

The above account has focused solely on the post-traumatic avascular necrosis as it occurs in the adult because it is found much more commonly in this age group and has therefore been studied more extensively than the equivalent condition in childhood.

Lam (1971) records an incidence of 17% avascular necrosis in a series of 75 cases of fracture of the femoral neck in children. Evidence regarding the relative importance of each blood vessel to the capital epiphysis is incomplete but the available information indicates that it is difficult to render a capital epiphysis ischaemic. It is also clear from observations on the natural history and histology of Perthes disease that an avascular and deformed secondary centre of ossification is often revascularized and structurally restored to a conditon very little different from normal. The articular cartilage of a child has much better regenerative potential than that of the adult and degenerative arthritis is a rare condition in childhood.

If good alignment and stability of the fracture fragments can be achieved there should be a low incidence of late and cirppling consequences following post-traumatic avascular necrosis in childhood. There is, however, a need for a long-term observation of these patients. There is very little information about the incidence and age of onset of degenerative arthritis in adults after femoral neck fracture in childhood, and without such data it is not possible to assess the relative merits of different forms of management.

PATHOLOGICAL FRACTURE

A pathological fracture is one which occurs through a bone of abnormal composition and in the absence of a major injury. The abnormality may be primarily in the marrow or surrounding soft tissue or primarily in the internal structure of the bone tissue. The latter group includes the 'metabolic' bone diseases, some of the developmental abnormalities and Paget's disease, which are discussed in Chapter 4.

Here we are concerned with those diseases which affect the periosteal and endosteal soft tissues first and produce a gross structural change in the bone. A list of the conditions which may be complicated by pathological fracture includes the following:

1. Congenital or development diseases
   (a) Fibrous dysplasia
   (b) Gaucher's disease
   (c) Neurofibromatosis
2. Infections
3. Tumour-like conditions
   (a) Simple bone cyst
   (b) Aneurysmal bone cyst
   (c) Enchondroma
   (d) Benign chondroblastoma
   (e) Angioma

4. Primary and metastatic tumours of bone
   (a) Osteosarcoma
   (b) Chondrosarcoma
   (c) Giant cell tumour
   (d) Fibrosarcoma
   (e) Angiosarcoma
   (f) Myeloma
   (g) Malignant lymphoma
   (h) Osteolytic metastases of carcinoma in adults and neuroblastoma in children
5. Post-irradiation necrosis

A complete exposition of each of these conditions would be inappropriate but there are aspects which are of particular importance in the context of fracture of the femoral neck and these are outlined below.

FIBROUS DYSPLASIA (Jaffe, 1958; p. 119)

This disorder is usually first manifest in childhood and may be monostotic or polyostotic in distribution. Femoral lesions and specifically lesions in the femoral neck occur in both varieties, and present real and difficult problems of both diagnosis and management. Most lesions are composed of fibrous tissue in which irregular bone trabeculae are deposited (Fig. 5.7). These present no serious problem in histological

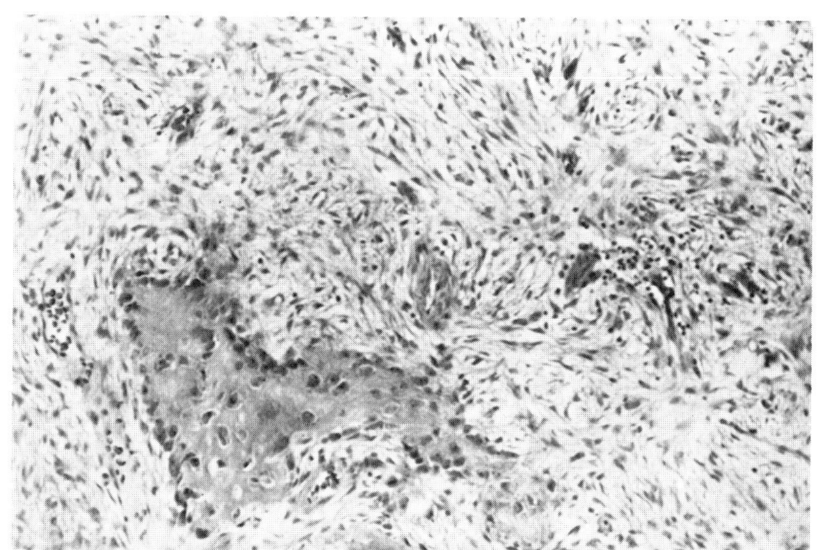

FIG. 5.7 Fibrous dysplasia; an isolated trabecula of immature bone forming in an area of well differentiated moderately cellular fibrous tissue.

interpretation and are often sufficiently diffuse and ossified to produce a distinctive radiographic change. The difficulties of histological diagnosis arise if there is little osseous differentiation and the predominantly fibrous lesion breaks down and becomes cystic or if the lesion changes in character and becomes neoplastic. If the former occurs, the lesion may be regarded as a simple bone cyst and if the latter the change may not affect the lesion uniformly and might be missed. Fortunately sarcomatous change in fibrous dysplasia usually occurs in adult life and one should therefore take special care with adult patients to obtain adequate tissue for histological examination and ensure that all the tissue is studied microscopically.

Benign lesions of fibrous dysplasia usually enlarge only whilst the skeleton is immature, but continued enlargement and the development of symptoms for the first time in adult life is not an absolute indication of sarcomatous change. The local growth potential of a lesion of fibrous dysplasia is highly variable and the extent of involvement of the femoral neck when fracture occurs is equally varied. Treatment should be aimed at complete excision to prevent further growth and repeated fractures. When the lesion involves the femoral shaft in addition to the neck such an aim cannot be realized. Such patients commonly suffer several fractures in childhood which unite but lead to an increasing deformity, characteristically resembling a shepherd's crook. Sarcoma arising from fibrous dysplasia is either a fibrosarcoma or an osteosarcoma and should be treated accordingly.

GAUCHER'S DISEASE

This is an uncommon condition and not all affected individuals have skeletal problems due to this disease. When the skeleton is sufficiently affected to produce symptoms the upper femur is commonly involved (Amstutz and Carey, 1966). Changes in the bone are secondary to an infiltration of the marrow by cells packed with lipids–Gaucher cells. The gross structure of the bone may be changed by expansion and thinning of the cortex and the internal structure by necrosis of bone. Both changes may contribute to the abnormal fragility and necrosis will delay or prevent fracture repair.

There is no specific treatment for the primary condition and management of the fracture is dictated by the severity of bone involvement.

NEUROFIBROMATOSIS (Harkin and Reed, 1969; p. 88)

Abnormalities of skeletal growth which occur in patients with neurofibromatosis can occur in any bone. The femur generally and the femoral neck in particular appears to fracture extremely rarely as a consequence of any abnormality. The histological appearances of the abnormal bone are non-specific and the diagnosis is dependant upon the clinical and radiograph features. Should non-union or fibrous union follow the fracture, the tissue forming around and between the fracture ends is remarkable for the absence of bony differentiation.

INFECTIONS

These are uncommon causes of pathological fracture of the femoral neck. Bacteriological examination of tissue from the fracture site is essential if an infective process is suspected, not only to identify the causative organism but more importantly, to select the appropriate antibacterial treatment.

SIMPLE BONE CYST (Jaffe, 1958; p. 64)

The femoral neck is in second place in order of frequency of distribution of these lesions and pathological fracture is the most common presenting feature. Although some fractures heal satisfactorily with conservative management the danger of recurrent fracture remains until the cyst is either removed or regresses spontaneously. Cysts occasionally disappear after the first fracture and usually stop enlarging as skeletal growth nears completion, but larger lesions in young children require surgical treatment if repeated fracture and disability are to be avoided. Tissue removed from these lesions after fracture will sometimes include reparative tissue which may be highly cellular or possibly of unusual appearance (Fig. 5.8).

ANEURYSMAL BONE CYST (Jaffe, 1958; p. 56)

The important characteristic of this lesion as regards biopsy and curettage is the tendency to severe haemorrhage and appropriate provision should be made to deal with that problem before operation is begun. Fracture healing following curettage and internal fixation may occur

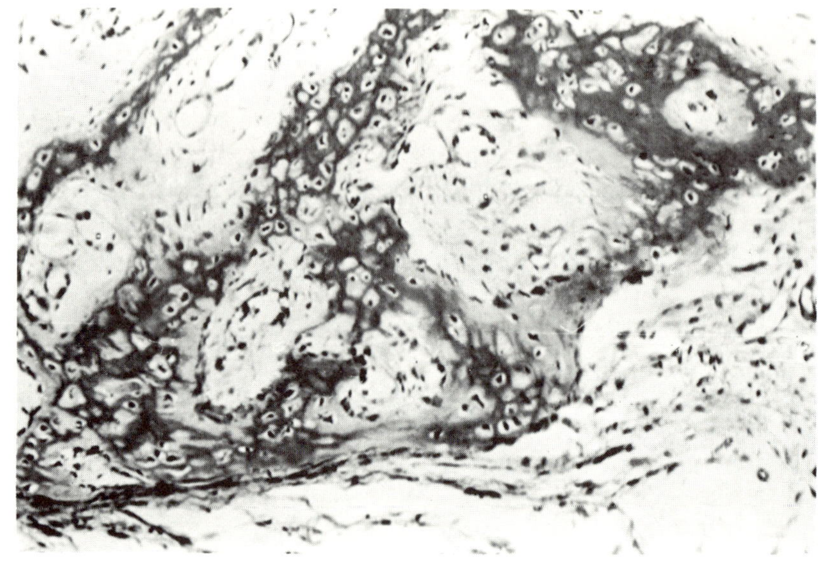

FIG. 5.8 Simple bone cyst 'callus' forming in cyst wall after fracture.

and the cyst re-ossify, or the cyst may recur after the fracture has united and lead to further fracture. There are no radiographic or histological appearances which enable one to predict the pattern of events.

ENCHONDROMA

An unusual cause of pathological fracture of the femoral neck and only to be considered as a possible cause in children.

BENIGN CHONDROBLASTOMA

Strictly speaking this lesion never leads to fracture of the femoral neck, but may cause collapse of the femoral head. The difficulties of histological diagnosis and possible confusion with a giant cell tumour or a malignant chondroblastic tumour have been reported (Jaffe, 1958; p. 52).

ANGIOMA

Lymphangiomatous lesions of bone are very rare in any part of the skeleton. Focal haemangioma producing an osteolytic defect large enough to cause fracture of the femoral neck is also rare. The condition of 'massive osteolysis' ('vanishing bone disease') may be a form of diffuse haemangiomatosis.

Extensive resorption of bone and the involvement of other bones in the same quadrant may be evident at the time of fracture or develop subsequently. The unpredictable natural history of the condition makes management difficult and the outcome uncertain. Lower limb lesions seldom spread to involve structures essential to life, but the frequent occurrence of fracture has been terminated in some patients only by disarticulation of the femur.

OSTEOSARCOMA (Jaffe, 1958; p. 256)

The femoral neck is one of the few sites where 'idiopathic' osteosarcoma and sarcoma secondary to Paget's disease or fibrous dysplasia all occur. The regime of treatment initiated is a matter of choice since the prognosis for patients with osteosarcoma in this site is no different to the general prognosis of the disease.

CHONDROSARCOMA (Jaffe, 1958; p. 314)

Malignant cartilage forming tumours of the femoral neck are not rare and pathological fracture is a common presentation of these lesions. The apparent size of the lesion may tempt the surgeon to try local excision and prosthetic replacement as a curative procedure. Intra- and extra-osseous infiltration of the tumour is usually impossible to delineate by radiographic techniques and by naked eye inspection at operation and local excision is often followed by 'recurrence'. The treatment most likely to effect cure is hind-quarter amputation.

GIANT CELL TUMOUR (Jaffe, 1958; p. 18)

As in the case of benign chondroblastoma, collapse of the femoral head is a more accurate description of the complication of giant cell tumour. The abnormal tissue commonly extends to and replaces the subchondral bone. If this has occurred and the prospect of joint disintegration is clear, resection of the lesion is indicated. A similar policy might have to be adopted if the size of the lesion does not allow secure internal fixation of the proximal fragment of the fracture.

Lesions which display unequivocal histological evidence of malignancy or have infiltrated the extra-osseous soft tissues are uncommon and have to be treated as other potentially metastasizing tumours.

FIBROSARCOMA (Jaffe, 1958; p. 304)

Fibrosarcoma in the upper end of the femur and femoral neck is not rare and may present difficulties. Diagnostic problems are due to the facts that the condition occurs in children and adults of all ages, has no distinctive radiographic features and may show great differences in cellular maturity and differentiation in different areas of one lesion. Small biopsy samples may not provide unequivocal evidence of malignancy and the diagnosis may remain in doubt until further growth of the lesion indicates the true state of affairs.

The limits of infiltration of fibrosarcoma are sometimes impossible to define and local resection is consequently an unsatisfactory method of treatment. Therapeutic irradiation may effectively destroy tumour tissue, but this is often at the expense of satisfactory union of the fracture. Radical excision which means hind-quarter amputation or disarticulation at the hip is required eventually in the majority of cases.

ANGIOSARCOMA (Jaffe, 1958; p. 341)

Malignant vascular tumours of bone are rare. They do not lead to any distinctive radiographic changes in bone and histological evidence is required to establish the diagnosis. The principles of management of intra-osseous sarcoma are applicable to this lesion.

MYELOMA

Although a relatively common form of primary intra-osseous malignant lesion, instances of large lesions leading to fracture of the femoral neck are infrequent (W.H.O. *Histological typing of Bone Tumours* Fig. 91A). The clinical and radiographic presentation may be indistinguishable from that of metastatic carcinoma. Apart from histological evidence, biochemical evidence of abnormal proteins in serum and urine will help to establish the diagnosis.

If the lesion appears to be solitary by virtue of there being no other osteolytic lesions detectable by radiography and no generalized marrow infiltration as judged by marrow aspirate examination, surgical ablation of the lesion might be considered as a curative procedure. Generalized disease leaves few alternatives to treatment which aims at stabilizing the fracture as well as possible and trying to eradicate the disease by a combined radio- and chemotherapeutic attack.

MALIGNANT LYMPHOMA (Jaffe, 1958; p. 402)

This term is used to cover lymphosarcoma, Hodgkins disease and reticulum cell sarcoma, all of which can occur as apparently primary tumours in bone and may destroy the femoral neck. The main problem of diagnosis is to differentiate reticulum cell sarcoma from other malignant lesions which are in a poorly differentiated state and from a Ewings tumour. In some patients no clear distinction will be made.

Malignant lymphoma occurs in all age groups, whereas Ewings tumour and metastatic tumours are unusual in the teens and early adult life.

Treatment of the primary condition is by irradiation and chemotherapy and the surgical contribution is towards stabilization of the fracture.

METASTATIC CARCINOMA AND NEUROBLASTOMA

Carcinomatous infiltration will probably be the most common localized disease process causing pathological fracture in adults encountered in orthopaedic practice. Those metastases which produce a net bone loss will be the most frequent offenders although, theoretically, any carcinoma may be responsible. In fact, one usually finds that the breast, bronchus or kidney are the site of the primary. The microscopic features are often sufficient to provide the correct suggestion as to the primary site, but poorly differentiated lesions may only be identified by systematic examination of all the possible sites of origin and sometimes only the later development of signs or symptoms will disclose the true state of affairs.

Metastatic neuroblastoma which, with occasional exception, affects preteenagers, presents a special problem because of the concept of 'Ewings tumour'. In spite of claims that Ewings tumour cells can be identified by special staining (Schajowicz, 1959) there is still no absolute method of distinguishing every case and the doubts expressed by Willis (1973) that metastatic neuroblastoma may not always be diagnosed for lack of complete and careful study are well grounded.

This lack of precision means that treatment cannot be organized on a rational basis since what might be reasonable in the case of primary tumours may be nonsensical if the tumour is a metastasis. The best compromise in this situation is to treat the local condition by irradiation whilst maintaining a watch for the appearance of other metastases. If the local lesion remains the only evidence of disease for an arbitary period, say six months, the advisability of surgical treatment can then be reconsidered in the light of the condition of the femur and the hip joint at that time.

IRRADIATION NECROSIS

Irradiation damage to the femoral head may result from treatment to an intra-osseous lesion or follow the intrapelvic implantation of radioactive substances. When this complication causes symptoms, it is usually because the femoral head has begun to collapse or fragment, but very occasionally a transcervical fracture will occur through necrotic tissue.

In the example of this condition which the author has seen, the bone trabeculae showed a variable loss of osteocyte nuclei and the marrow a variable degree of fibrous replacement; changes similar to those depicted in Fig. 5.4.

REFERENCES

AMSTUTZ, H.C. and CAREY, E.J. (1966). *J. Bone Jt. Surg.* **48A**, 670.
BOYD, H.B. and CALANDRUCCIO, R.A. (1963). *J. Bone Jt. Surg.* **45A**, 445.
CATTO, M. (1965*a*). *J. Bone Jt. Surg.* **47B**, 749.
CATTO, M. (1965*b*). *J. Bone Jt. Surg.* **47B**, 777.
GARDEN, R.S. (1961). *J. Bone Jt. Surg.* **43B**, 647.
GARDEN, R.S. (1971). *J. Bone Jt. Surg.* **53B**, 183.
GORHAM, L.W. and STOUT, A.P. (1955). *J. Bone Jt. Surg.* **37A**, 985.
GREEN, J.T. (1960). *Inst. Course. A.A.O.S.* **17**, 94.
HARKIN, J.C. and REED, R.J. (1969). *Tumours of the Peripheral Nervous System.* Armed Forces Institute of Pathology, Washington, D.C.
HARRISON, M.H.M. (1962). *J. Bone Jt. Surg.* **44B**, 858.
HODGES, P.C. (1954). *Am. J. Roentg.* **71**, 925.
JAFFE, H.L. (1958). *Tumours and tumorous conditions of the Bones and Joints.* Henry Kimpton, London.
LAM, S.F. (1971). *J. Bone Jt. Surg.* **53A**, 1165.
MCGINNIS, A.E. *et al.* (1958). *Missouri Med.* **55**, 31.
MCLEAN, F.C. and URIST, M.R. (1953). *Am. J. Surg.* **85**, 444.
NELSON, C.L. and HAYNES, D.W. (1970). *Calc. Tiss. Res.* **6**, 260.

PHEMISTER, D.B. (1947). *J. Bone Jt. Surg.* **29**, 946.
PRICE, E.R. (1962). *J. Bone Jt. Surg.* **44B**, 854.
SCHAJOWICZ, F. (1959). *J. Bone Jt. Surg.* **41A**, 349.
SEVITT, S. (1964). *J. Bone Jt. Surg.* **46B**, 270.
SEVITT, S. and THOMPSON, R.G. (1965). *J. Bone Jt. Surg.* **47B**, 560.
SHERMAN, M.S. and PHEMISTER, D.B. (1947). *J. Bone Jt. Surg.* **29**, 19.
TRUETA, J. and HARRISON, M.H.M. (1953). *J. Bone Jt. Surg.* **35B**, 442.
WILLIS, R.A. (1973). *The Spread of Tumours in the Human Body*. 3rd Edn., Butterworths, London, p. 248.
WOODHOUSE, C.E. (1962). *Surg.* **52**, 55.

Chapter Six

FRACTURES OF THE FEMORAL NECK–CHILDREN

J. Cockin

Incidence ~ Types of fracture ~ Clinical presentation ~ Treatment ~ Complications ~ Results

Fractures of the femoral neck in children are rare injuries. The first recorded case was in 1885 (Cromwell) of a fracture in a child and in 1899 Russell reported two cases and suggested that they were apparently rare because they were mistaken for other diseases such as tuberculosis. This mistake is easily understood when one remembers the high proportion and severity of the complications following this fracture and the all too common end point of a grossly damaged hip.

The fracture of the femoral neck in the child is totally different from that in the adult. The forces involved, the prognosis and methods of treatment are all entirely different.

INCIDENCE

The true incidence of this fracture is difficult to determine since most of the reported series in the literature have been obtained by the collection of cases from many centres. Ratliff (1962) quoted a comparable incidence, comparing the fractures of the hips seen in the adult to those in the child, as being 130 : 1. In his series of 70 fractures occurring under the age of 17 years, there was a peak incidence at the age of 11–12.

Our experience at the Accident Service in Oxford demonstrates a similar incidence. In the period 1969–1973 there were six femoral neck fractures in children. The adult : child femoral neck fracture

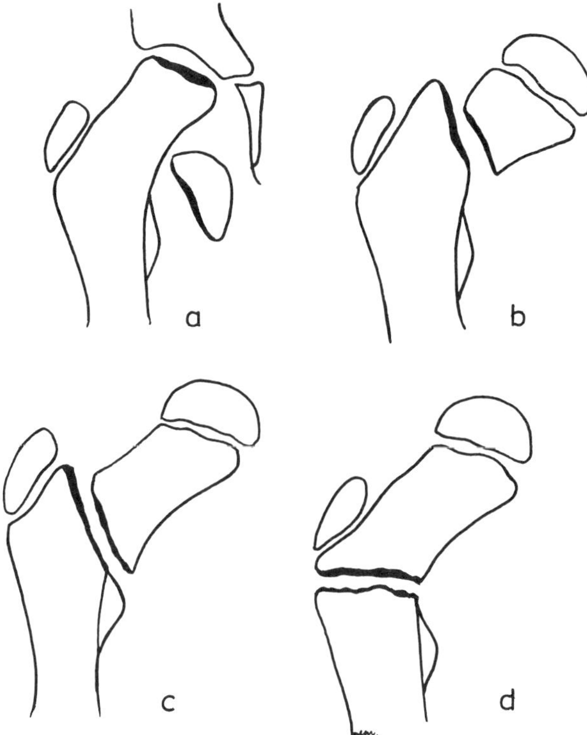

FIG. 6.1 Classification of femoral neck fractures in children (after Ratliff, 1962). (*a*) Trans-epiphyseal; (*b*) trans-cervical; (*c*) basal; (*d*) pertrochanteric.

ratio was 139: 1. These fractures in children comprised 0.03% of all admissions and 0.004% of all new Accident attendances.

TYPES OF FRACTURE

Various classifications have been described based on the anatomical level of the fracture and of the degree of displacement. A very acceptable classification is that described by Ratliff (1962) and it agrees very closely with that used by Colonna in 1929.

TRANS-EPIPHYSEAL FRACTURES (Fig. 6.1*a*)

Ratliff (1962) reported two fractures out of a total of 70 in this group. In 1973 Ratliff reported nine cases of this type. These fractures are all produced by very severe violence. They are accompanied by gross displacement and premature fusion of the upper femoral epiphyseal plate is common.

TRANS-CERVICAL FRACTURES (Fig. 6.1*b*)

This group was the commonest one in Ratliff's (1962) series with 38 out of 70 fractures. 50% of this type go on to produce avascular necrosis of the capital epiphysis.

BASAL FRACTURES (Fig. 6.1*c*)

This group was the second most common; there being 26 out of 70. They develop less incidence of avascular necrosis than the overall group, avascular necrosis occurring in 25% of basal fractures as compared with 42% of the total group and as compared to a little over 50% for the trans-cervical group (Ratliff, 1962).

PERTROCHANTERIC FRACTURES (Fig. 6.1*d*)

This is a relatively uncommon group with only 4 out of 70 fractures in Ratliff's series. It is, however, important to recognize the difference in this fracture when it occurs in childhood from when it occurs in adults. McDougall (1961) pointed out that avascular necrosis of the capital epiphysis in children occurred in trochanteric fractures and basal fractures as well as cervical ones. In adults this is an extremely uncommon occurrence following a trochanteric fracture.

CLINICAL PRESENTATION

A common feature of fractures of the femoral neck in children is the severe degree of violence which is necessary to produce the fracture. It has been stressed by all authors writing on the subject and in Ratliff's (1962) series of 70 fractures, 54 had been sustained by severe violence. In view of this fact it is not surprising that a number of these fractures occur in children as part of multiple injuries, and fractures of the pelvis associated with this fracture are not uncommon. This makes the diagnosis and treatment more difficult. Fardon (1970) reported a patient with a fracture of the femoral neck and a fracture of the shaft of the femur on the same side.

The history, therefore, is of a fall from a height or a road traffic accident; the common feature being severe violence to the leg and pelvis area. This presentation should be compared with the clinical presentation of the majority of adult femoral neck fractures where the degree of violence is minimal and where the fracture is basically a pathological fracture predisposed to by osteoporosis, osteomalacia or metastatic bone deposits.

The clinical presentation of the limb, however, is similar to that in the adult with true shortening of the leg which lies in an adducted, externally rotated position. X-rays confirm the fracture of the hip and it is essential to obtain lateral pictures in order to determine the degree of displacement accurately.

TREATMENT

The principles of fracture treatment are the same in this fracture as any other: being that of achieving a reduction of the fracture and maintaining reduction until the fracture is united. Treatment is frequently complicated by a fracture of the pelvis which may have associated visceral injuries which will make the treatment of the fractures difficult. Associated fractures of the pelvis or fractures of the femoral shaft can also complicate management.

The serious problems and complications of this fracture are non-union and avascular necrosis of the femoral head. Delayed union and deformity are common. Avascular necrosis is similarly common. Modern authors writing on this condition have found it useful to base their treatment on the degree of displacement at the fracture.

UNDISPLACED FRACTURES

Lam (1971) and Ratliff (1962) recommended a single hip spica for the undisplaced fracture (Fig. 6.2); the spica being retained for 6–12 weeks. It is important to verify the position of the fragments by check X-ray after 1 or 2 weeks to see that no displacement has occurred. However, too frequent X-ray examination is to be avoided in children.

DISPLACED FRACTURES

Lam (1971) recommended a closed manipulation and reduction under anaesthetic followed by internal fixation using multiple Moore's pins.

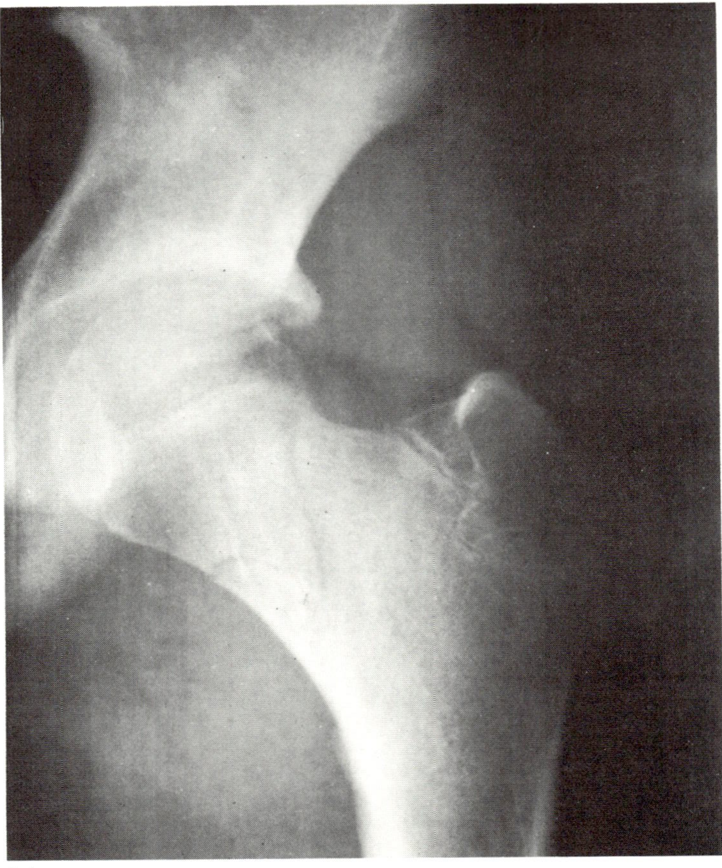

(*a*)

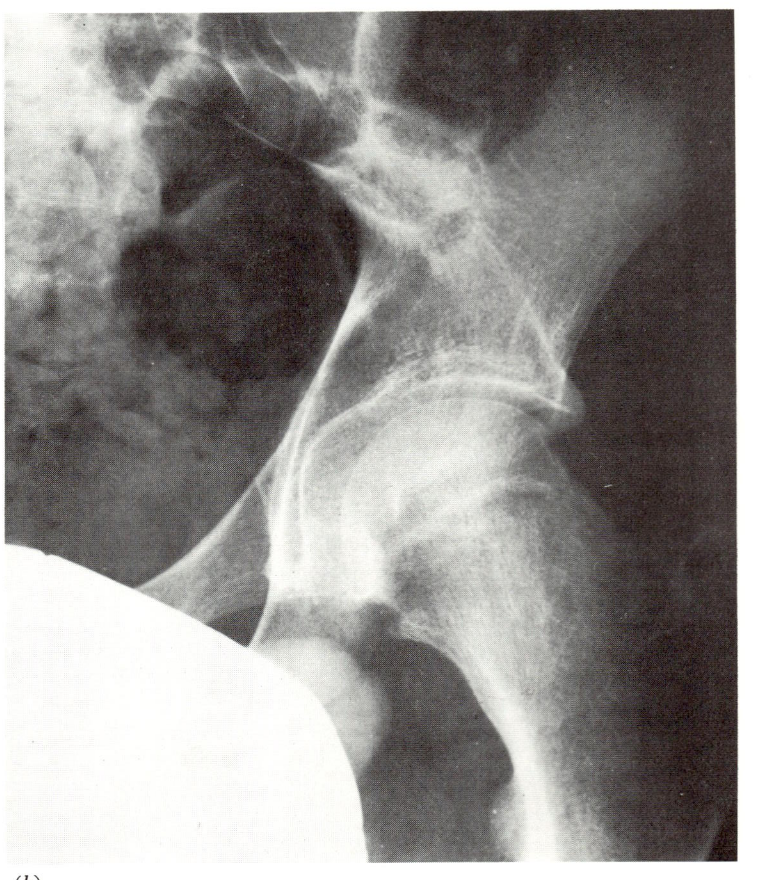

(*b*)

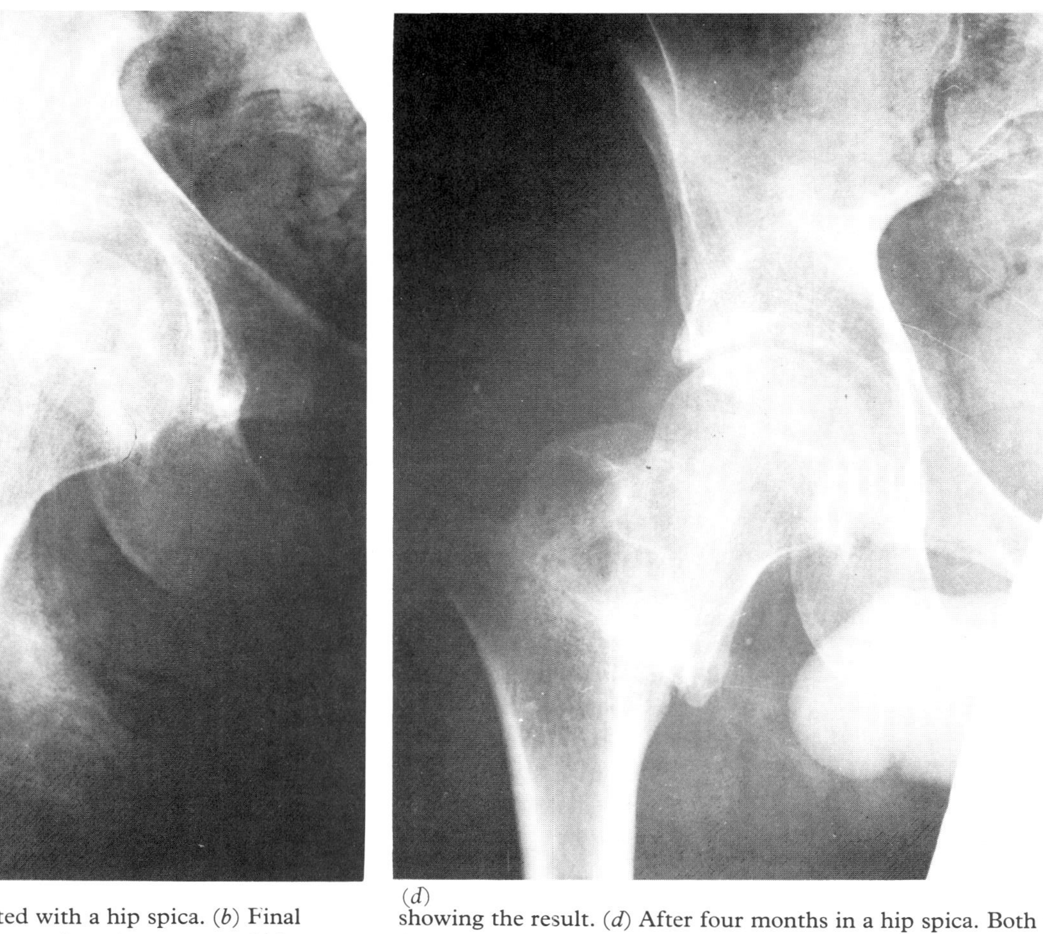

(*c*) (*d*)

FIG. 6.2 (*a*) Type B fracture treated with a hip spica. (*b*) Final result one year later. (*c*) Type C fracture in a sixteen year-old boy showing the result. (*d*) After four months in a hip spica. Both were fractures with minimal displacement and the end-results were excellent.

Ratliff (1962) did not favour a manipulation and plaster hip spica since of 19 patients treated this way 15 were unreduced or had displaced following the initial reduction.

Of the ones manipulated and treated by internal fixation less than 50% had a good result. Ratliff further reported the results of a primary subtrochanteric osteotomy on the displaced group and although the series was small with only four patients treated this way, they were all good results.

Based on this Ratliff suggested that the treatment of the displaced fracture occurring under the age of ten years should be by a primary displacement osteotomy. In the patient over ten years a manipulation and reduction under anaesthetic should be attempted and if the reduction is successful then the fracture should be internally fixed. If the manipulation is unsuccessful in achieving a reduction then a primary osteotomy should be carried out.

McDougall (1961) stressed the importance of keeping the patient non-weight-bearing for at least twelve months. He pointed out that there was a degree of plasticity at the fracture site which persisted for a long time, even after apparent union of the fracture. This led on to the problem of resultant deformity of the femur with shortening occurring due to coxa vara. He further stressed the importance of using Moore's pins or Knowle's pins rather than a Smith-Petersen trifin nail. Bone density in the child is considerable and having achieved a reduction it is almost impossible to insert a Smith-Petersen nail without redisplacing the fracture or without producing distraction at the fracture site when using a large trifin nail.

COMPLICATIONS

The incidence of complications from this particular fracture are extremely high. This fact has been stressed by all writers and is well recognized by anyone dealing with this problem. As in the adult these problems are related to the anatomical and physiological considerations affecting the blood supply to the femoral head and neck.

Trueta (1957) described the blood supply to the femoral head and neck at different ages and in particular he stressed the vulnerability of the capital epiphysis and diaphysis of the neck of the femur between the ages of four and eight. At this age the capital epiphysis derives its blood supply almost entirely through the lateral epiphyseal group of vessels with very minor contributions via the ligamentum teres and the medial epiphyseal group. It is seen therefore at this age that the femoral head is at great risk from avascular necrosis even more so than in the adult.

AVASCULAR NECROSIS

Avascular necrosis is the major problem in this fracture. McDougall (1961) pointed out that this complication occurred not only in transcervical fractures, but also could occur following basal and intertrochanteric fractures in children. Ratliff (1962) found that avascular necrosis occurred in 42% of the series. The majority of these followed transcervical fractures with 25% following basal fractures.

The radiological evidence of avascular necrosis occurred early and was usually visible within one year (Fig. 6.3). Avascular necrosis was

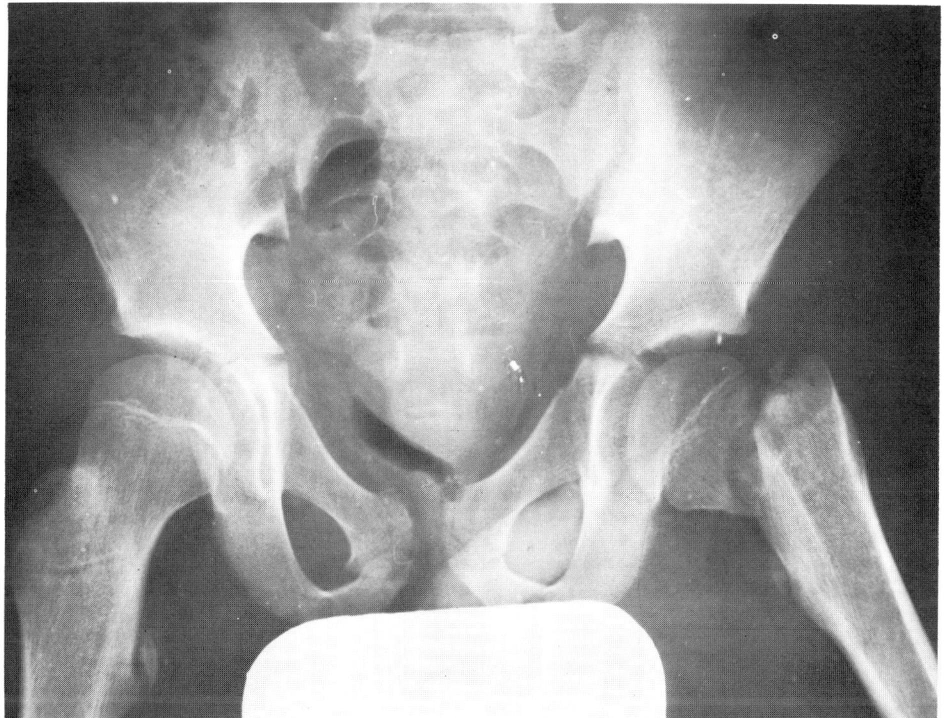

(*a*) FIG. 6.3 (*a*) Fractured femoral neck with displacement which was treated by reduction and attempted pinning; three months later (*b*) shows early avascular necrosis [more obvious in (*c*) 1 year later].

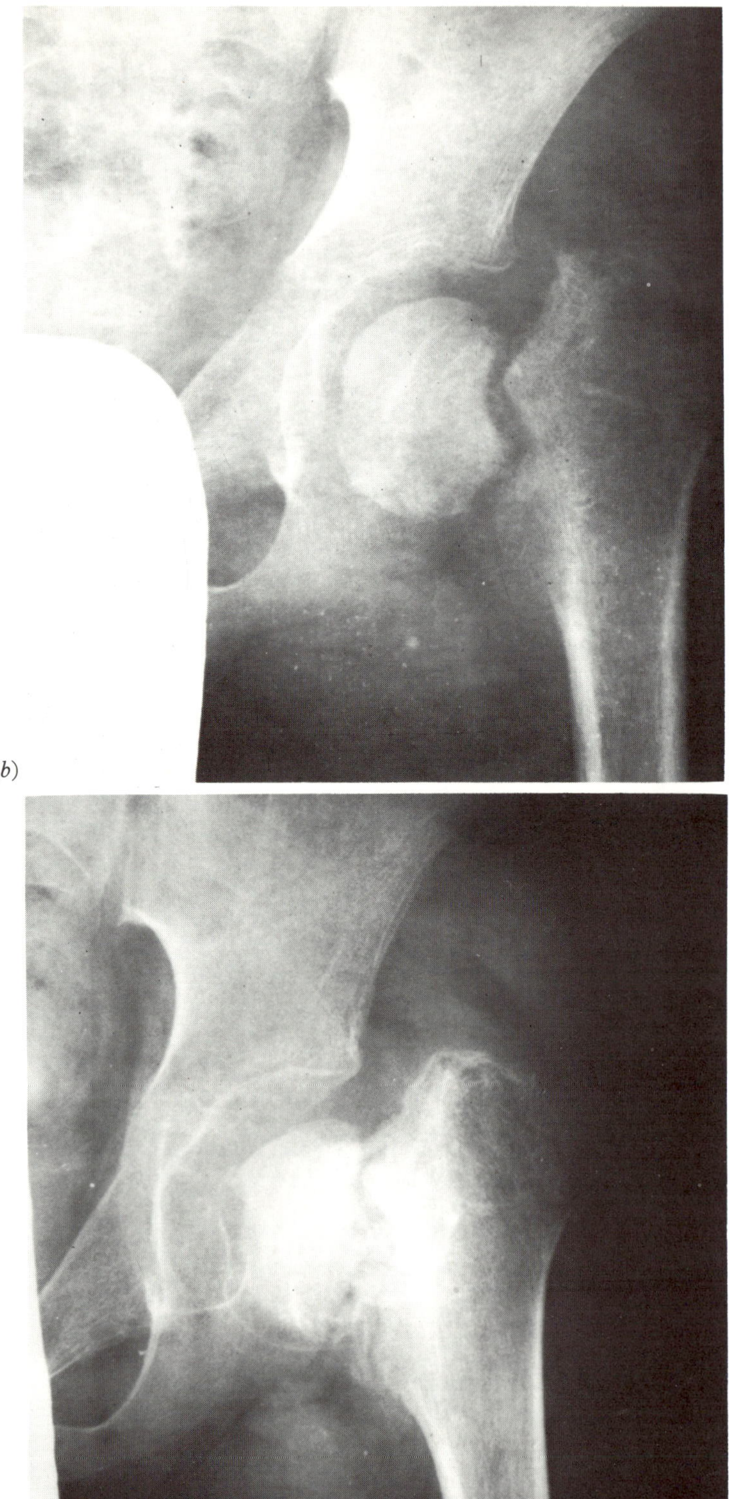

(b)

(c)

uncommon in the undisplaced fractures, but nevertheless it did occur in four out of thirteen cases.

Ratliff (1962) described three types of avascular necrosis. The commonest type involved the whole of the femoral head and neck down to the fracture site. This he called type I and related it to possible damage to the lateral epiphyseal group prior to its division. Type II involved a portion of the supero–lateral epiphysis and metaphysis. He correlated this with damage to the lateral epiphyseal group after its entry into bone (Fig. 6.4).

A smaller number were type III which involved the diaphysis of the bone down to the fracture site, but with sparing of the epiphysis. This later group occurred in children of eleven years or less and was not seen in older children. He correlated this with damage to the vessels actually at the fracture site in transcervical fractures and therefore the lateral epiphyseal group remained undamaged so that the epiphysis retained its blood supply.

Durbin (1959) described three cases of avascular necrosis complicating undisplaced fractures and suggested that the diaphyseal vessels of the femoral neck played an important role in the blood supply of the capital epiphysis. He deduced that this was the reason for avascular necrosis occurring following undisplaced fractures.

All authors have stressed the need for a guarded prognosis in these injuries as regards avascular necrosis.

DELAYED UNION

Delayed union has been defined by Ratliff (1962) as 'no visible sign of union on X-ray at five months'. He discovered 17 out of his 70 patients with delayed union and 7 out of 70 went on to a non-union This group were associated with difficult internal fixation and also with a closed reduction which had displaced.

PREMATURE FUSION OF THE UPPER FEMORAL EPIPHYSIS

This is extremely common following traumatic separation of the upper femoral epiphysis. It occurred in 8 out of 15 patients described by Ratliff (1973). Taking the group as a whole this occurred in some 10% of all femoral neck fractures, just over half occurring following avascular necrosis. In Lam's group 17% developed premature epiphyseal closure. This, of course, is one of the reasons for shortening following this fracture. The other major cause of shortening was due to coxa vara deformity.

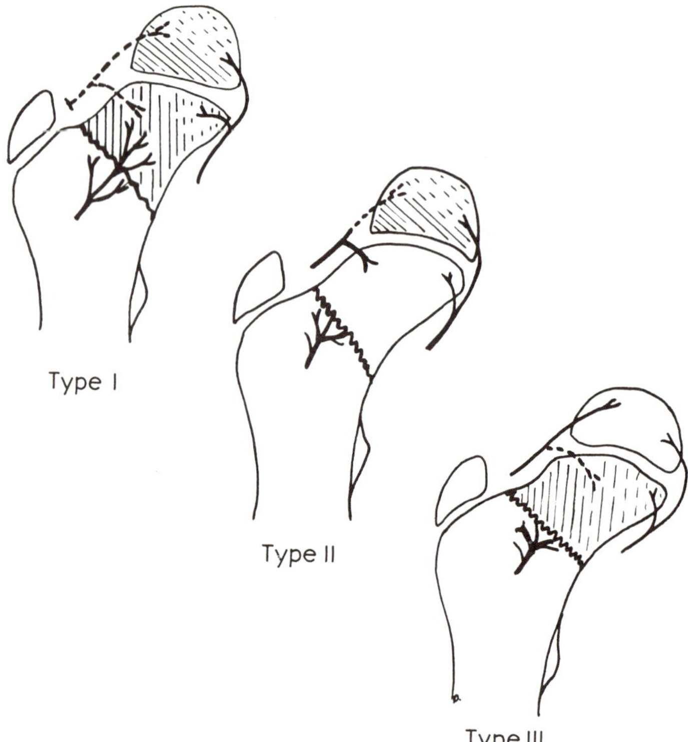

FIG. 6.4 Types of avascular necrosis. Type I shows injury to lateral epiphyseal group prior to division; type II shows damage as vessels enter the bone; type III shows damage at fracture site with sparing of the epiphysis.

DEFORMITY

Coxa vara is the major deformity following this fracture. This is a common complication and was felt in part to be due to a degree of plasticity at the fracture site which persisted for a considerable time and after the fracture has united. In Lam's (1971) series of 75 fractures this occurred in 32% and was a significant cause of shortening.

Blockey (1969) felt that some cases of infantile coxa vara were due to trauma in the newborn and felt that this was a possible cause of infantile coxa vara. He described four cases, two of which had occurred in injuries to children at birth, and all were the result of severe trauma.

RESULTS

It can be seen from the list of complications that the results in this type of fracture are depressing. The injuries are severe ones caused by severe trauma with a significant number of complications. Some of these problems being difficulties in achieving a reduction and then in maintaining it. Problems are associated with avascular necrosis, due to damage to the blood supply to the head and neck of the femur, and to delayed union. Following on this damage, premature closure of the upper femoral epiphysis occurs in some 15–17% and a coxa vara deformity occurs in approximately 33% of the cases as end results.

The results described by McDougall (1961) with 33% having normal hips, 50% having a bad result and 10% having good function, but complicated by avascular necrosis or coxa vara, is probably an average result with this type of fracture. Ratliff's suggested line of treatment is based on the analysis of results of different modes of treatment and appears to be the most logical plan of treatment. It may be that with the utilization of Ratliff's programme and with more use being made of primary osteotomy the future end results may be improved. Any one surgeon's experience of this type of fracture is inevitably bound to be small in view of its rarity and it is only by the careful collation of records to produce a sufficiently large series that advances will be achieved. This has been Ratliff's major contribution in the study of this particular type of fracture.

REFERENCES

BLOCKEY, N.J. (1969). *J. Bone Jt. Surg.* **51B**, 106.
CROMWELL, B.M. (1885). *North Carolina Med. J.* **15**, 309.
DURBIN, F.C. (1959). *J. Bone Jt. Surg.* **41B**, 758.
FARDON, D.F. (1970). *J. Bone Jt. Surg.* **52A**, 797.
LAM, S.F. (1971). *J. Bone Jt. Surg.* **53A**, 1165.
MCDOUGALL, A. (1961). *J. Bone Jt. Surg.* **43B**, 16.
RATLIFF, A.H.C. (1962). *J. Bone Jt. Surg.* **44B**, 528.
RATLIFF, A.H.C. (1973). *Proc. 12th Congress SICOT*, p. 869. *Pub. Exc. Med.* 1973.
TRUETA, J. (1957). *J. Bone Jt. Surg.* **39B**, 358.

Chapter Seven

DISLOCATION OF THE HIP AND ACETABULAR FRACTURES

J. Kenwright

Introduction ~ Classification of injuries ~ Mechanism of injury ~ Methods of diagnosis ~ Treatment and expected results ~ Complications and their management

INTRODUCTION

According to Brav (1962) dislocation of the hip comprises 5% of all traumatic joint dislocations. There are many patterns of injury with varying degrees of dislocation and fracture and one surgeon's experience in each type is usually limited. Therefore difficulty is often encountered when deciding upon the most effective treatment for each particular injury.

There are many excellent and extensive reviews of long term follow-ups in the literature but there still remains controversy concerning certain important issues. This applies particularly to:

(1) The most useful classification of the injuries.

(2) The best method of management of dislocations with fracture of the acetabulum and the place of surgical reduction in these types of injuries.

(3) The importance or not of the post-reduction care in relation to the development and progress of avascular necrosis of the head of the femur.

(4) The management of the dislocation presenting late.

(5) The management of unusual problems such as dislocations in children, combined injuries involving dislocation of the hip and fracture of the neck or shaft of the femur, and recurrent dislocation.

The following sections are written predominantly concentrating upon these controversial issues.

CLASSIFICATION OF INJURIES

The ideal system of classification should have the following features:

(1) Embrace most of the injuries seen in practice.

(2) Be simple and convey to others the nature of the injury.

(3) It should be easy to classify a patient early after injury from simple clinical and X-ray examination i.e. from information rapidly and conveniently available.

(4) Classification should be related to treatment and prognosis.

Many reviewers have concentrated upon either assessing the results of anterior or posterior dislocations (with or without fractures of the acetabulum) or upon fractures of the acetabular floor including central dislocation. There is a considerable overlap between these different groups and it is valuable to look at all groups together. The classification which has been used in many studies, and will be discussed here when comparing results of different forms of treatment, is that of Thompson and Epstein's (1951) method for posterior dislocations. In this classification dislocations are divided into five types;

Type 1. Without fracture or with no more than a minor fracture.

Type 2. With a large single fracture of the posterior acetabular rim.

Type 3. With a comminuted fracture of the posterior rim of the acetabulum.

Type 4. With a fracture of both the acetabular rim and the floor.

Type 5. With fracture of the femoral head with or without other fractures.

Many reviewers have used this classification or the one described by Brav (1962) for fractures which are predominantly associated with a posterior dislocation. These methods do not elaborate upon the acetabular floor component which is so important nor do they include central dislocation.

Rowe and Lowell (1961) classified injuries according to fracturing of the acetabulum into the following groups:

(1) Linear undisplaced fractures;

(2) Fractures of the posterior portion of the acetabulum;

(3) Inner wall fractures;

(4) Superior acetabular and bursting fractures.

They divided each group into sub-groups according to the severity of the injury. Judet *et al.* (1964) stressed the importance of the surgical anatomy of the acetabulum. Their study of 173 patients included 129 who were treated surgically and this classification was therefore devised

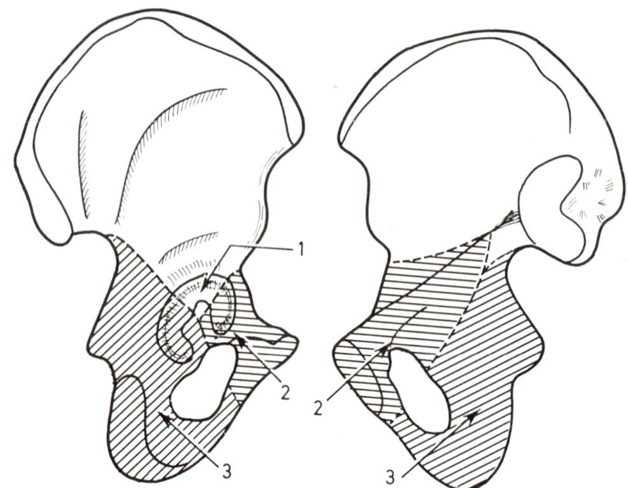

FIG. 7.1 Arch and two columns of the acetabulum are depicted. (1) roof; (2) ilio-pubic column; (3) ilio–ischial column. Medial (right) and lateral (left) aspects. (After Judet *et al.*, 1964.)

from both the radiographic evidence and the operative findings. It is a classification which enables more accurate assessment of the pattern of the acetabular fracture.

The acetabulum lies in the cavity of an arch formed by two columns of bone (Fig. 7.1). The posterior or ilio-ischial column is thick and strong and passes from the ischial tuberosity through the vertical portion of the ischium to that portion of the ilium immediately above the ischium. On its antero-lateral surface lies the posterior part of the articular surface of the acetabulum. The anterior or ilio-pubic column consists of the pubic bone and a short segment of the ilium extending up as far as the anterior inferior spine of the ilium. On the postero–lateral surface of this column is the anterior portion of the articular surface of the acetabulum. These two columns converge and meet in a thick and compact zone of bone which is always spared by fractures of the acetabulum, according to Judet. He describes the assessment of fractures from the radiographs taken in three standard projections and divides injuries into four elementary types:

(1) Fractures of the posterior lip of the acetabulum.
(2) Fractures of the ilio-ischial column.
(3) Transverse fractures.
(4) Fractures of the ilio-pubic column.

Each group is sub-divided into further groups but many injuries are complex and may even embrace several of the elementary groups. However, 111 of the 173 fractures Judet examined fell into one of the four basic groups and nearly all injuries could be embraced within the classification. Other excellent classifications have been described by Stewart and Milford (1954), Pearson and Hargadon (1962) and Eichenholtz and Stark (1964).

A modification has been presented here as a method of classification based upon three main types (A, B and C) easily recognizable on the initial radiograph (see Table 7.1). The sub-groups (Fig. 7.1) are really a combination of those of Judet *et al.* and of Thompson and Epstein. The acetabular roof and floor fractures are sub-divided according to the concept of the acetabulum being set within posterior and anterior columns and fractures involving primarily one of these. However, it is important to have a definite sub-group (Type C, 5) which includes fractures with displacement of the superior weight-bearing segment of the acetabulum (Fig. 7.2). It is in this group that most investigators have found poor results if accurate reduction is not obtained. Also with a fracture–dislocation an assessment must be made of the degree of displacement of the fragments, and of the head of the femur, as well as the degree of comminution of fragments. These additional factors are most important when considering surgical reduction.

TABLE 7.1 Classification of hip dislocations and fractures of the acetabulum.

Type A	Anterior dislocation
Type B	Posterior dislocation: (1) With no fracture or small fragment (2) With large, single, posterior acetabular rim fracture (3) With comminuted fracture of posterior rim
Type C	Dislocation with acetabular roof and/or floor fracture: (1) Posterior ilio-ischial column (2) Anterior ilio-pubic column (3) Transverse fracture (4) Combination of 1–3 (5) 1–3 plus fracture displacement of superior weight bearing segment of acetabulum (6) 1–5 with fracture of the head of femur
	Add to description: (1) Degree of displacement of fracture elements and of head of femur (2) Degree of comminution

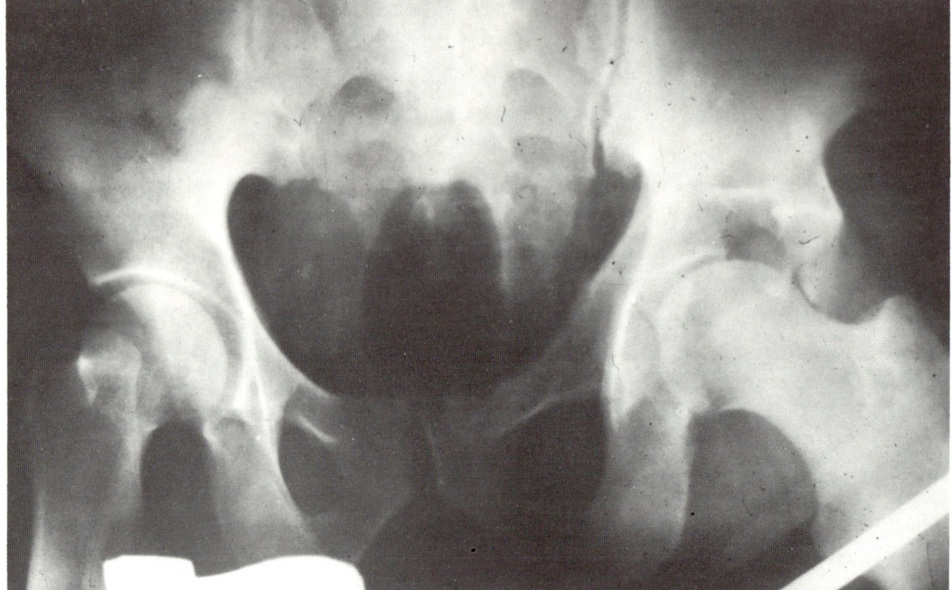

FIG. 7.2 A fracture of the superior weight-bearing segment of the acetabulum.

MECHANISM OF INJURY

The studies of Pearson and Hargadon (1962) and Hunter (1969) have shown that in civilian practice the major cause of hip fracture–dislocation is the road traffic accident. Studies on cadavers showed that acetabular floor fractures involving the anterior or posterior columns, with or without central dislocation, were almost always caused by a direct, violent, lateral force upon the trochanteric region. Of considerable interest in this study was their finding that fractures of linear type of the anterior column involving the inferior and superior pubic rami always entered the hip joint itself (Fig. 7.3). This was seen at dissection even although the acetabular fracturing could not be seen on radiographs.

Most other conclusions about the mechanism of injury have been inferred from the nature of the accident and the supposed line of acting force. It is supposed that anterior dislocation of the hip is caused by a force applied to the knee region with transference of an extension, abduction and lateral rotation force to the hip joint. Watson Jones (1955) describes posterior dislocation of the hip being caused by the

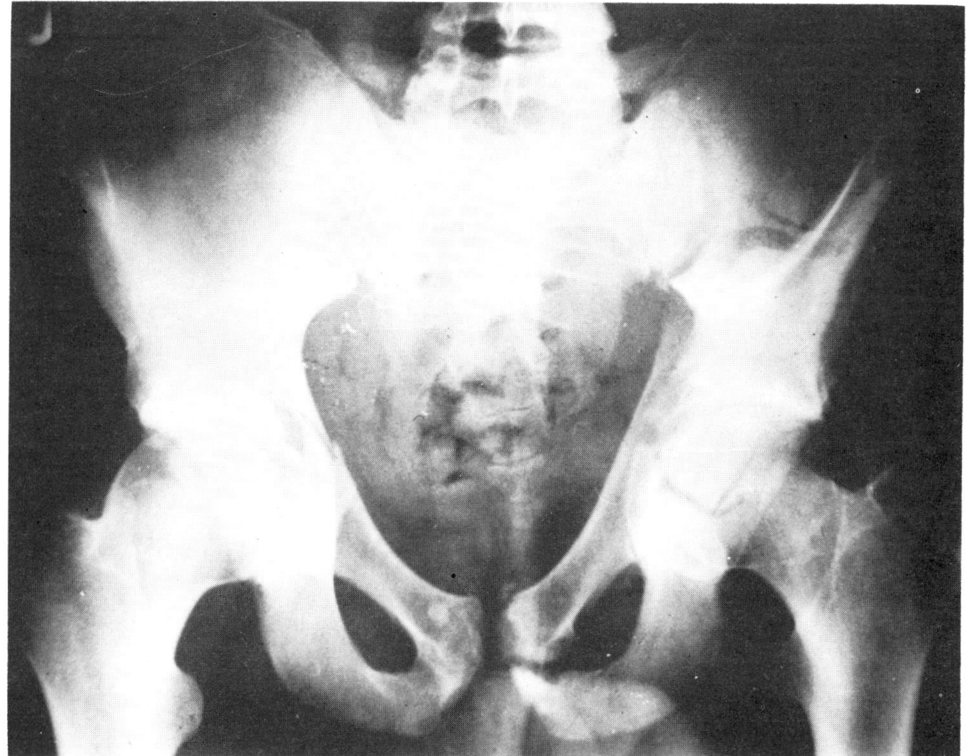

FIG. 7.3 Bilateral fractures extending into the acetabular fossa: on the right a linear fracture and on the left a comminuted fracture.

femur being driven back with the thigh flexed and adducted. The more adducted the thigh the less the risk of fracture of the posterior wall. Judet *et al.* (1964) follow this argument further, describing a close correlation between the type of injury seen and the assumed type of force acting. The different angles of action lead to the many varieties of fracture–dislocation.

METHODS OF DIAGNOSIS

Clinical examination

This is most important. The rotatory deformity with shortening of the limb in the anterior and posterior dislocations is very characteristic. There are usually few diagnostic difficulties. However, every year

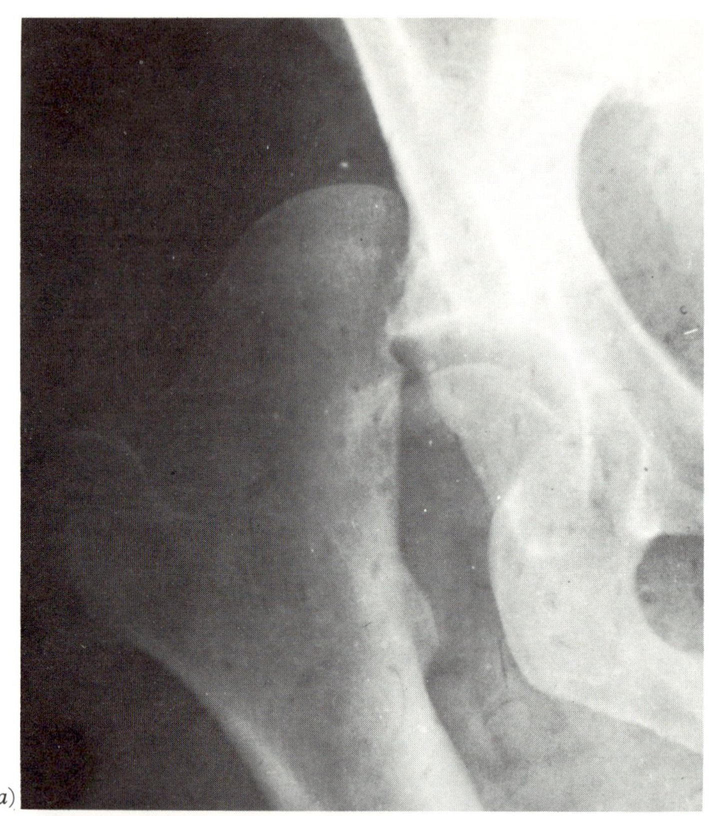
(a)

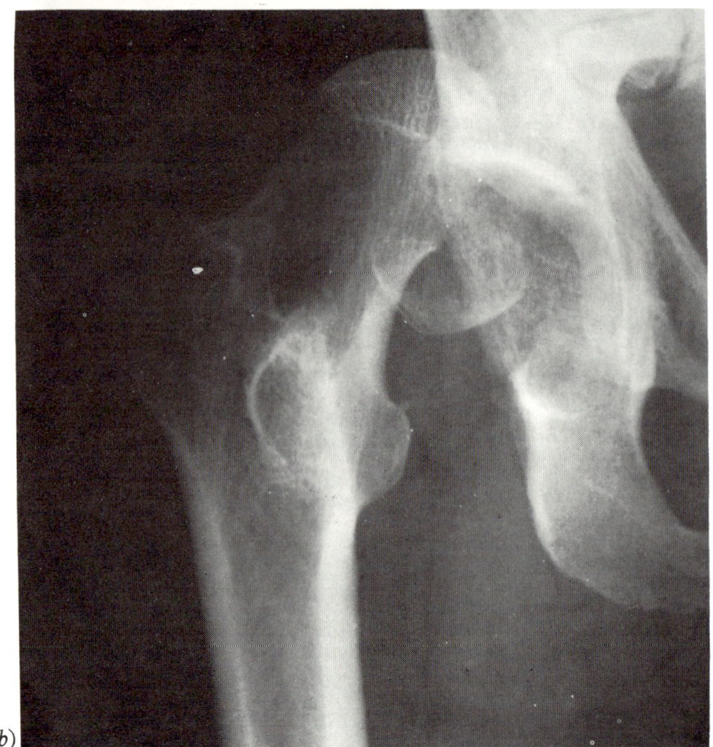
(b)

(d) (c)

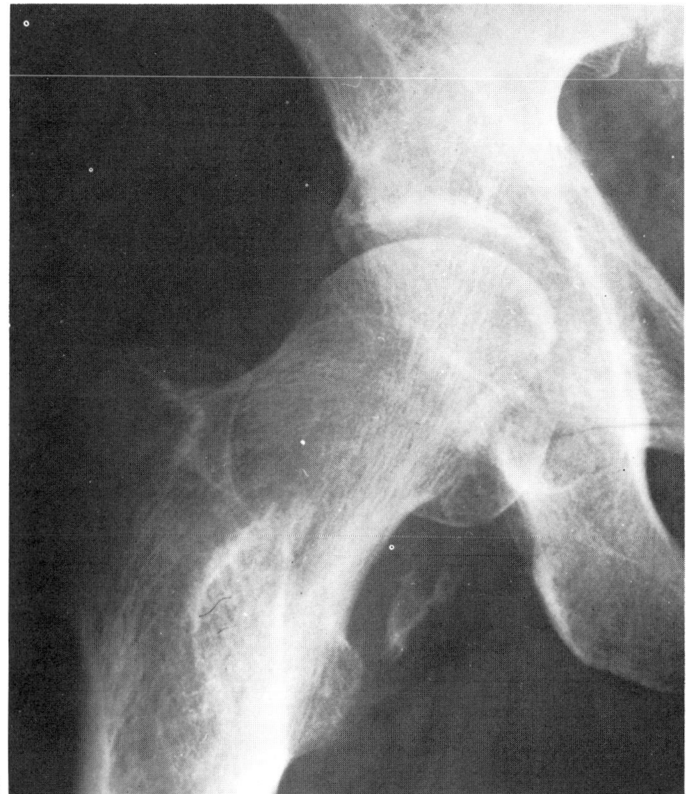

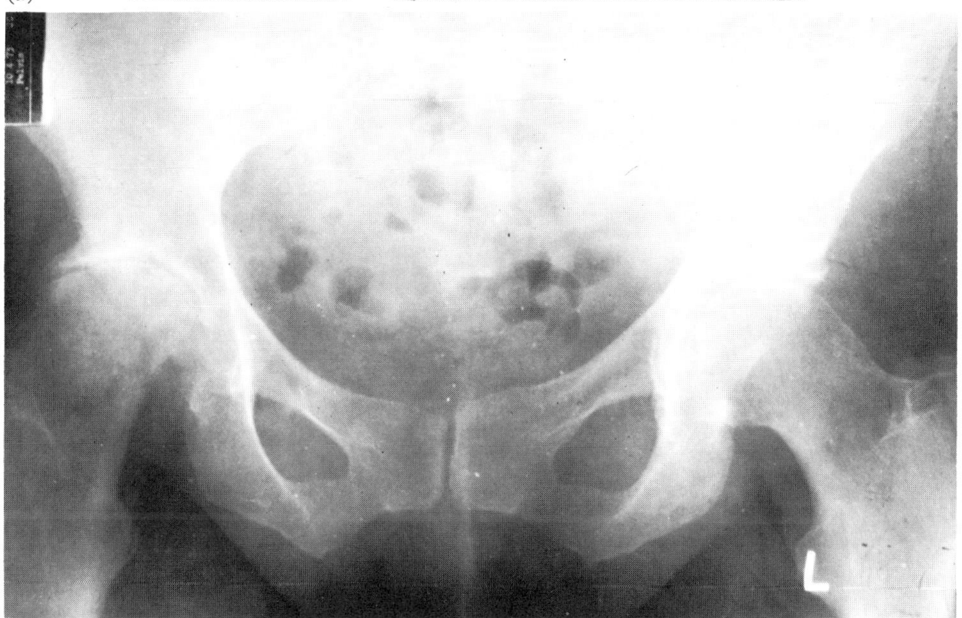

FIG. 7.4 (*a*) Antero–posterior view of the pelvis showing a dislocation of the femoral head and an adducted proximal segment. (*b*) The adduction has been corrected. (*c*) The head is reduced into the acetabulum. (*d*) Avascular changes have occurred 2 years later.

(a)

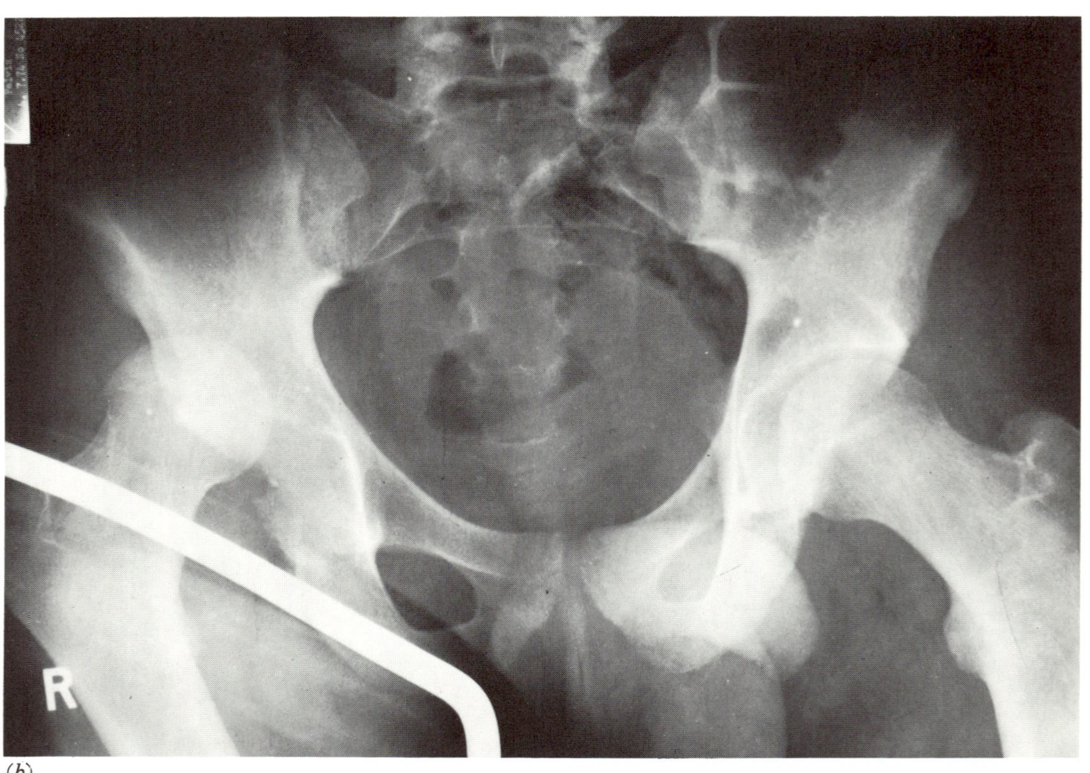

(b)

FIG. 7.5 A fractured shaft of femur (*a*) and the hip is dislocated on the same side (*b*).

dislocations of the hip are missed in association with a fractured shaft of femur. Helal and Stevis (1967) have stressed the importance of X-raying the ipsilateral hip joint in all patients with fracture of the shaft of the femur and particularly the association of an adducted proximal segment of the femur with a dislocated hip (see Figs. 7.4 and 7.5).

All multiple injuries should have an X-ray of the pelvis even if there is no clear-cut clinical evidence that this has been injured. It is very easy to miss a fracture of the pelvis on clinical examination and the predicted blood loss from the patient may be under-estimated and the chance to treat the joint injury early is lost.

Clinical examination of sciatic nerve function and examination to exclude pelvic organ damage is important. Patients with anterior column fractures often cause confusion because of rising haematoma formation in the anterior abdominal wall which may suggest an intra-peritoneal haemorrhage.

Radiographic examination

Antero–posterior radiographs should be taken immediately of the

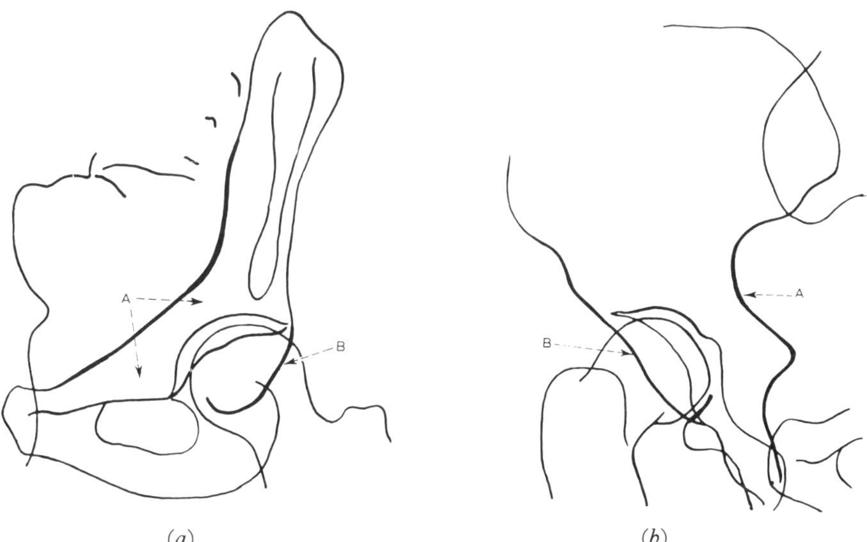

FIG. 7.6 (*a*) Three-quarter internal oblique view of the hip (with the patient supine and rotated 45° away from the injured side. (A) ilio–pubic column; (B) posterior lip of the acetabulum. (*b*) Three-quarter oblique view of the hip (patient supine and rotated 45° towards the injured side). (A) posterior lip of the ilium; (B) anterior lip of the acetabulum. (After Judet *et al.*, 1964.)

whole pelvis. Such a view is enough in the emergency room. A later more detailed assessment of the injury is important. If there is a posterior fragment associated with a posterior dislocation of the hip oblique views must be taken to assess the size of this fragment. Such fragments are easily missed altogether if no oblique views are taken and the size may be grossly under-estimated on an antero–posterior view as the fragment may be seen on its long axis. It is particularly important to have adequate radiographs if surgery to the acetabulum is to be considered. The oblique views described by Judet are recommended. These are described as three-quarters oblique and one-quarter oblique (Fig. 7.6).

TREATMENT AND EXPECTED RESULTS

The specific types of injury will be discussed in the following order:

(a) Anterior dislocation (type A injury).

(b) Posterior dislocation (type B).

(c) Fractures and dislocation involving the acetabular floor and roof including central dislocation (type C).

(d) Fracture dislocations in children.

(e) Associated injuries.

The general care of the patient is very important as frequently these patients have sustained multiple injuries. The patients should be placed on one trolley throughout and X-rays using standard projections should be taken without moving the patient. Adequate blood replacement is needed and it is very easy to under-estimate the loss.

ANTERIOR DISLOCATION (TYPE A INJURY)

This is an uncommon injury (Fig. 7.7) and has been estimated as making up between 9 and 12% of dislocated hips when considering anterior and posterior dislocations. The limb is shortened and lies in external rotation and often in abduction. The head is dislocated into pubic, obturator or perineal positions. It is essential to reduce the hip within the first few hours in order to prevent avascular necrosis. The hip can usually be reduced by applying longitudinal traction on the

FIG. 7.7 An anterior dilocation of the hip [antero–posterior view (*a*) and lateral (*b*)].

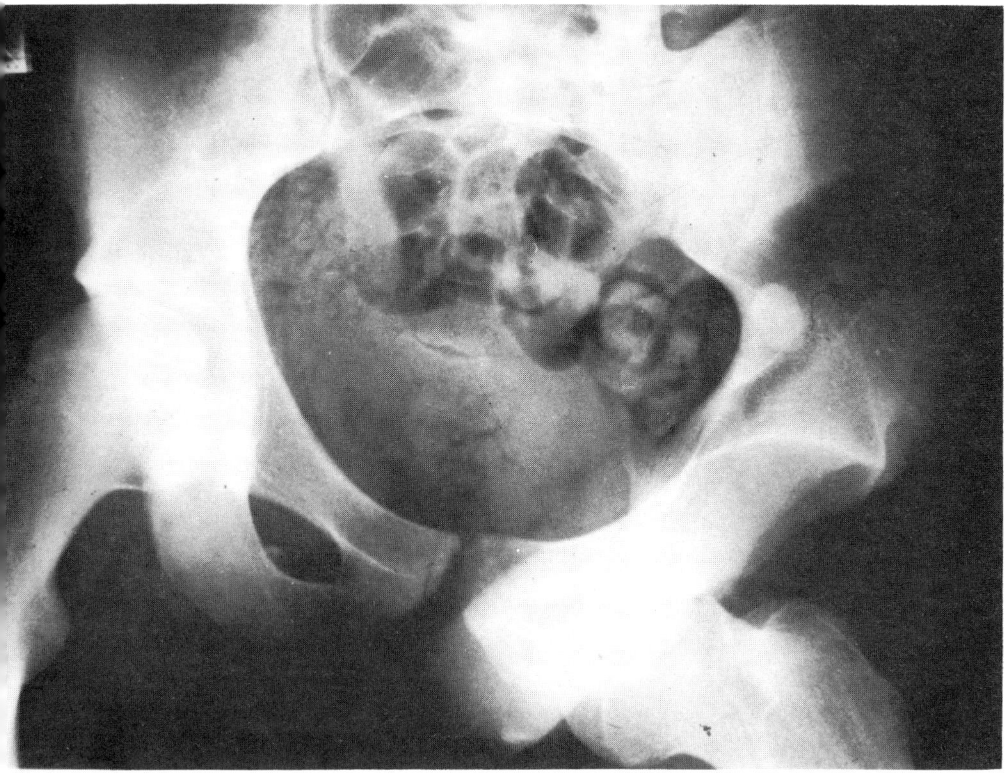

(a)

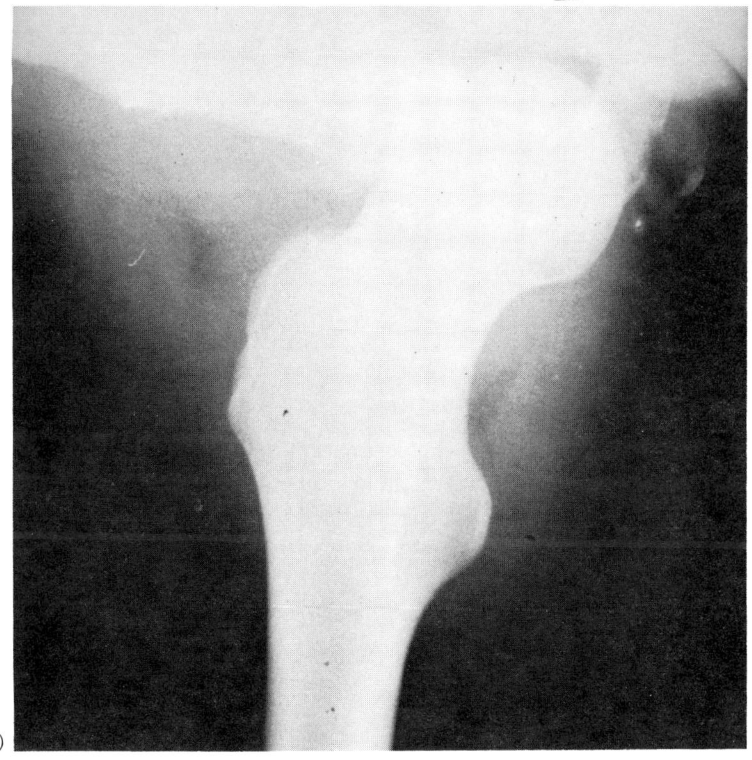

(b)

thigh with a flexion, adduction and internal rotation force. Stewart (1971) describes the use of a canvas sling around the proximal thigh upon which a lateral force is applied together with longitudinal traction at the same time pushing the femoral head towards the acetabulum. In the absence of a fracture it is most unusual not to be able to reduce the hip by closed means but if failure occurs open reduction must be performed through an anterior approach.

Post-operatively the hip is nearly always stable and the risk of redislocation very small. Skin traction for three weeks followed by mobilization – non-weight-bearing on crutches for another six weeks– is the compromise regime suggested. The question of when to weight-bear after injuries where there is a risk of the development of avascular necrosis will be discussed later. Avascular necrosis follows anterior dislocation in approximately 10% of patients. However, so few anterior dislocations have been seen and reviewed that definite conclusions really cannot be made. The complications following these injuries are few and most patients proceed to a good or an excellent result.

POSTERIOR DISLOCATION WITH OR WITHOUT POSTERIOR LIP FRACTURE (TYPE B INJURIES)

In this group there are those with only a very minor fracture; those with a large, single acetabular rim fragment which is displaced (Fig. 7.5*b*); and those with a comminuted acetabular rim fracture. The limb classically lies shortened, flexed, adducted, and in internal rotation. The rotatory deformity may not always be present. Early reduction is vitally important to reduce the incidence of avascular necrosis of the head of the femur. Nearly all investigators have found that avascular necrosis, when seen, was in those cases where there had been delay in reduction. Stewart and Milford (1954) found poor results when reduction was delayed for 24 hours.

Ideally, reduction should be performed within the first hour or two. A general anaesthetic is necessary and then reduction can be obtained using the method described by Watson Jones (1955) in which the patient lies supine and the hip is flexed and vertical traction applied. The Bigelow method using flexion, traction and circumduction is equally effective. If necessary the patient can be placed upon the floor on a mattress, the assistant pressing on the anterior superior iliac spines while the manipulator performs the appropriate reducing manoeuvre.

In most series reduction by closed means is obtained in over 90% of posterior dislocations. After manipulation, whilst examining under anaesthetic, the manipulator should make an assessment of the stability of the hip and should also have a check radiograph to confirm reduction has occurred and that the head lies concentrically within the acetabulum. Occasionally the head is not concentric because a small fragment from the acetabular rim or the head itself lies within the joint.

There is controversy concerning the post-operative care for uncomplicated posterior dislocations. How long should the patient be immobilized on traction and for how long should weight-bearing be prevented?

If the reduction is clinically stable redislocation is extremely uncommon. Liebenberg and Dommisse (1969) felt that inadequate immobilization was occasionally a cause for redislocation but this complication is very rare. It would seem rational, however, to keep patients in bed on skin traction for at least three weeks in order to obtain sound capsular healing and to allow the haemarthrosis to absorb. The issue of when to allow weight-bearing is more controversial. There are those who feel that early weight-bearing predisposes to avascular necrosis although there is no direct evidence for this (Banks, 1941; Nicholl, 1952; Brav, 1962). Banks advocated non-weight-bearing for four to six months in order to avoid avascular necrosis.

The incidence of avascular necrosis in type B dislocations and fracture – dislocations is in the order of 10%. It does not usually appear on X-ray for at least three months and it is difficult to predict which patients will develop the complication unless there is a delay in initial reduction. It is suggested here that the best method of post-reduction care for the uncomplicated posterior dislocation is three weeks in bed on skin traction and then mobilization with protected weight-bearing for a further six weeks. The latter period is to facilitate repair of cartilage which must always be damaged in these injuries. If reduction is delayed for more than six hours from the time of injury then there is a higher risk of avascular necrosis and partial protection from weight-bearing should be prolonged for a further eight weeks. For all patients it is important to make sure that radiographs are taken of the hip at two to four weekly intervals at least six months after injury. In this way the late onset of avascular necrosis can be recognized and the patient treated by restriction of weight-bearing in order to prevent collapse of the femoral head.

Indications for surgery in posterior dislocation of the hip

The main indications for operative intervention are:

Failed closed reduction

It may not be possible to reduce the dislocation because some structure such as the edge of the torn capsule may be wrapped around the femoral neck. The sciatic nerve has occasionally been found looped around the neck of the femur. There may be a small fragment from the femoral head or from the acetabulum blocking reduction. If the head cannot be reduced, open reduction is necessary using a direct posterior approach.

A large posterior fragment

This is associated with either instability of the reduction or with loss of the articular congruity. The fragment must be assessed by oblique radiography both in relation to its size and comminution. The emergency closed reduction should be performed but a delay of several days can be allowed before reconstructing the posterior rim. Of great interest were the results shown in a recent investigation by Epstein (1974) reviewing 242 posterior dislocations. He noted better results in those with posterior lip fractures with a large fragment following early open reduction and internal fixation of the fragment; with closed reduction only 32% had a good result whereas with delayed open reduction 54% had good results, and 87% if open reduction was performed during the first few days.

Open reduction should be performed through the posterior approach splitting the gluteus maximus and dividing the common tendon of the piriformis, obturator internus and gemelli muscles. The anterior approach should not be used since the dislocation will have injured the posterior blood supply. It is best to approach the hip through the injured area thus maintaining intact anterior structures. An important step is to wash the joint of small fragments. The triangular fragment of bone from the rim of the acetabulum is then reduced and fixed with one or two screws. Care should be taken that the screws do not protrude through the articular surface.

Loose fragments within the joint

The presence of loose fragments within the joint as seen on an X-ray is an indication for operation, as also is a small fracture of the head

(Fig. 7.4*a*) preventing concentric reduction. Epstein (1974) found that the results were markedly improved by surgical intervention and that at operation much debris was frequently found within the joint even although it could not be seen on an X-ray. He strongly advocates operation in order to lavage the joint thus removing these loose fragments and feels his improved results are due to this.

Sciatic nerve lesion

If there is a sciatic nerve lesion associated with a significant fragment displacement an operation should be performed because the fragment may cause direct pressure upon the nerve. When there is no fragment with a sciatic nerve lesion then conservative treatment can be utilized. This is a somewhat unusual situation.

The results to be expected after this type of injury have been well described by Hunter (1969). 95% of those with simple posterior dislocations produced good or excellent results and 75% of those with a fracture of major degree of the posterior lip had good or excellent results. Epstein's (1974) figures are similar although better results are shown after primary open reduction. The major cause of the poor results was delayed reduction with or without the development of avascular necrosis. Patients over 50 do less well than younger patients and if there has been fracture of the head, acetabular floor or weight-bearing segment then the percentage of good results dropped dramatically.

DISLOCATION WITH ACETABULAR ROOF AND/OR FLOOR FRACTURE (TYPE C INJURIES)

This comprises a large spectrum of injuries from linear fractures of the acetabular floor to major central dislocations (Fig. 7.8). There is considerable overlap between the many classifications but the one shown in Table 7.1 will embrace most other classifications. It is in the field of treatment of such injuries that there is the most controversy.

In the past most of these injuries have been treated by conservative means using closed reduction. It has been held that after a severe fracture of the acetabulum osteoarthritis is inevitable; that surgical reduction was hazardous due to complications and unfruitful with regard to reconstructing the normal anatomy. Most were treated by traction and many surprisingly good clinical results were obtained despite poor X-ray appearances of the hip.

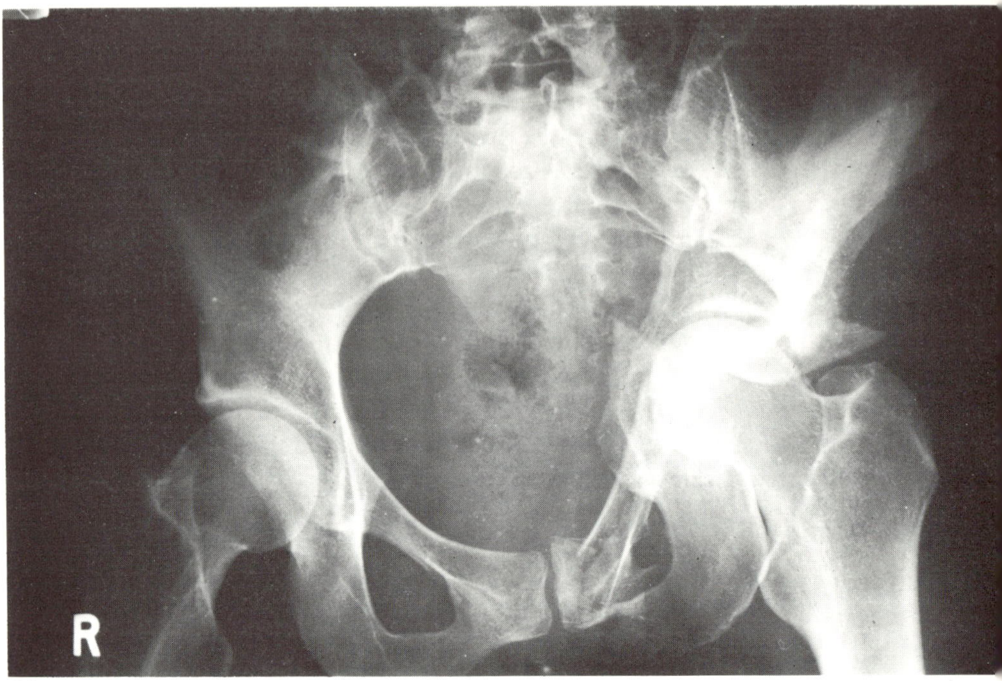

(a)

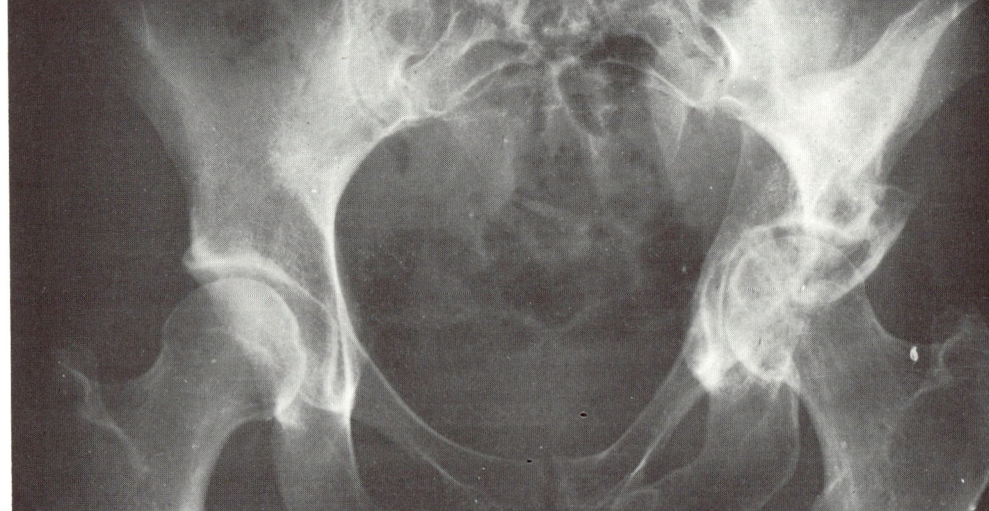

(b)

Treatment of these type C injuries will be described under the two headings of 'undisplaced fracture' and 'displaced fractures'.

Undisplaced fractures

Fractures of the anterior ilio-pubic column with linear fracture into the acetabulum require only bed rest until there is pain-free mobility in the hip joint. The patient should then be mobilized with protection from weight-bearing until six to eight weeks after the injury in order to allow fibro-cartilage repair. In old patients it is frequently necessary to ignore this last point and mobilize with early weight-bearing.

Displaced fractures and dislocations

The more accurate the reduction the better the chance of a satisfactory end result. It is of particular prognostic importance for the head of the femur to be in perfect relationship with the superior weight-bearing segment of the acetabulum. The radiographs must be adequate enough to assess accurately the displacements of the fractures, the degree of dislocation and the presence of fragments within the hip joint from the head or acetabulum. If there is any significant central or other displacement, attempt at manipulation under anaesthetic should be made. This should be performed as early as possible and certainly within the first few days. A general anaesthetic is given, a tibial Steinman's pin is inserted and longitudinal traction applied, following which a check radiograph is taken. If reduction is poor in central dislocations an antero–posterior Steinman's pin is also inserted through the trochanteric region and lateral traction applied under the same anaesthetic. This traction (in two directions, if necessary) should be maintained for a period of several weeks. In this way the head can usually be pulled out of the pelvis and maintained in its correct relationship to the acetabular floor. Post-operatively it is then important to restrict weight-bearing until union is well advanced. A period of bed rest for six to eight weeks is needed followed by at least another four weeks non-weight-bearing, and during this period it is important to encourage early mobilization. Stewart and Milford (1954) have stressed the

---

FIG. 7.8 Central dislocation of the hip in a 40 year-old woman (*a*) treated by traction; (*b*) result one year later.

importance of this early mobilization in converting a possible poor result into a good result.

There is a place for surgery in certain types of type C injury. Judet *et al.* suggest that most of these injuries with displacement should be subjected to surgery to obtain an anatomical reduction. Most clinicians although agreeing with these excellent aims find that the technical difficulties prevent them from achieving these aims in most cases. The following is a suggested line of approach to such problems:

(*a*) After resuscitation and within the first 24 h a serious attempt should be made at conservative closed reduction of the fracture dislocation under general anaesthesia.

(*b*) The patient should then be observed and allowed to recover from the acute phase of his trauma.

(*c*) Within the first week a complete X-ray examination must be made so that the complete picture of the anatomy of the fracture can be made and the injury classified according to Table 7.1 assessing the many factors described.

Loose fragments or an incorrect relationship between the femoral head and the superior weight-bearing surface of the acetabulum are absolute indications for open operation. Disruption of the acetabular floor with radiographs showing fracturing within the limits of accurate surgical reduction and stabilization is a relative indication for open reduction depending upon the patient and the exact nature of the injury.

When surgery is used a careful selection of the correct incision is essential and should be planned according to the anatomy of the fracture. Judet *et al.* (1964) advocates a posterior approach (when appropriate) with splitting of the gluteus maximus. A wide exposure is needed and he also describes cutting the sciatic spine at its base in order to obtain access to the inner aspect of the acetabulum. Anteriorly, he describes an approach extending along the anterior half of the iliac crest and extending anteriorly beyond the antero-superior iliac spine, along the lateral border of the sartorius. The abdominal muscles are detached from the iliac crest and the inner aspect of the pelvis exposed from the sacro-iliac joint to the ilio-pectinate protruberance. For the more complicated mixed injuries he advocates both the anterior and posterior approach. Fractures are fixed with screws, plates, or occasionally with staples.

The results after this type of injury have been described in many excellent reviews. Rowe and Lowell (1961) and Eichenholtz and Stark (1974) have described surprisingly good results with conservative therapy even in those with a major degree of central dislocation of the head of the femur or with fragmentation of the inner acetabular wall. Most investigators, however, have found that poor results were obtained in those in whom there was a displaced fracture of the superior acetabular weight-bearing segment so that the femoral head was not in its correct relationship to this segment. Poor results will also usually follow if there is an associated fracture of the head of the femur with a fragment left within the hip joint. The figures from the large number of patients reviewed by Epstein (1974) show that in this group of dislocations with fractures of the acetabular floor plus a fracture of the head, closed treatment led almost always to poor results. Closed initial treatment plus delayed open reduction led to 31% good results; and primary open reduction and removal of fragments from the joint led to 56% good results.

However, Rowe and Lowell showed 90% good or excellent results in inner wall acetabular fractures on a six year (average) follow up period treated by conservative methods; and 58% similarly good results even in the superior and bursting type of acetabular fractures. Operative treatment with its inevitable complications both at and after operation must show a clear advantage over these figures before it becomes the generally accepted treatment.

FRACTURE DISLOCATIONS IN CHILDREN

These are most unusual injuries but several investigators have collected relatively large series from different centres and some conclusions have been reached upon the patterns of injury and the difficulties encountered. Funk (1962) reviewed 40 patients of whom 37 had sustained posterior dislocations and grouped them according to age:

Group I 2–5 years;
Group II 6–10 years;
Group III 11–14 years.

Fractures were excluded. He found, as also did Glass and Powell (1961), that those in group I frequently sustained relatively minor trauma whereas those in groups II and III occurred, as in adults, after major trauma. The reason for this pattern of injury in group I is not clear for there was no evidence of any underlying hip dysplasia which might predispose to dislocation. The group I dislocations were easy to reduce and did not lead to problems later nor apparently to a risk of redislocation.

The group II and III injuries were sometimes associated with difficulty in closed reduction but once reduced the injuries were stable. Those injuries occurring in the older age groups, associated with major trauma, had a significant incidence of complications. Avascular changes occurred in approximately 10%, rising to 25% in those aged 10 years or more. A coxa magna may develop.

The several reviews differ in their conclusions upon the best post-reduction care. The method suggested here is to keep the patient in bed non-weight-bearing until the soft tissues have healed (after about three weeks) and then to mobilize partially weight-bearing on crutches for another six weeks.

Fracture–dislocations with a severe degree of damage to the acetabulum are very unusual in children but when they occur a poor result often follows.

ASSOCIATED INJURIES

Fractures and dislocations of the hip joint are frequently associated with multiple injuries. Injuries to the ipsilateral knee are particularly common but in this section the following associated injuries will be discussed:

(a) Associated fractures of the head and neck of femur;
(b) Ipsilateral fracture of the shaft of the femur;
(c) Intra-pelvic injuries;
(d) Sciatic nerve lesion and plexus injuries;

Fractures of the head and neck of the femur

Fracture of the head is a severe complication of fracture–dislocation of the hip joint with a bad prognosis. Commonly the fracture is in the inferior portion of the head and, if small, may be satisfactorily reduced after the manipulation of the dislocation and may well unite. If closed methods are used, it is essential to confirm that the fragment is absolutely reduced with adequate X-rays taken from various angles. If there is any doubt about the position of the fragment or if it is a large fragment then early surgery should be performed, usually to remove the fragment. A large fragment will become avascular and must predispose to a poor result. Epstein (1974) noted poor results after conservative methods with the figures improving to 56% with good results after primary open operation.

If there is an associated fracture of the femoral neck either caused at injury or during the manipulation under anaesthetic then primary fixation of this will be needed.

Ipsilateral fracture of the shaft of the femur associated with dislocated hip

In 1823 Astley Cooper first described this combination of injuries. Fig. 7.5 shows the classical situation. There is a transverse fracture of the mid-shaft of the femur with a markedly adducted proximal fragment. This feature strongly indicates a posterior dislocation of the hip proximal to the fractured shaft of femur. It is axiomatic that all long bone fractures, particularly those of the femur, must have adequate antero–posterior radiograph of the hip and knee joints. Despite this being fairly common knowledge, dislocated hips proximal to fractured shafts of femur are frequently missed.

The associated dislocation is usually posterior and urgent reduction of the dislocated hip is required in order to prevent avascular necrosis. This should be done within the first hour or so after admission to hospital. Frequently closed manipulation of the dislocated hip can be performed. In the patient seen in Fig. 7.5 closed reduction was followed by open reduction with Kuntscher fixation of the femoral shaft fracture under the same anaesthetic. Difficulties may be encountered in reduction of the hip joint. Helal and Stevis (1967) suggest opening the femoral fracture when it should be possible at operation to control the proximal fragment of the femur and reduce the hip. Watson Jones (1955) describes open reduction of the femoral shaft fracture, its fixation, and following this reduction of the hip. If this method is used then several hours may be lost before the hip joint is reduced. Lyddon and Hartman (1971) and others have suggested the use of a threaded screw or Steinman's pin which is placed into the trochanteric region in order to reduce the hip dislocation.

The most important factor however is not to miss the diagnosis. It is salutory that Lyddon and Hartman (1971) described the incidence of delayed diagnosis of the dislocated hip as being present in 50–54% of patients with this dual condition of fracture of the shaft and dislocation.

Intra-pelvic injuries

These are much more common in fractures of the pelvis associated with disruption of the pelvic ring. They do, however, also occur in central dislocation of the hip. Such complications are uncommon but injury to the bladder or major vessel injury is possible. The tracking of blood within the anterior abdominal wall associated with anterior column fractures makes the interpretation of physical signs difficult. It is not appropriate in this chapter to discuss the management of intra-pelvic injuries.

Sciatic nerve lesion and plexus injuries

The incidence of sciatic nerve involvement after fracture dislocation of the hip has usually been assessed as varying between 10 and 20%. The complication arises with varying frequency for the differing types of injury; it being more common in those with a marked posterior displaced dislocation with significant fracturing of the acetabular rim and less common in those with no fracture. It is, however, just as frequent a complication of acetabular floor or roof fractures without displacement of the hip.

Injuries to the peroneal element of the sciatic nerve are more frequent than total sciatic nerve lesions involving peroneal and tibial elements by a ratio of 2 to 1. Various theories have been put forward to explain this predominance of peroneal nerve injury. The sciatic nerve emerges from the pelvis distal to the piriformis muscle but sometimes the two divisions are separate throughout their extra-pelvic course. In this case the common peroneal division pierces the belly of piriformis (Seddon, 1972). If there is high separation like this then one nerve may be more liable to injury than the other. The tibial division is also much thicker than the common peroneal division and therefore less likely to be totally damaged at injury. Sunderland (1968) also felt that lack of effective post-operative care was more likely to lead to damage of the dorsiflexors than of the plantarflexors.

The prognosis for partial nerve injury is good. Most of the lesions associated with simple dislocations and dislocations with posterior fragment avulsion proceed to a state of recovery where no caliper is needed and an almost normal gait is achieved. Less good results are seen in those with severe fracturing of the acetabular roof or floor with associated nerve injury. In this group significant residual nerve dysfunction is likely to persist in over half of those with nerve injury (Epstein, 1974).

It is not possible here to cover all the aspects of the care of those patients with sciatic nerve injury. The following are important principles of treatment.

(a) Early reduction is of great importance if there is any sciatic nerve involvement particularly if the dislocation is posterior and associated with rotation of the leg.

(b) If there is a large posterior acetabular fragment with displacement and an associated sciatic nerve lesion, this is an indication for open operation and replacement of the fragment. Such fragments are frequently in direct contact causing pressure upon the nerve. Seddon (1972) has also recommended open operation even for those where the injury is predominantly a central dislocation of the hip if it is considered that a displaced fragment of bone may be pressing upon the nerve.

(c) In other patients with nerve injury and post-reduction in those treated as in (a) and (b) above, objective observations are made at intervals to assess recovery. The leg is rehabilitated with care for the skin and prevention of contractures, and the appropriate splintage is applied to allow walking. If progressive recovery does not occur then surgical exploration must be considered. Most patient recover sufficient function to have protective sensation and adequate walking function except for their having perhaps to wear a toe-raising device. Seddon (1972) has stressed the lack of correlation between neurological and functional recovery as applied to the sciatic nerve with much better total function than anticipated by neurological examination. Most of the lesions seen are partial, there being nearly always protective sensation, and any permanent disability is usually small. Surgical reconstruction of the nerve is unlikely to enable the patient to dispense with the toe-raising spring. In partial lesions it is best to await the fullest recovery that is going to occur and then consider either tendon transplant or stabilization of the foot and ankle.

Very occasionally there will be a complete sciatic nerve lesion with no objective signs of recovery even after several months. In such instances exploratory operation is warranted and should be performed at a time when the hip joint function is at an advanced stage of recovery, the fracture soundly healed with mature callus and the scars in the soft tissues well healed. Very few patients will require this type of treatment.

(d) Occasionally post-operative pain may be due to sciatic nerve irritation. The patient whose X-rays are seen in Fig. 7.8 had post-operative pain in the leg of sciatic distribution with minor motor changes in the foot. The main complaint was of severely painful paraesthesia. At an operation, two years after the initial injury, the sciatic nerve was found to be completely flattened and adherent to a large posterior fragment which had healed in poor position. The sciatic nerve was freed by neurolysis and the fragment excised although maintaining stability of the hip. Pain was immediately relieved.

COMPLICATIONS AND THEIR MANAGEMENT

Complications following fracture dislocations of the hip will be discussed under the following headings:

(a) Late presentation of dislocation;
(b) Recurrent dislocation;
(c) Myositis ossificans;
(d) Avascular necrosis;
(e) Osteoarthritis.

LATE PRESENTATION OF DISLOCATION

There is little reference in the literature to the management of the patient with a dislocation presenting late. This may be due either to missed diagnosis or to a dislocation associated with severe acetabular fracturing which has been accepted at an earlier stage in a patient with severe multiple injuries endangering life.

If the posterior dislocation presents late, with or without a posterior acetabular fragment, it is most important that a major attempt be made to reduce the fracture dislocation and stabilize the hip by surgery. This applies however long the delay between the injury and the diagnosis. If reduction is accomplished it is often possible to obtain a painless, stable, functioning hip although degenerative arthritis of the hip may ensue later. This arthritis, however, can be more easily treated by replacement arthroplasty if the normal anatomical relationship between the femur and the pelvis has been restored.

It is more difficult to know how to approach the problem when major central dislocation of the hip has persisted, or if a posterior or superior subluxation associated with fracturing of the floor or roof of the acetabulum has persisted. Coventry (1974) advocates an aggressive surgical approach to such problems. He reports a small series of patients in whom the problem has been treated in two stages. In the first stage, the head of the femur was removed and reduction and internal fixation of the acetabular fragments performed. This was successfully accomplished in the patients described and after a period of five to eight weeks a second stage procedure was performed on the now stable acetabular floor in which a total hip arthroplasty was inserted. In certain cases these two stages were performed together.

RECURRENT DISLOCATION

This is a most unusual complication and Brav (1962) estimated that it occurred in 1.5% of posterior dislocations or fracture dislocations.

The factors predisposing to this problem are as follows:

(a) The commonest factor is major acetabular fracturing which leads to loss of posterior stability. This may well be an indication for open reduction and fixation of the fragments in order to restore stability. If total stability is not gained by operation then the patient should be kept for six weeks on traction with the hip in extension.

(b) Inadequate immobilization has been described as a major cause of redislocation by Liebenberg and Dommisse (1969). This complication is, however, rare and redislocation will only occur if very early mobilization occurs in an unstable situation with fracturing.

(c) There have been various case reports in the literature referring to recurrent anterior and posterior dislocations being associated with a large pouch found in the posterior capsule or anterior capsule. Plication of the capsule and removal of the pouch has led to satisfactory stability.

MYOSITIS OSSIFICANS

This problem does occur following fracture dislocations of the hip but has little effect upon the clinical end-result. The overall incidence of radiological ectopic bone formation is about 15% the problem being much more common in those treated by open reduction. Rowe and Lowell (1961) estimated its incidence as being 34% in those acetabular fractures treated by open operation.

AVASCULAR NECROSIS

The incidence of this problem has been variably described and most of the reviews quoted in this paper have estimated the incidence. A review of the literature shows that on average avascular necrosis occurs in about 10% of the fracture – dislocations of the hip (Fig. 7.4).

There are certain diagnostic problems associated with avascular necrosis. It is rarely seen on radiographs before three months after injury. Usually it is seen at some time between three months and two years after injury. However, many patients with dislocated hips are not followed for this length of time with serial X-rays. Such serial observations should be made as the finding of late avascular changes on X-ray may lead to modifying the treatment.

There is controversy about the factors which are said to affect the incidence and outcome of avascular necrosis.

(a) Delayed reduction is universally blamed as the major cause for the occurrence of avascular necrosis. It is difficult to define delay but reduction of the posterior dislocation until 24 h after injury predisposes strongly to the development of avascular necrosis. Reduction within four hours of injury should be the priority of treatment. Stewart and Milford (1954) stressed this fact in showing that there were no good results in their series of patients with posterior dislocations in whom reduction was delayed 24 h.

(b) Repeated reductions are said to predispose to avascular necrosis. This seems a reasonable supposition but has not been proven.

(c) There is great controversy as to whether weight-bearing or the lack of it affects the incidence and outcome of avascular necrosis. This was discussed in the section on the treatment of posterior dislocations. Morton (1959) wrote that he did not know the answer to this question and this is probably the present state of knowledge. The problems concerning protection from weight-bearing are that avascular necrosis is relatively uncommon and it is difficult to predict which patients will develop it. The diagnosis will probably not be made on X-ray until over three months after injury. In practice, it is advocated therefore that only patients in whom there is a high risk should be subjected to prolonged non-weight-bearing (i.e. those in whom reduction is performed later than 12 h after injury). Although it has also never been proven that protection from weight-bearing prevents an avascular head from collapsing, if a diagnosis of avascular necrosis is made then protection from weight-bearing would seem to be reasonable empirical treatment. There are several controversial issues regarding avascular necrosis but two clear issues (a) its development is one of the major causes of a poor end result; (b) in the posterior dislocations and fracture dislocations its development is a largely preventable entity by early reduction.

OSTEOARTHRITIS

The major factors predisposing to the development of osteoarthritis in the hip joint are as follows:

(a) The severity of the initial injury and particularly the fracture. The results described by Brav for 264 long-term follow-ups are very typical.

Type of injury	*% of osteoarthritis seen on X-ray*
Posterior dislocation without fracture	26.4
Posterior dislocation with fracture of the posterior lip of the acetabulum	50.5
Posterior dislocation with fracture of the acetabulum or femoral head	72.4

(b) The nature of the acetabular fracture. If the superior weight-bearing dome of the acetabulum is damaged and particularly if the relationship of this part of the acetabulum to the head of the femur is disturbed, then the risk of development of osteoarthritis is very high.

(c) Avascular necrosis. If this later develops then the risk of subsequent osteoarthritis is very high.

The management of the osteoarthritis when it has once developed has been the subject of several studies and the details cannot really be discussed in this chapter. Frequently the patients with unsatisfactory results following fracture dislocations of the hip are young and there may well be a place for cup arthroplasty as described by Harris (1969). Coventry (1974) has more recently described the use of total hip replacement for old fracture dislocations and the use of this method must have increasing indications in patients with painful and unsatisfactory results.

However, it is upon the prevention of the development of osteoarthritis that surgeons should be concentrating. At present the two main factors which can be influenced by the surgeon which may prevent the development of this complication are:

(a) Prevention of avascular necrosis by early reduction of the dislocation.

(b) Reconstitution of a normal acetabular contour and a normal relationship between the femoral head and this acetabulum. In certain instances where careful pre-operative clinical and radiographic assessment indicates that the goal of perfect anatomy can be achieved technically and that the risk of the development of complications from surgery is small, then a radical surgical approach to accurate reduction should be undertaken.

REFERENCES

BANKS, S.W. (1941). *J. Bone Jt. Surg.* **23**, 753.
BRAV, E.A. (1962). *J. Bone Jt. Surg.* **44A**, 1115.
COVENTRY, M.B. (1974). *J. Bone Jt. Surg.* **56A**, 1128.
EICHENHOLTZ, S.N. and STARK, R.M. (1964). *J. Bone Jt. Surg.* **46A**, 695.
EPSTEIN, H.C. (1974). *J. Bone Jt. Surg.* **56A**, 1103.
FUNK, F.J. (1962). *J. Bone Jt. Surg.* **44A**, 1135.
GLASS, A. and POWELL, H.D.W. (1961). *J. Bone Jt. Surg.* **43B**, 29.
HARRIS, W.H. (1969). *J. Bone Jt. Surg.* **51A**, 737.
HELAL, B. and SKEVIS, X. (1967). *J. Bone Jt. Surg.* **49B**, 293.
HUNTER, G.A. (1969). *J. Bone Jt. Surg.* **51B**, 38.
JUDET, R., JUDET, J. and LETOURNEL, E. (1964). *J. Bone Jt. Surg.* **46A**, 1615.
LIEBENBERG, F. and DOMMISSE, G.F. (1969). *J. Bone Jt. Surg.* **51B**, 632.
LYDDON, D.W. and HARTMAN, J.T. (1971). *J. Bone Jt. Surg.* **53A**, 1012.
MORTON, K.S. (1959). *Canad. J. Surg.* **3**, 67.
NICOLL, E.A. (1952). *J. Bone Jt. Surg.* **34B**, 503.
PEARSON, J.R. and HARGADON, E.J. (1962). *J. Bone Jt. Surg.* **44B**, 550.
ROWE, C.R. and LOWELL, J.D. (1961). *J. Bone Jt. Surg.* **43A**, 30.
SEDDON, H. (1972). *Surgical Disorders of the Peripheral Nerves.* Churchill Livingstone, Edinburgh, London.
STEWART, M.J. and MILFORD, L.W. (1954). *J. Bone Jt. Surg.* **36A**, 315.
STEWART, M. (1971). *Campbell's Operative Orthopaedics.* Vol. I, Mosby Co., St. Louis.
SUNDERLAND, S. (1968). *Nerves and Nerve Injuries.* Livingstone, Edinburgh.
THOMPSON, V.P. and EPSTEIN, H.C (1951). *J. Bone Jt. Surg.* **33A**, 746.
WATSON JONES, R. (1955). *Fractures and Joint Injuries.* Livingstone, Edinburgh.

Chapter Eight

FRACTURES AND DISLOCATIONS OF THE PELVIS

J. W. Goodfellow

General considerations ~ Types of fracture and their management

GENERAL CONSIDERATIONS

Functionally the pelvis can be regarded as a rigid ring of bones bound together by the dense ligaments of the symphysis pubis anteriorly and the sacro-iliac ligaments posteriorly. In the erect position this ring carries the load of the body's weight from the lumbar spine to the hip joints (Fig. 8.1). Through the ring passes the termination of the intestinal, urinary and genital tracts; and the main trunks of the vessels and nerves to the lower limbs are closely related to it. For these reasons, mere preoccupation with the appearances of a fracture on an X-ray plate, always a dangerous approach in the management of the injured, is in the case of the fractured pelvis more than ordinarily hazardous.

The clinical examination of any person who has been involved in a serious fall or in a motor car or motor cycle crash is incomplete without careful assessment of the possibility of a pelvic injury, even if no specific complaint is made to draw attention to that part. Unstable fractures of the pelvis are the third commonest cause of death following road traffic accidents, and a mortality rate of 25% has been recorded (Froman and Stein, 1967). If the clinical examination is even suggestive of such injuries X-ray examination of the pelvis should be made as soon as circumstances allow. So easy is it to overlook pelvic injuries in those who have suffered multiple trauma that it is wise to include an antero–posterior radiograph of the pelvis in the preliminary screening examination of such cases, although positive physical signs to suggest these injuries are lacking. The presence of a pelvic fracture always

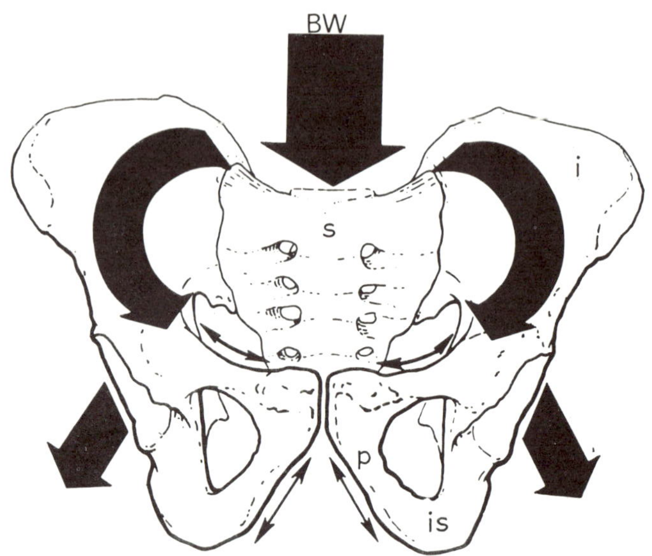

FIG. 8.1 Stress lines in the pelvis; BW = body weight. (After Peltier, 1965.)

demands examination specifically to exclude associated injuries to those structures which traverse or lie adjacent to the pelvic ring.

CLINICAL DIAGNOSIS

The examiner looks for bruising, particularly of the perineum, and for bleeding from the anus, vagina or urethra. Palpation of the subcutaneous surfaces of the bones is the most useful method of detecting the presence of a fracture in the ilium, both pubic rami, the ischium and the sacro-iliac joints. Tenderness at any site demands X-ray examination. 'Springing' of the pelvis will certainly reveal the presence of grossly unstable fractures of the pelvic ring, but a negative result by no means excludes less serious fractures.

RADIOLOGICAL DIAGNOSIS

Most pelvic fractures are revealed by a simple antero–posterior radiograph. Supplementary views, including lateral and lateral-oblique films, may be necessary to reveal minimally displaced fractures and those occurring in the region of the sacro-iliac joint. Two further X-ray views have been described: the inlet view taken with the patient supine and the X-ray source directed 25° caudad displays the brim of the true pelvis in outline; with the patient in the same position films may be taken with the X-ray source directed 35° cephalad to demonstrate rotation of the hemipelvis in the antero – posterior plane.

TYPES OF FRACTURE AND THEIR MANAGEMENT

AVULSION FRACTURES

The pelvic ring offers attachment to the muscles of the abdominal wall and to those of the proximal part of the lower limb and avulsion of their origins can result from vigorous muscle action. The anterior-superior and anterior-inferior iliac spines are sometimes detached in this way, and the hamstrings can avulse the epiphysis of the ischial tuberosity in the immature pelvis (Fig. 8.2*a*, *b*). Such injuries occur usually in young people during sporting and athletic activities. There is a sudden and disabling pain at the affected site, and the injury is readily confirmed by X-ray examination. Reduction of the displaced fragments is not possible by closed methods, but open reduction is not necessary. Symptomatic treatment requires rest until the pain subsides, and then gradual resumption of activity as union progresses. Even if bony union fails, firm fibrous union is almost always adequate for full functional recovery.

STABLE FRACTURES OF THE PELVIC RING

Some fractures do not transgress the pelvic ring and by no means all the fractures which do so render it insecure, although all should be viewed with suspicion until their stable character has been established. Of 115 patients with pelvic fractures reported by Dunn and Morris (1968) 77 fell into the category of stable fractures.

Fractures of the wing of the ilium

Those fractures which involve only the wing of the ilium, although often comminuted and with the fragments displaced, present no serious structural problems (Fig. 8.2*a*). The muscles which invest the ilium on both sides maintain the general shape of the bone which requires neither reduction nor fixation. However, such fractures may cause serious haemorrhage. They are always associated with rigidity of the abdominal muscles (which take origin from the iliac crest), a

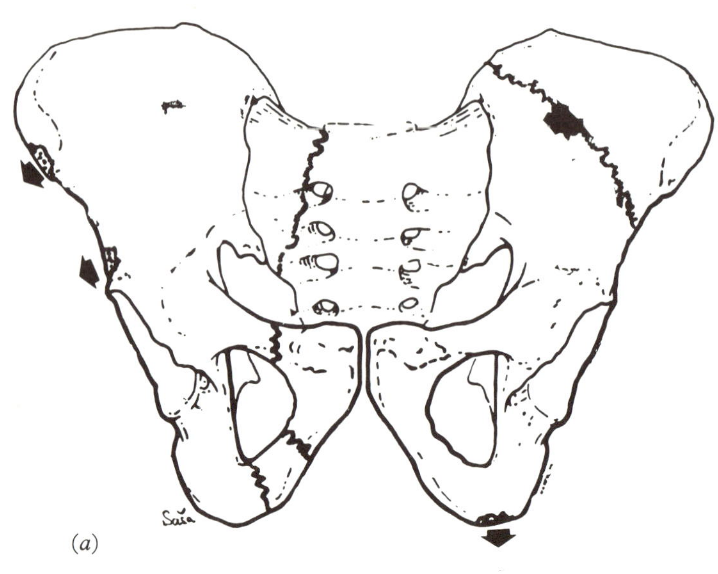

(*a*)

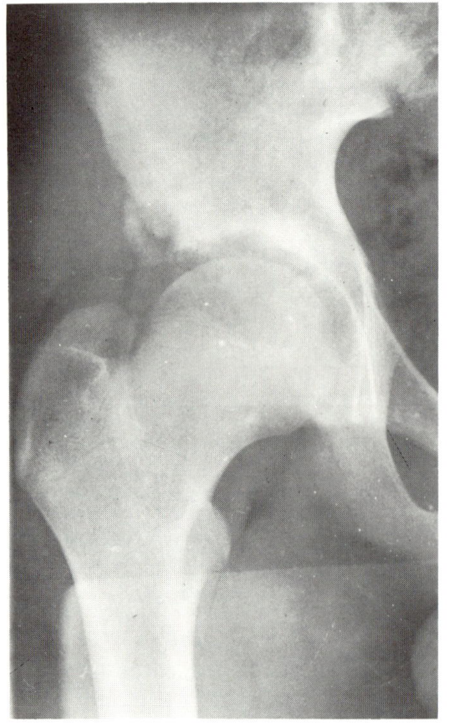

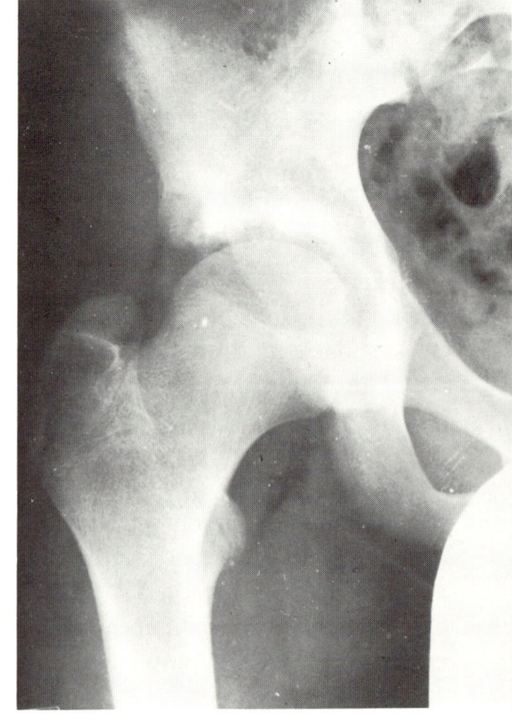

(*b*)

circumstance which may suggest visceral damage. In fact visceral injury is rarely associated with this type. Management consists of careful observation to detect the local and general signs of serious haemorrhage, and rest in bed either recumbent or sitting, whichever is the more comfortable. Ambulation is allowed as the pain subsides, usually in two or three weeks. The fragments are usually stable and largely painless within three to four weeks, and union occurs.

Fractures of the pubic rami

Although the pubic rami complete the pelvic ring anteriorly, fractures of these bones do not produce significant instability (Fig. 8.2). When standing the body's weight is borne through the posterior elements of the pelvis from the spine to the acetabuli, and thence via the femora to the ground. Since the sacro-iliac joints are substantially immobile, the posterior half of the ring remains stable despite discontinuity anteriorly. Of course, this is true only if the sacro-iliac joints are intact. If the force that broke the pubic rami also dislocated one or other of the sacro-iliac joints then pelvic stability is lost. Instability of a sacro-iliac joint can be diagnosed from the X-ray plate only if displacement was present at the time the film was taken. The distinction between stable and unstable fractures of the pubic bones can therefore only be made with certainty after careful clinical examination. Pain, or appreciable movement on 'springing' the pelvis, or tenderness over one or other of the sacro-iliac joints, implies instability even if the X-rays of the posterior part of the pelvic ring appear normal.

Stable fractures of one or more of the pubic rami account for about one-third of all fractures of the pelvis, and in most of these the fractures are unilateral. They are common in old people, whose osteoporotic bones may fracture from relatively trivial injury. In these patients, the physical signs often mimic a fracture of the neck of the femur and can only be distinguished by X-ray examination. Serious haemorrhage

---

FIG. 8.2(*a*) Common fractures of the pelvis and sacrum. Avulsion fractures are indicated by arrows at the anterior superior and inferior spines, and ischial tuberosity.

FIG. 8.2(*b*) An avulsion of the anterior iliac spine sustained while hurdling treated by restricted mobilization for three weeks. X-ray six weeks after injury showed healing of the injured area.

and visceral injury are uncommon. Treatment requires usually no more than bed rest until the pain subsides, usually in two to four weeks.

In contrast to the above, bilateral pubic rami fractures are often the result of severe trauma. They are often associated with sacro-iliac disruption and visceral damage and they are dealt with under the heading of unstable fractures.

UNSTABLE FRACTURES AND DISLOCATIONS

It is the main purpose of the classification of injuries to assist the clinician in deciding upon the appropriate treatment. All unstable fractures of the pelvis result from severe trauma, and all are associated with a high risk of soft tissue injury. They require some form of immobilization in their management. Displacement of the elements of the pelvic ring requires accurate reduction if eventual disability is to be avoided; potential displacement requires prolonged protection from weight-bearing. Reduction and immobilization of the fragments is a matter of urgency if haemorrhage from the bone ends is to be controlled and further laceration of adjacent soft tissues avoided.

Several classifications of the unstable injuries of the pelvis are described (Pennal and Sutherland, 1961; Peltier, 1965) based upon the pattern of fractures. But since there are innumerable ways in which the bones may break, no classification on these lines can accommodate all injuries without becoming unwieldy. We shall adopt here a functional rather than an anatomical classification based not upon the pattern of fractures visible radiologically but upon the displacements of the fragmented pelvic ring. Such a classification is simpler and of more practical value, since it is the displacements which require reduction.

For a segment of the rigid pelvic ring to become unstable requires that the ring be disrupted at two sites – either by two fractures, each transgressing the ring, or by one such fracture accompanied by a dislocation at the sacro-iliac joint or the symphysis pubis. If the ring is broken in three places, then the two segments become unstable in relation to one another as well as in relation to the vertebral column.

An unstable section of the pelvis initially displaces in the direction of the force applied at the time of injury, but its eventual position depends more upon the direction of pull of the muscles attached to it and on the effects of gravity. Since these forces persist they need to be counteracted by appropriate forces applied either directly to the fragments, or indirectly through the lower limb. The correcting force must be maintained until union has become established in a stable ring.

Unilateral fractures and dislocations of one hemipelvis

In these injuries one half of the pelvic ring breaks free (Fig. 8.3). Firstly, it is detached from the vertebral column either by disruption of its sacro-iliac joint or by a fracture adjacent to the joint. Secondly, it is detached from the other half of the pelvis either by disruption of the symphysis pubis or by fractures adjacent to the pubis. The commonest fracture pattern is a combination of dislocation of the sacro-iliac joint on one side and contra-lateral fractures of both pubic rami, but there are many other combinations of fracture and dislocation which produce an essentially similar mechanical failure.

The free segment of pelvis has one lower limb attached to it through the hip joint, and the origins of most of the muscles which control the hip. However, the fragment remains attached to the axial skeleton through the medium of the powerful abdominal muscles. Thus, in the recumbent position the weight of the lower limb tends to rotate the free segment of the pelvis laterally and the unopposed action of the abdominal muscles tends to displace the fragment upwards towards their origins on the vertebral column and the thorax. External rotation of the hemipelvis can be controlled by a pelvic sling which applies a

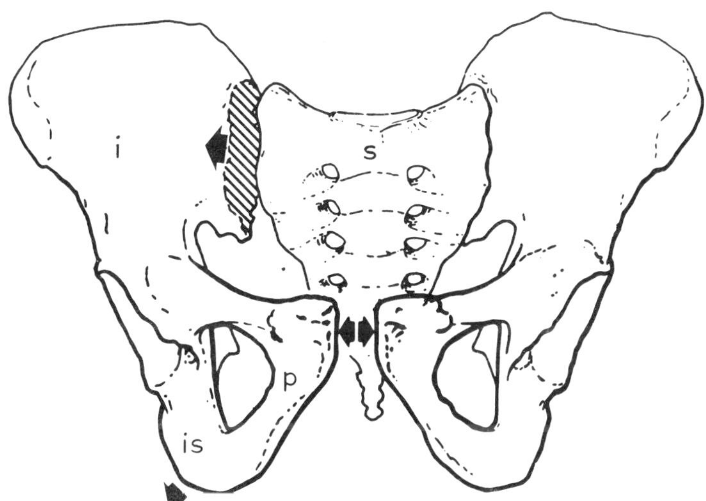

FIG. 8.3 Unilateral dislocation of the pelvis. (After Peltier, 1965.)

correcting force directly to the iliac bone. Upward translation of the hemipelvis can be corrected by applying traction in the long axis of the ipsilateral limb through the medium of a Steinman pin in the upper tibia.

By the judicious application of one or other of these techniques, or both, it is possible to reduce most hemipelvic displacements and to maintain reduction during the several weeks which must elapse before repair is secure. Balanced methods of traction with weights and pulleys are employed both for the pelvic sling and the limb traction, so that the manoeuvres necessary in nursing the patient can be accomplished without occasioning redisplacement. It takes about eight weeks for union of these fractures to render the pelvis stable in recumbency and twelve weeks before the repair is sufficiently strong to withstand the forces of weight-bearing. Frequent X-ray examination of the pelvis is necessary during the first weeks of treatment, and adjustment of the corrective forces is needed from time to time to maintain accurate reduction.

Bilateral fractures and dislocations of the hemipelvis

In this type of injury both hemipelves displace in relation to the vertebral column and to one another. For this to occur, fracture adjacent to, or dislocation of, both sacro-iliac joints is required in addition to disrup-

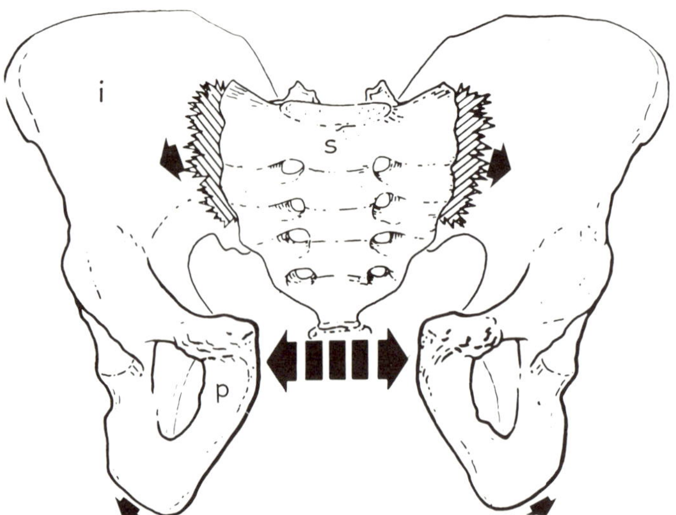

FIG. 8.4 Bilateral dislocation of the pelvis. (After Peltier, 1965.)

tion of the pelvic ring anteriorly (Fig. 8.4). Both hemipelves are then subject to the deforming forces described under the previous heading, and the problem of achieving and maintaining an acceptable reduction is much more difficult. It may require application of a pelvic sling and bilateral skeletal leg traction. The direction of pull upon the hemipelvis can be modified by abducting or rotating the appropriate limb.

These methods may fail to reduce displacement because of impaction of one or other of the fractures. Direct manipulation under anaesthesia may then be required, and the appropriate traction is applied thereafter to maintain the position.

Bilateral pubic rami fractures (straddle fracture)

A different kind of instability arises when the pelvic ring breaks in two places anteriorly, while its posterior part remains intact. The free segment, consisting of the pubic bones bound together by their symphysis is pulled upwards by the rectus abdominis muscles and falls inwards. Displacement can be minimized by nursing the patient in the semi-sitting posture. Accurate reduction is not essential for full functional recovery since the structural integrity of the posterior pelvic ring is intact.

The injury is, however, a serious one and it is often associated with intra-pelvic haemorrhage and damage to the viscera, especially the urethra.

RESIDUAL DISABILITY

The eventual prognosis in stable fractures of the pelvis is uniformly good. Discomfort may persist for months or even years, but disability is usually slight.

In unstable fractures the prognosis is also favourable for those who survive the initial hazards from the soft tissue complications and associated injuries. If accurate reduction has been achieved and maintained until repair is sound, full recovery of function can be expected. In this context it is to be remembered that fractures heal more certainly than do dislocations of the sacro-iliac joints. The commonest complaint is of persistent pain in the sacro-iliac region, and this can often be attributed to failure of primary reduction or to the too early resumption of weight-bearing which results in secondary subluxation.

COMPLICATIONS OF PELVIC FRACTURES

Vascular injuries

The commonest and most serious complication of pelvic fractures is haemorrhage. Bleeding occurs from the ends of the broken bones and from lacerated soft tissues adjacent to them and the symptoms are those of oligaemic shock, abdominal pain and back-ache. The retroperitoneal space can accommodate several litres of blood without there developing a palpable mass [2.5–3 l have been reported (Peltier, 1965)], and the possibility of haemorrhage into this space should always be borne in mind. Ecchymosis in the scrotum, along the inguinal ligaments and in the buttocks suggests intra-pelvic haemorrhage (Braunstein *et al.*, 1964).

While rupture of major vessels with catastrophic haemorrhage can occur, the bleeding is more usually from small vessels in the bone or branches of the internal iliac artery. Although the rate of blood loss may be moderate, it often continues for many hours to achieve eventually massive proportions. Exploration to ligate bleeding vessels may be unrewarding, Bayliss *et al.* (1962) reported only one successful ligation in 25 laparotomies. Thus, the replacement by infusion of whole blood and immediate immobilization of the broken pelvis to avoid repeated damage to soft tissues usually controls the haemorrhage. There are, however, occasions when bleeding continues and is so severe as to demand an attempt at ligature of the ruptured vessel. If, as has frequently been reported, no specific bleeding point can be found ligature of the internal iliac artery is advised (Horton and Hamilton, 1968). The procedure carries a small, and in the circumstances, acceptable hazard of ischaemia of the sigmoid colon when performed on the left side.

Damage to intra-pelvic viscera

Injuries of the bladder or urethra complicate about 10% of fractures of the pelvic ring (Hartmann, 1955; Zorn, 1960). In a series of 46 genito-urinary injuries, 19 had a ruptured urethra, 14 had a ruptured bladder, 2 a ruptured bladder and urethra, and 9 urethral injuries coexisted with rectal damage (Froman and Stein, 1967). Bruising in the perineum or bleeding from the urethral meatus indicate urethral damage, but absence of these signs gives no reassurance, and urinary tract injury must be positively excluded. A rectal examination should always be performed, since rupture of the posterior urethra produces a palpable haematoma and rectal trauma may also be found. If the patient has passed clear urine since his accident all is well, but if he has not then the passage of a soft urethral catheter should be attempted. This is better than pressing the patient to void urine when the danger of extravasation becomes great. If there is any obstruction to its passage or any clinical sign to suggest urethral damage, urethrography should be performed by injecting 20 ml of 30% urographin through the catheter.

If the urethra is intact the catheter is passed on into the bladder. A flow of clear urine excludes bladder injury. If no urine flows, or it is blood-stained, a further 20 ml of urographin is injected for cystography. Lateral as well as antero–posterior X-rays are necessary to exclude leakage (Froman and Stein, 1967). The presence of blood-stained urine in the bladder is not pathognomonic of a rupture of that organ, for contusion of the bladder wall without rupture can cause haematuria, as can damage to a kidney sustained at the time of the pelvic fracture.

The cystogram may also demonstrate displacement of the bladder or distortion of its outline from the presence of a retroperitoneal haematoma. Even if no damage to the urinary tract has been sustained the catheter may with advantage be left in the bladder so that urinary output can be estimated, a useful measurement in patients who are liable to severe haemorrhage.

Nerve injuries

Damage to the lumbo-sacral plexus may result from fractures involving the sacrum (Bonnin, 1945; Patterson and Morton, 1961), and by avulsion of the lumbo-sacral nerve roots in dislocations of the sacro-iliac joint (Harris *et al.*, 1973). In these injuries peripheral nerve function must be carefully tested if nerve lesions are not to be overlooked. Also the femoral, sciatic, obturator and lateral cutaneous nerve of the thigh may be directly involved by a bone fragment or by a traction injury. When the peripheral nerves are torn surgical repair can be carried out. An important, and often forgotten feature of nerve damage in association with pelvic injuries, is the coincidental injury to the sympathetic and parasympathetic plexuses. Trafford (1955) reported that 25% of patients with severe pelvic fractures may become impotent.

Associated injuries

Fracture of the pelvis is very commonly but one component of a multiple injury. It is particularly associated with injury to the thorax in those cases in which crushing force has been applied to the whole trunk [in these circumstances there may be an associated rupture of the diaphragm (Levine and Crampton, 1963)], and with fractures of the femur and tibia in road traffic accidents and falls from a height. Rectal and vaginal injuries required excision and suture, with a defunctioning colostomy in the case of severe rectal trauma. Occasionally, the pregnant uterus poses complications. Fractures of the pelvis have been shown to have a detrimental effect on child development (carrying a high foetal mortality (Speer and Peltier, 1972), and labour may be difficult due to malunion or non-union in the case of recent fractures. A Caesarian section may be required.

REFERENCES

BAYLISS, S.M., GLAS, W.W. and LANSING, E.H. (1962). *Am. J. Surg.* **103**, 477.

BRAUNSTEIN, P.W., SKUDDER, P.A., MCCARROLL, J.R., MUSOLINO, A. and WADE, P.A. (1964). *J. Trauma* **4**, 832.

BONNIN, J.G. (1945). *J. Bone Jt. Surg.* **27**, 113.

DUNN, W. and MORRIS, H.D. (1968). *J. Bone Jt. Surg.* **50A**, 1639.

FROMAN, C. and STEIN, A. (1967). *J. Bone Jt. Surg.* **49B**, 24.

HARRIS, W.R., RATHBUN, J.B., WORTZMAN, G. and HUMPHREY, J. (1973). *J. Bone Jt. Surg.* **55A**, 1436.

HARTMANN, K. (1955). *Arch. klin. Chir.* **201**, 147.

HORTON, R.E. and HAMILTON, S.G.I. (1968). *J. Bone Jt. Surg.* **50B**, 376.

LEVINE, J. and CRAMPTON, R.S. (1963). *Surgery Gynec. Obstet.* **116**, 223.

PATTERSON, F.P. and MORTON, K.S. (1961). *Surgery Gynec. Obstet.* **112**, 702.

PELTIER, L.F. (1965). *J. Bone Jt. Surg.* **47A**, 1060.

PENNAL, G.F. and SUTHERLAND, G. (1961). Motion picture available from the Film Library of the American Academy of Orthopaedic Surgeons.

SPEER, D.P. and PELTIER, L.S. (1972). *J. Trauma* **12**, 474.

TRAFFORD, H.S. (1955). *Br. J. Urol.* **27**, 165.

ZORN, G. (1960). *Beitr. klin. Chir.* **201**, 147.

Chapter Nine

SLIPPED UPPER FEMORAL EPIPHYSIS

E. W. Somerville

Aetiology and pathology ~ Clinical examination ~ Treatment ~ Complications

AETIOLOGY AND PATHOLOGY

Slipping of the upper femoral epiphysis is a relatively uncommon condition which occurs in children between the ages of ten and fifteen years but occasionally it is seen in younger or older subjects. The cause of the slip has never been determined with certainty but about 70% of patients show evidence of endocrine abnormality. Trauma alone will not cause displacement, the femoral neck will fracture first. It is also not uncommon for the opposite hip to displace at a later date and the history suggests either a minor degree of trauma or no trauma at all. Thus for displacement to occur there must be some pathological softening of the epiphyseal plate. That there is some pathological change is supported by the fact that closure of the growth plate occurs rapidly after slipping is manifest, even following a good reduction. The exception is seen in the young child in whom the epiphyseal plate may remain open and growth continue (Figs. 9.1–9.6; Table 9.1).

The cause of the softening has never been established but often there is evidence of endocrine abnormality. Most of the patients are overweight and a small number are exceptionally tall, while some show evidence of pituitary disturbance. Nevertheless there are the remainder who appear to be perfectly normal children in whom there is no obvious reason.

Howarth (1941) has suggested that there is chronic synovitis which causes vascular changes leading to softening with osteoporosis. Rennie (1959) believes that before the actual slip occurs there is increased

TABLE 9.1 X-ray classification

I	Preslipping phase	Epiphyseal plate widened and irregular, areas of demineralization in metaphysis adjacent to plate. Bulging of joint capsule with effusion
II	Mild slipping	Displacement less than one-third diameter of femoral neck. Initially epiphysis migrates posteriorly on metaphysis with no inferior displacement. Oblique or lateral view to reveal slip. Minimal inferior displacement on antero–posterior film accentuated by drawing line along upper border of femoral neck. In normal hip a small but definite segment is seen above line. With slipping, no part or a very small area projects above this line (Kline's line)
III	Moderate slipping	Slipping from one to two-thirds of the diameter of the femoral neck. Abnormalities in both antero–posterior and lateral views
IV	Severe slipping	From two-thirds to complete dislocations of the epiphysis. Many acute cases in this category. Treatment essentially same for moderate and severe slips
V	Residual stage	Closure of epiphyseal plate with malunion. Degenerative arthritis, avascular necrosis, or cartilage necrosis may be seen

lengthening of the anterior part of the neck of the femur due to injury to the posterior part of the growth plate by repeated trauma and that it is only then that the acute slip occurs. An interesting observation relating to this fact is that in the typical child in whom a slip may be a strong possibility – the fat child with thick tapering legs – it will be found frequently that there is an increase in the arc of rotation laterally but a decrease in the medial rotation even though no split ever occurs.

Whatever the cause of the slipping it may occur either as

(a) An acute slip;
(b) An acute slip superimposed on a chronic slip; or
(c) A chronic slip.

CLINICAL EXAMINATION

The clinical features will differ considerably according to whether the slip has taken place acutely or gradually.

FIG. 9.1(*a*) Slipped (left) upper femoral epiphysis in girl aged eight.

FIG. 9.1(*b*) Reduced and pinned: eight years later, the epiphyseal plate did not undergo premature closure.

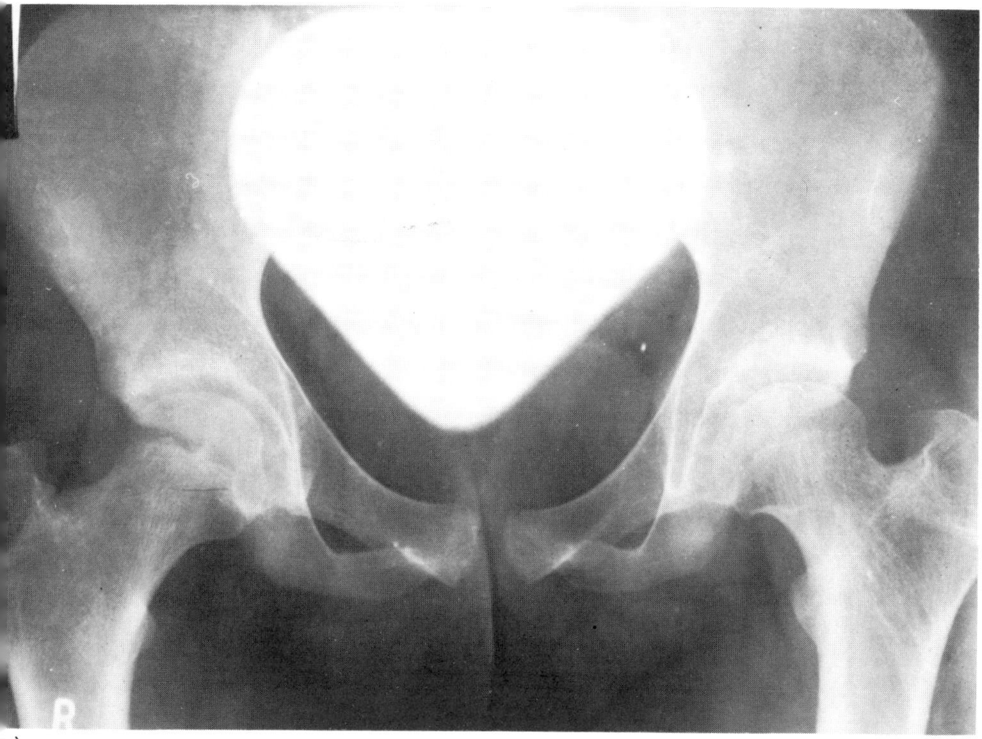

a)

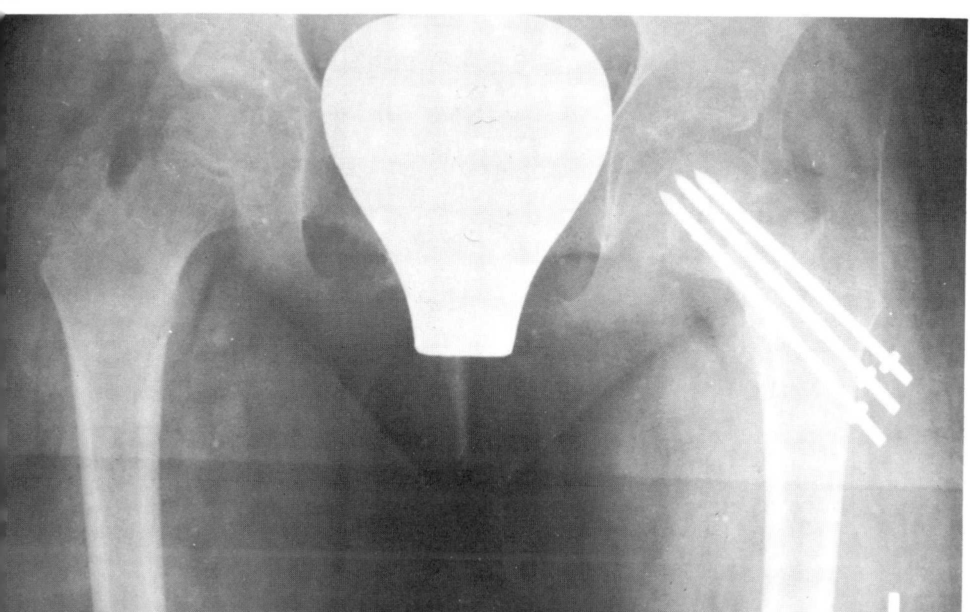

b)

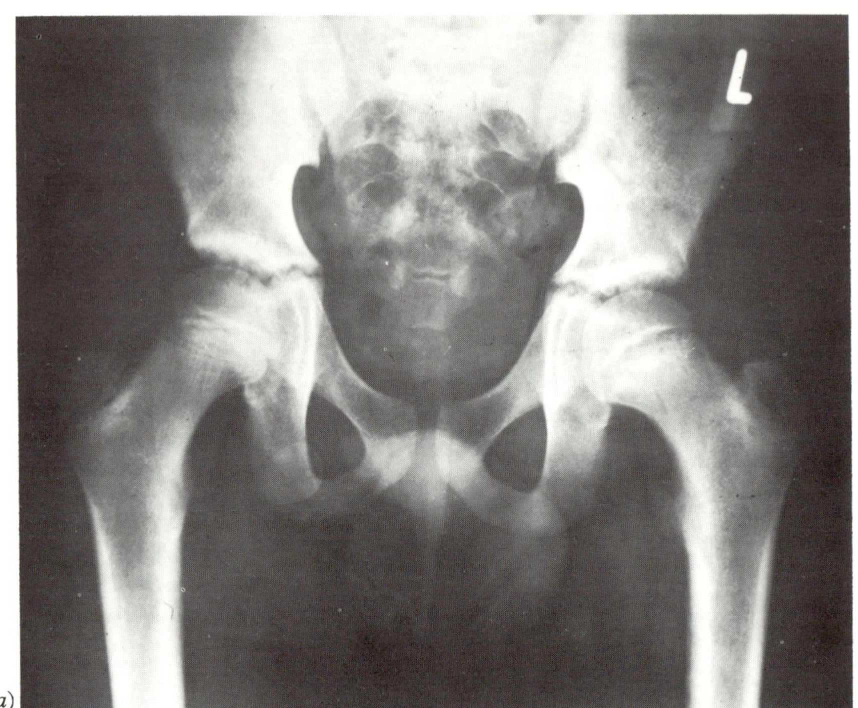

(a)

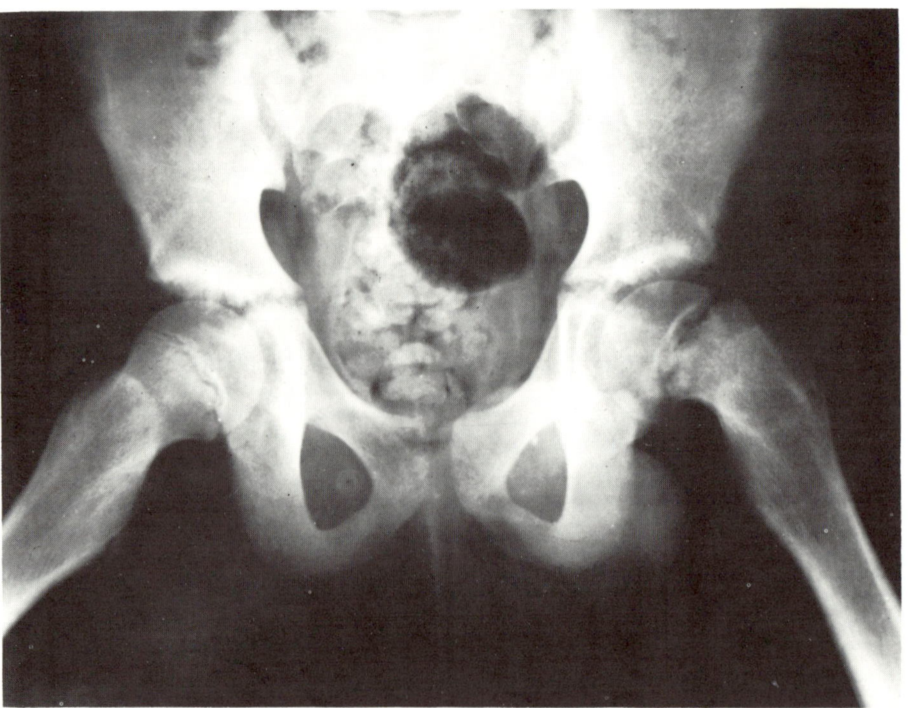
(b)

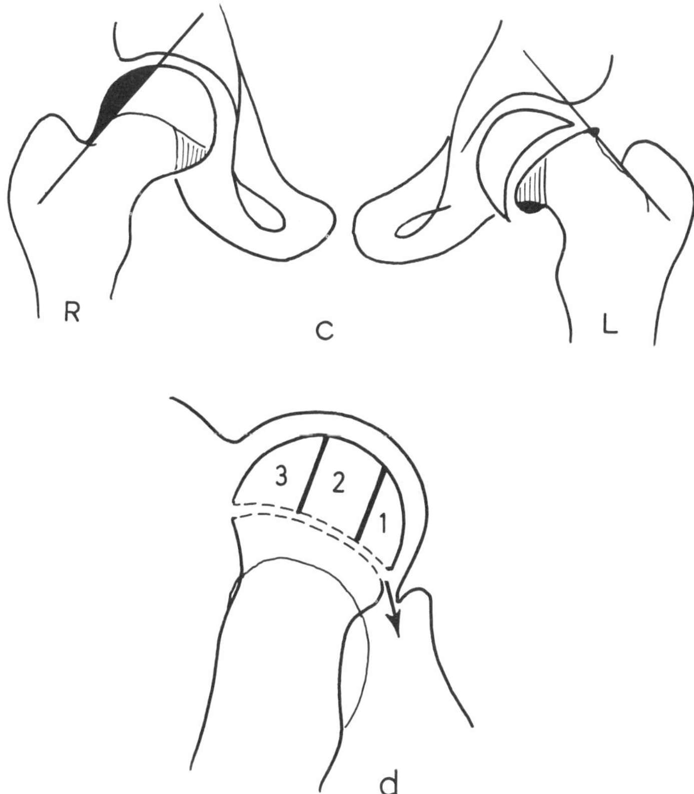

FIG. 9.2 Slipped epiphysis: male aged thirteen years. Five week history of pain. Gross limitation of internal rotation of the left hip. In (*a*) Antero–posterior film showing a wide radio-lucent zone in the line of the epiphyseal cartilage and the absorbed metaphyseal zone. Reactionary radio-density in the diaphysis of the neck. Lateral longitudinal area of femoral capital epiphysis shorter than on right. (*b*) The lateral film is shown. Metaphyseal zone disintegrated and with epiphyseal cartila constituting a wide zone of translucency. Reactionary changes in the diaphysis confirmed. (By permission of F.H.Kemp) (*c*) Diagram showing that a line projected along the upper surface of the femoral neck does not transect the femoral head on the left side, and there is extrusion of the medial third of the metaphysis with remodelling. (*d*) Lateral projection, each area represents the grade of slipping of the head on the neck.

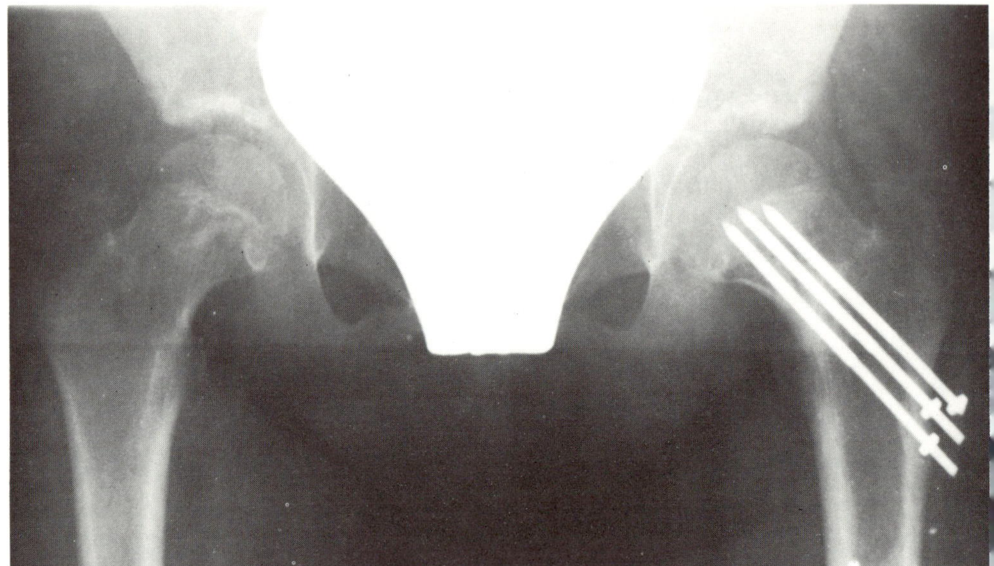

FIG. 9.3 Growth continued but further slipping did not occur when the pins were no longer any use.

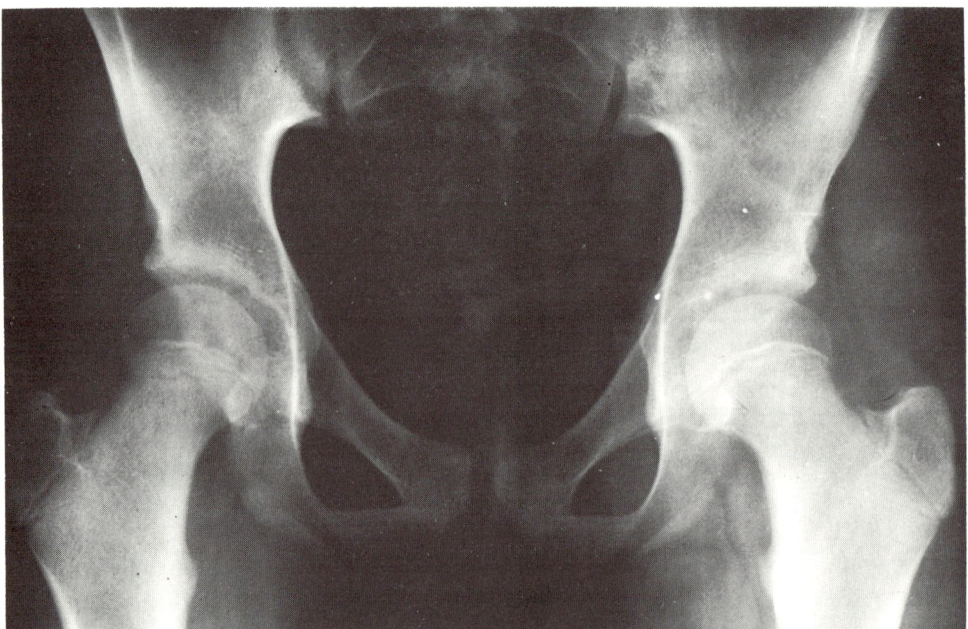

FIG. 9.4 In the antero–posterior view the X-ray of both hips is within normal limits.

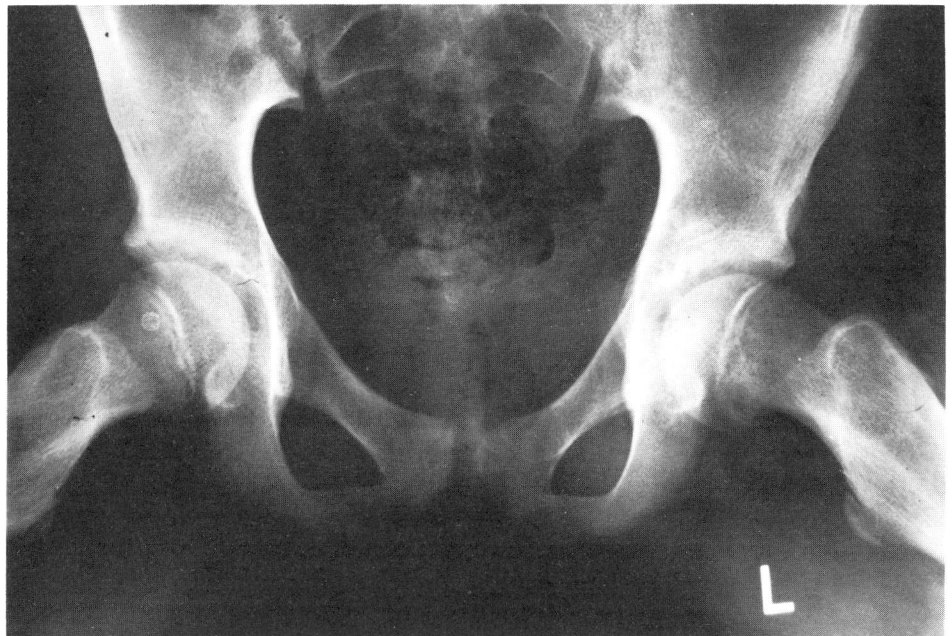

FIG. 9.5 The later view shows posterior slipping of the left epiphysis.

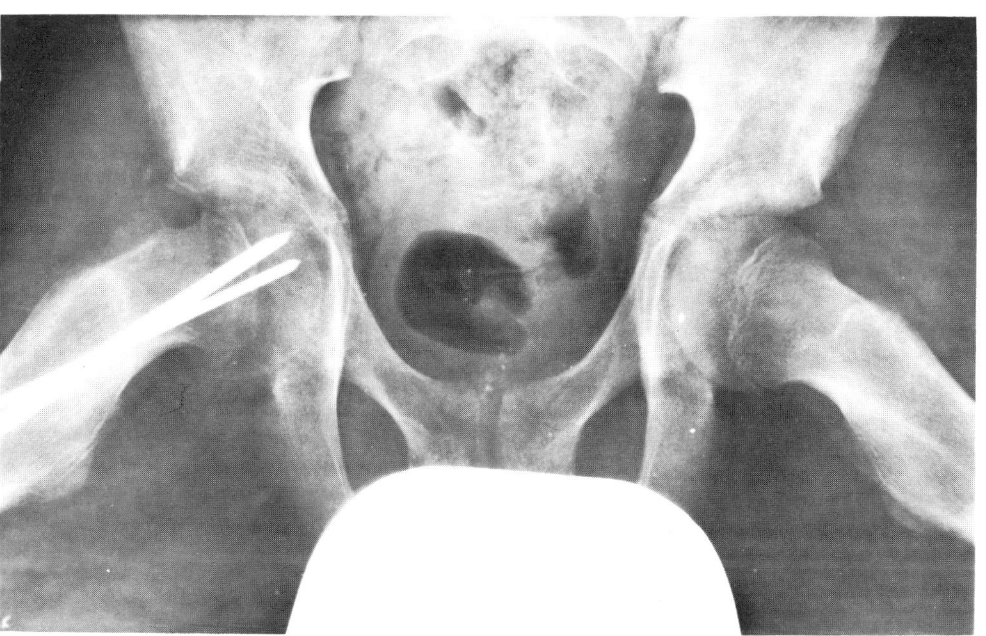

FIG. 9.6 Shows small slip right, the extent of which is to some degree disguised by the moulding of the neck. This position is acceptable.

Acute slip

As a rule there will be some story of trauma although it will be of a minor nature only and in some there will be no history of injury at all. Sometimes there will be a story of a fall or trip but on close questioning it will appear that something happened in the hip first to cause the fall. Pain in the hip and an inability to walk will be features of the complaints. As is so common in children with hip problems the pain may be referred to the knee, and sometimes the only complaint will be of knee pain which may lead to a faulty diagnosis.

On examination it will be noticed that the leg will be lying externally rotated and possibly adducted giving an appearance of shortening. There will be tenderness around the hip and movements will cause pain. Pain will probably exclude further examination which should not be attempted.

Acute on chronic slip

Sometimes following an acute slip, a history will be obtained of minor symptoms in the hip or knee for several weeks or even months often associated with a limp which may have been intermittent. Clinically the picture will be the same as is found when there has been an acute slip.

Chronic slip

A history will be obtained of intermittent discomfort in the hip or knee with occasional exacerbations of more severe pain. The symptoms will tend for a while to increase and the associated limp will become more marked. If no treatment is undertaken the limp will persist but the symptoms of pain will decrease.

On examination it will be seen that there is usually a severe limp of the positive Trendelenberg type. The leg will lie externally rotated and adducted and there will be both real and apparent shortening which in severe cases may be considerable. On palpation around the hip tenderness may be present but is not consistent; however, prominence of the femoral neck anteriorly will be obvious. Movements will usually be much restricted. There will be fixed adduction and external rotation deformities. Flexion is sometimes grossly restricted but when possible will be associated with external rotation. The range and arc of movement will depend on the degree and direction of the slip.

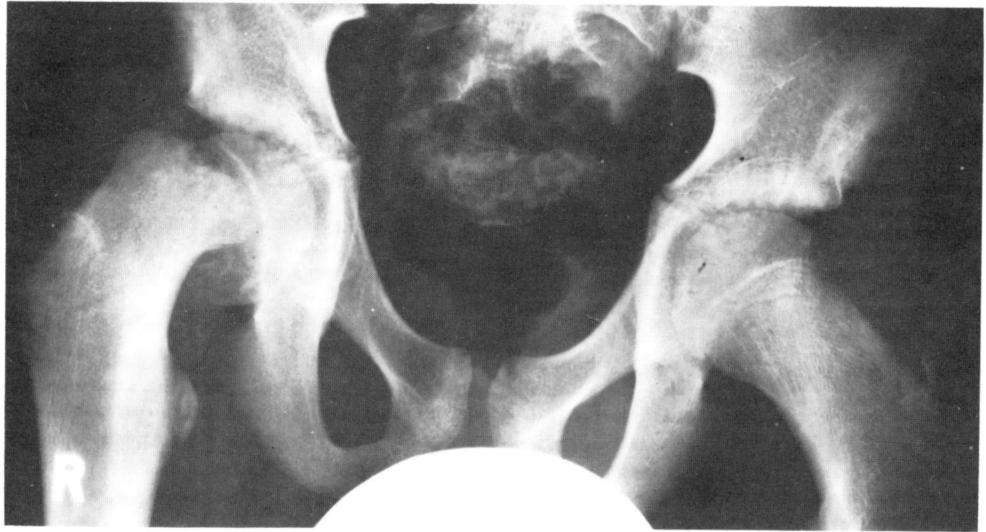

FIG. 9.7 Acute slip of more than 50% will require correction.

THE DISPLACEMENT

While there is the academic point of whether the epiphysis slips on the shaft or the shaft slips on the epiphysis, for the purposes of description it will be considered that the epiphysis slips on the shaft.

The displacement is similar to that of a fracture of the neck of the femur. The epiphysis is displaced mainly posteriorly but to a small extent inferiorly, which is why the leg lies externally rotated and adducted. The extent of the displacement may vary considerably, from only a few degrees to a severe slip with almost complete displacement (Fig. 9.7).

When the displacement is slight (Fig. 9.1) the radiological appearance may be misleading. In the antero–posterior view it may not be possible to detect any abnormality. In any case in which the clinical examination suggests the possibility of slipping, it is essential that a lateral view be taken because it is often only in this view that minor degrees of displacement can be seen (Fig. 9.5).

A preslipping stage has been described in which porotic changes can be seen in the metaphyseal region before a slip actually occurs.

TREATMENT

Treatment nowadays is always surgical with internal fixation of one form or another after reduction of the displacement, if this is necessary. There is no longer any place for conservative treatment and it cannot be over-emphasized that treatment in all those cases where closure of the epiphyseal line has not taken place is a surgical emergency necessitating the patient's immediate admission to hospital for reduction and fixation. Fixation is simple. It is reduction which is difficult.

In many hips the amount of displacement will be only of a minor degree and reduction will not be necessary. It is generally accepted that a slip of up to one-third of the width of the neck does not require correction. This does not mean that in the case of an acute slip, gentle correction should not be carried out with a one-third slip, but that if a one-third displacement remains this is acceptable, and it is quite possible to carry out internal fixation with this amount of displacement.

REDUCTION IN THE ACUTE OR ACUTE ON CHRONIC SLIP

In these cases the epiphysis may still be mobile and it may be possible to produce adequate correction.

Manipulation

This may be either acute or gradual. There has always been disagreement as to whether an acute manipulation under anaesthetic prior to internal fixation is a safe procedure or not. If it is carried out it must be done very gently and no force must be used. First of all gentle but firm traction is applied to the leg with gentle internal rotation. If the epiphysis is very loose reduction will occur but the procedure may be assisted by carrying out the manoeuvre in some flexion because of the element of extension which is present in many cases.

If full correction cannot be obtained easily, a decision must be made as to whether the position is acceptable or whether surgical correction will be necessary. The temptation to improve the position further by a little force must be resisted.

Traction

An alternative to an acute manipulation, and much safer, is gradual reduction with traction and internal rotation. This is best applied through a Steinman pin through the lower end of the femur with balanced traction. Because of the posterior displacement it may be wise to carry out the traction in some flexion. The amount of traction should not exceed 15 lb and this is combined with a rotational force through the pin. If obvious improvement has not been obtained within one week the manoeuvre should be discontinued because improvement will not take place after this and the risk of producing stiffness will increase. It is often very difficult to be certain that improvement has occurred and a very critical assessment of the X-rays must be made.

OPEN REDUCTION OF THE DEFORMITY

This may be carried out at the epiphyseal line, through the neck of the femur or in the subtrochanteric region.

Open reduction through the epiphyseal line

This procedure was first carried out by Whitman (1909) and was later revived by Klein *et al.* (1948). While this operation has the great attraction of correcting the deformity at the right place it has always been criticized because of the considerable risk of damage to the blood supply to the epiphysis with resulting avascular necrosis and it has been considered that the incidence of this serious complication is too high. Newman (1960) suggests that the operation is successful in only two-thirds of cases.

The blood supply to the head of the femur is through two leashes of vessels, one postero-lateral and the other postero-medial; the blood supply through the ligamentum teres is of little importance and is inconstant. The important point is that both main leashes of vessels are slightly posterior so that when the epiphysis displaces posteriorly these vessels are carried backwards with the synovium covering them and their integrity is preserved (Fig. 9.7). The great danger is that the vascular pedicle quite quickly undergoes adaptive shortening and at the same time the neck of the femur increases in length by growth and the formation of callus. Any attempt at reduction in these circumstances will result in the pedicle being put on the stretch with damage to the blood vessels (Fig. 9.8).

Dunn (1964) has made use of these observations in carrying out open reduction before the epiphyseal line has closed with bone (Figs. 9.9–9.11). The hip joint is approached through a lateral incision and

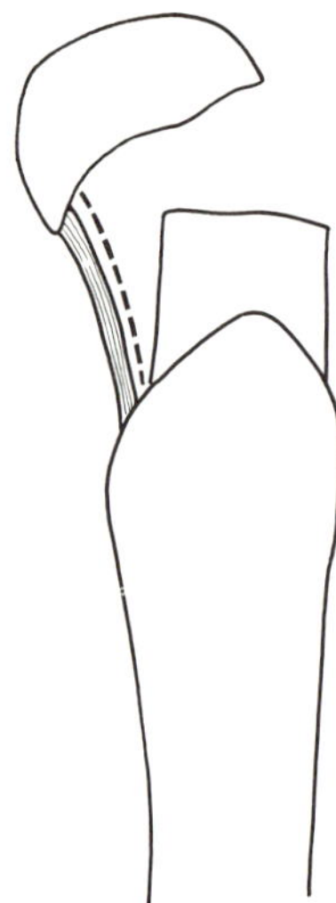

FIG. 9.8 Line drawing showing the synovial pedicle attached to neck and head containing vessels.

the great trochanter is divided at its base and turned up with the attached abductor muscles. The capsule is opened by a T-shaped incision. The synovial pedicle containing the blood vessels is very gently separated from the posterior aspect of the neck of the femur and unless it is completely loose the epiphysis is eased from the neck with a gouge. All of this must be done with great care so that the blood supply is not damaged. The raw surface of the epiphysis is curetted gently and the fact that the blood vessels are intact can be confirmed by the presence of bleeding from the cancellous bone. The neck of the femur is then shortened sufficiently to allow the head of the femur to be replaced on the end of it without putting the pedicle on the stretch. Fixation is by means of three or four pins of the Moore or Newman type. The pins are inserted under direct vision and the position is then confirmed radiologically (Fig. 9.10).

Post-operative care consists of light balanced traction of the Russell type which will allow movements to be started as soon as the post-operative reaction has settled. This is continued for six weeks after which the patient is allowed up, non-weight-bearing on crutches for a further two months. When bony union is demonstrably present radiologically partial weight-bearing and finally full weight-bearing is allowed. Fig. 9.10 shows the result five years after treatment when the pins have been removed.

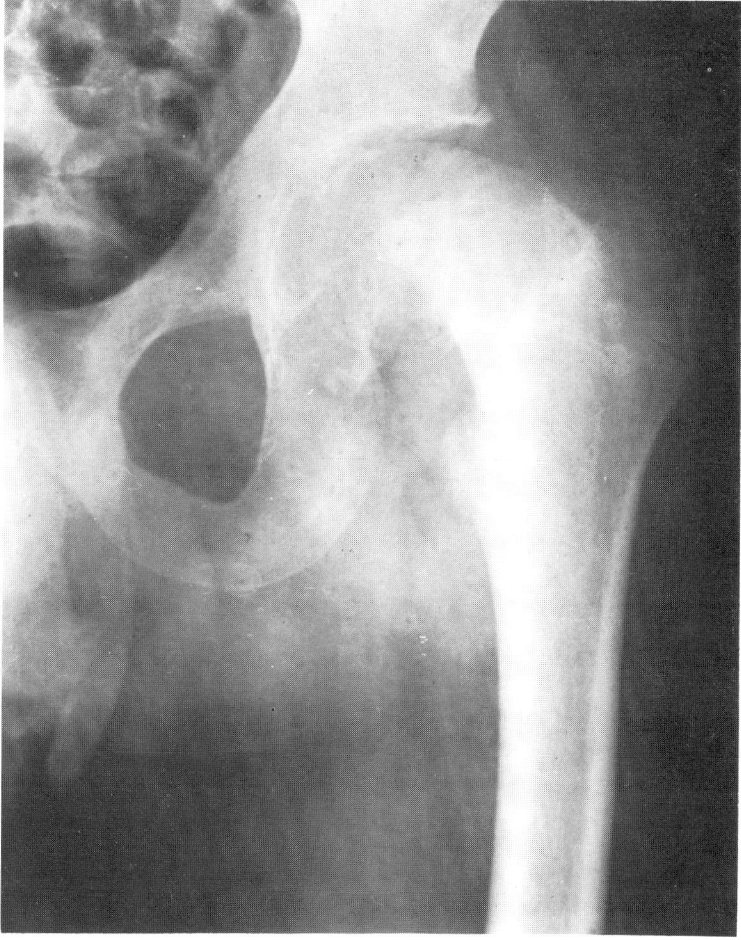

FIG. 9.9 Severe displacement with probably fibrous union. Correction is only possible with open operation.

Osteotomy through neck of femur

For those cases in which the epiphysis is already fused to the neck by bone with an unacceptable degree of deformity which is seriously affecting function, Foley (1946) described an osteotomy of the neck of the femur. He approached the hip through an anterior Smith-Petersen incision, and making no attempt to produce correction at the site of the deformity removed a wedge from the neck of the femur. The base of the wedge was situated antero–superiorly and was taken in such a

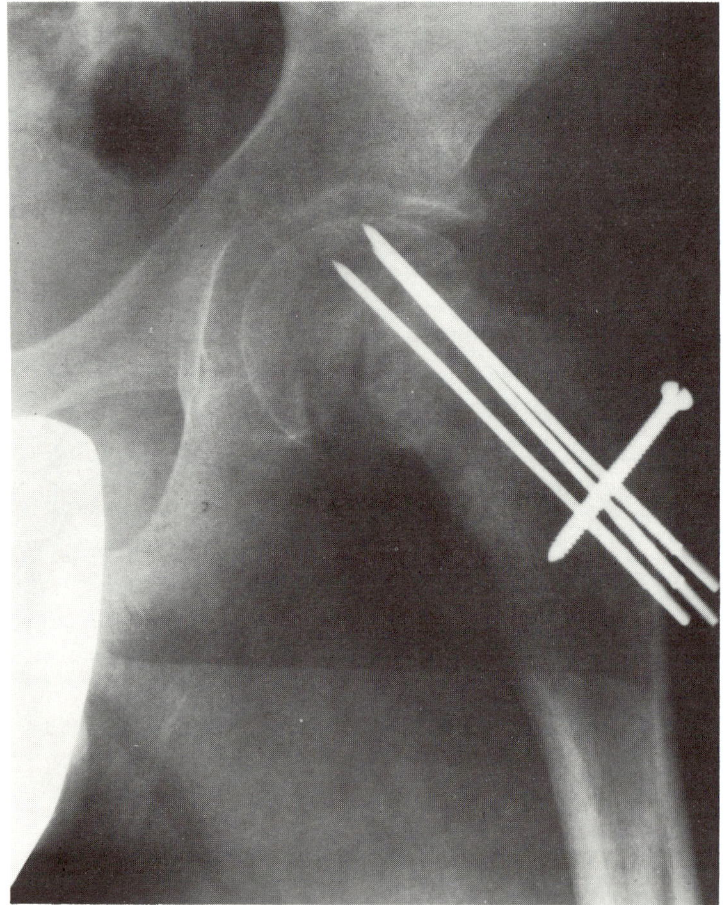

FIG. 9.10 Position after correction as described by Dunn. Fixation with Adam's pins.

way so as to produce shortening of the neck (Fig. 9.12). In removing this wedge great care had to be taken to avoid damage to the vascular pedicle which was lying posteriorly. Foley used a Smith-Petersen nail for securing internal fixation but multiple pins are to be preferred.

Subtrochanteric osteotomy

As already mentioned all open reductions carry with them a high risk of vascular damage with the serious complication of avascular necrosis and such operations should only be carried out by those with some

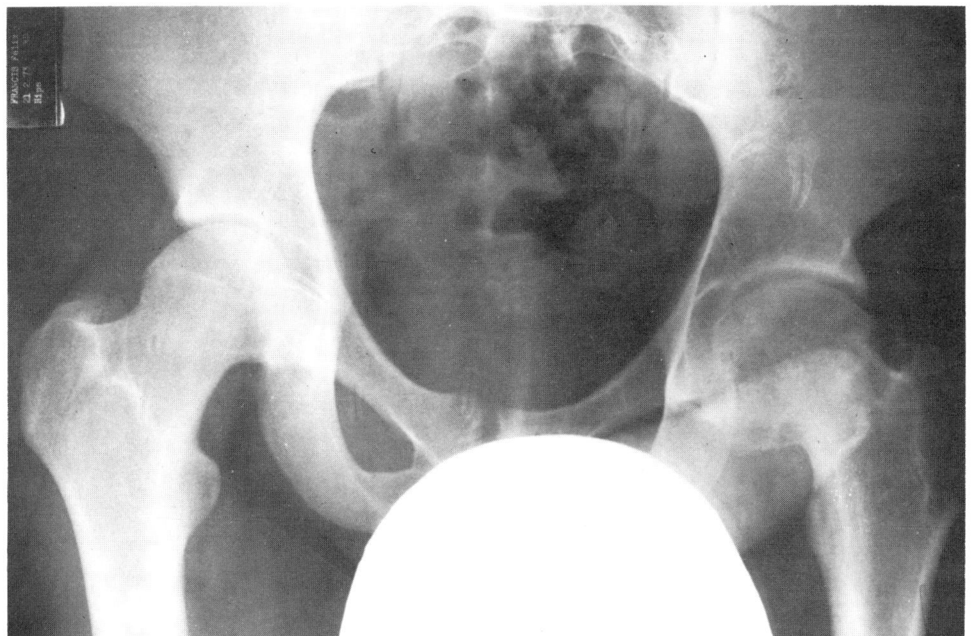

FIG. 9.11 The final result five years later.

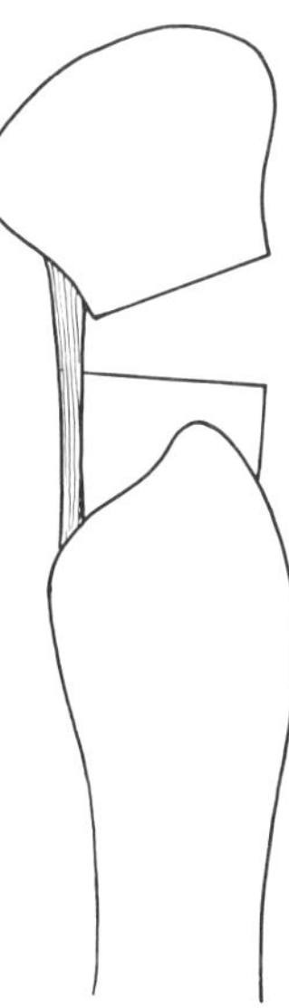

FIG. 9.12 Correction of extension, adduction and external rotation by osteotomy.

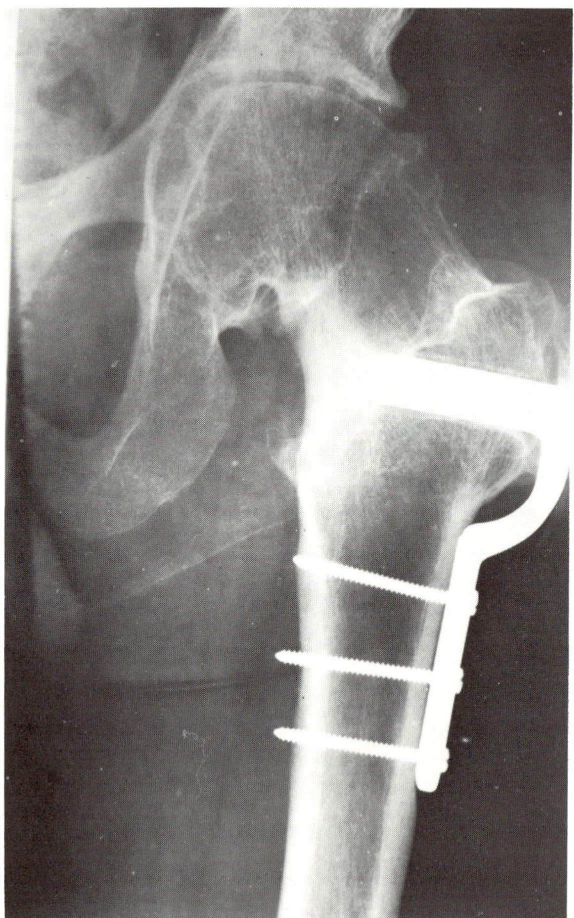

FIG. 9.13 Sub-trochanteric osteotomy with Müller–Harris spline.

knowledge of this type of surgery. A far safer procedure is subtrochanteric osteotomy. The anatomical result is less good from this operation but the functional result is satisfactory and the risks are much less.

The upper end of the femur is approached through a lateral incision as when carrying out a nailing for a fracture of the neck of the femur. The deformities which have to be corrected are extension, adduction and internal rotation. The extension/adduction can be corrected by removing a wedge with its base anterior and lateral. The size of the wedge and its siting is best estimated on clinical rather than radiological grounds. In order to render the location of the wedge as simple as possible and to enable the rotational deformity to be corrected, it is wisest to remove the wedge from the proximal fragment, the distal fragment being cut transversely. In this way when rotation is carried out the mechanics of the wedge will not be altered, as would be the case if the wedge had been removed from the lower fragment or worse still from both. Internal fixation may be either by a nail-plate or by a Müller-Harris spline (Fig. 9.13). Whichever is used it is often helpful to assess the correction before doing the osteotomy and introduce the spline or nail into the intact femur, then to remove it leaving its track ready for its reinsertion when the correction has been carried out.

INTERNAL FIXATION

Internal fixation presents few problems. In the earlier cases it was common practice to use a Smith-Petersen nail (Fig. 9.14). This affords good fixation but has certain disadvantages. In a young patient the head of the femur is often extremely hard and it may require great force to knock the pin in. This in itself may cause vascular damage and it is not unknown for the head of the femur to be knocked off producing

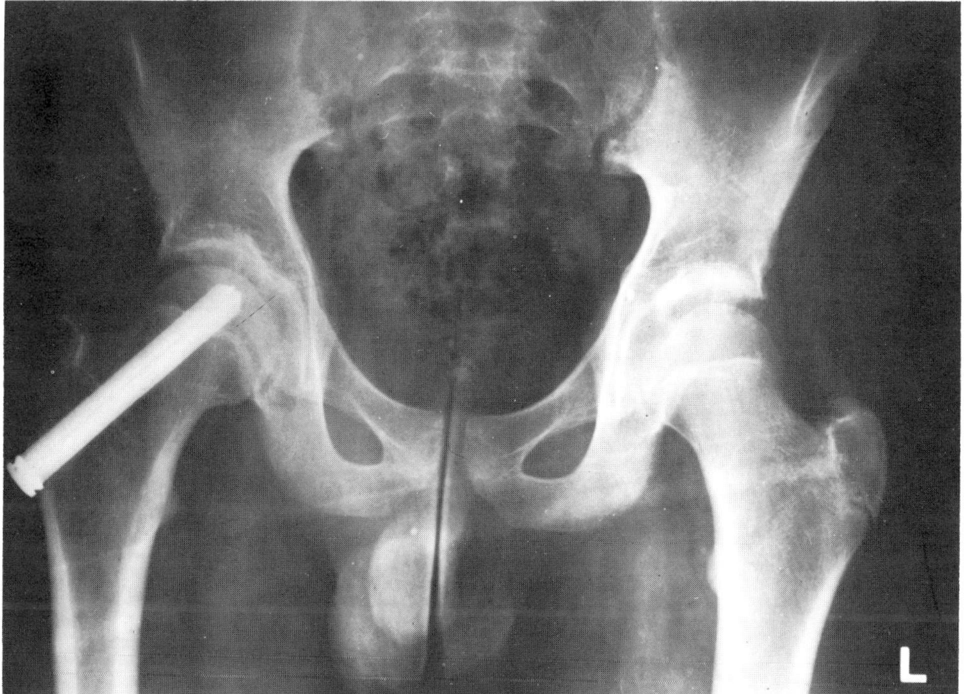

FIG. 9.14 Internal fixation with a Smith-Petersen nail.

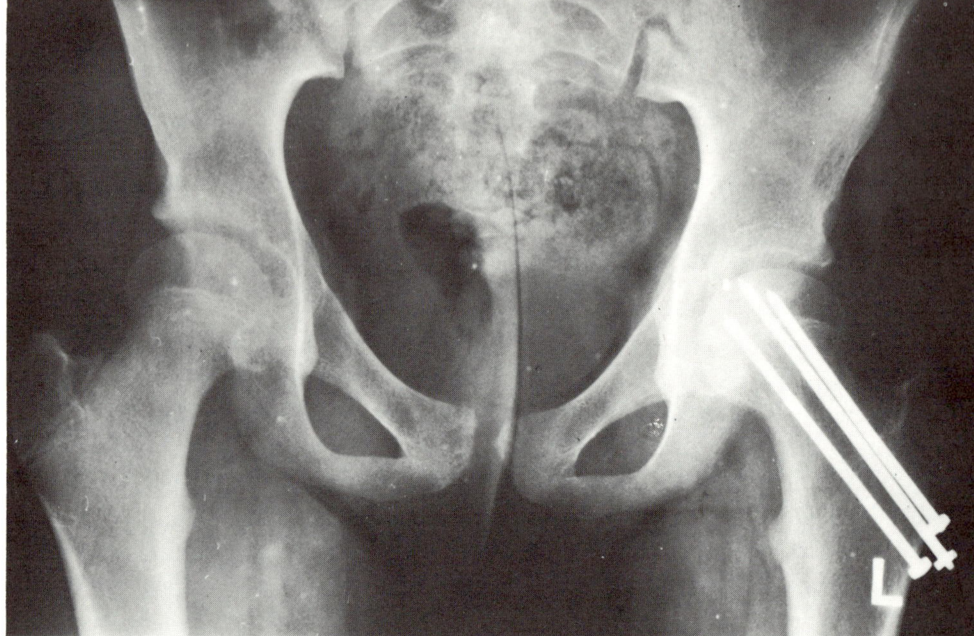

FIG. 9.15 Internal fixation with Moore's pins.

wide separation at the epiphyseal line with resulting avascular necrosis.

For this reason it is better to use multiple pins. These can be of different types. Probably Moore's pins are most commonly used (Fig. 9.15). These pins provide excellent fixation, and having a thread on half the shaft can be screwed in with great accuracy. Only three pins are necessary. They have the great disadvantage that they can be very difficult to remove. The pins described by Newman or Adams do not have this disadvantage and may be preferred.

It is advisable to remove all pins or nails when the epiphysis is closed at about the end of one year. If when removing Moore's pins it is necessary to ream around them because they are so firmly embedded the bone may be substantially weakened and it is not unknown for spontaneous fractures to occur. Post-operatively it is wise to insist on partial weight-bearing with crutches for at least one month.

The other hip

Some degree of slipping may occur in the other hip in about 25% of cases although some authors have put the incidence higher than this.

This is not sufficiently high to warrant prophylactic pinning but it is very important to watch the other hip until the epiphysis is fused so that if a slip occurs it can be fixed as early as possible.

COMPLICATIONS

Complications result from vascular damage and from persistent deformity. The fact that it is in the hips which are the most seriously displaced and that they rarely occur in untreated hips indicates the importance of undertaking treatment only with the greatest care.

The causes of avascular necrosis of the head of the femur have already been discussed (Chapter 5). The changes may become apparent during treatment but it is not uncommon for them to be unseen for some months after all treatment has been completed. Radiologically the epiphysis becomes dense, the joint space becomes narrow, the bone collapses and gradually disintegrates resulting inevitably in osteoarthritis. In many hips the clinical picture of slight spasm, some loss of movement and discomfort with a limp lasting longer than might be expected will suggest that all is not well, often long before the X-ray confirms the diagnosis. No treatment will improve the hip and the best result that can be expected is an arthrodesis. Such children are young for any form of arthroplasty.

Lowe (1961, 1970) has described the development of cartilage necrosis. This condition develops quite separately from avascular necrosis with which it seems to have no connection. The hip becomes stiff and painful with much spasm and on X-ray it is seen that the articular cartilage is degenerating. Although in many cases the condition leads in the end to arthrodesis, in a certain number, spontaneous recovery will occur aided by gentle non-weight-bearing exercises.

The longer term complications are associated with persistent deformity leading to arthritis, although it is surprising how long a hip even with severe deformity will continue to work well and give very little trouble even in the presence of gross deformity. It is also found that an appreciable number of arthritic hips appearing in later life without known cause have the origin of arthritis in a minor slip in adolescence which has passed undetected.

REFERENCES

DUNN, D.M. (1964). *J. Bone Jt. Surg.* **46B**, 621.
FOLEY, W.B. (1946). *Proc. R. Soc. Med.* **39**, 201.
HOWARTH, M.B. (1941). *Surgery Gynec. Obstet.* **73**, 723.
KLEIN, A. JOPLIN, R.J. and REIDY, J.A. (1948). *J. Am. med. Ass.* **136**, 445.
LOWE, H.G. (1961). *J. Bone Jt. Surg.* **43B**, 688.
LOWE, H.G. (1970). *J. Bone Jt. Surg.* **52B**, 108.
NEWMAN, P.H. (1960). *J. Bone Jt. Surg.* **42B**, 280.
NEWMAN, P.H. (1964). *J. Bone Jt. Surg.* **46B**, 155.
RENNIE, A.M. (1959). *J. Bone Jt. Surg.* **41B**, No. 3.
WHITMAN, R. (1909). *Med. Rec.* **75**, 1.

Chapter Ten

MEDICAL FACTORS

H. C. Burbidge, D. S. Muckle, R. A. Griffiths

PRE-OPERATIVE ASSESSMENT AND PREMEDICATION

PRE-OPERATIVE ASSESSMENT

On average, elderly patients present no particular problem to the anaesthetist and tolerate operations, especially those with which we are concerned, very well indeed. However, the effects of drug therapy (including anaesthetics) may vary greatly for individual patients depending on their general condition and the state of shock. Also the autonomic nervous system may be slow or deficient in response to the calls made on it, and cardiovascular atherosclerosis may adversely impair the response of the heart or the central nervous system to medicaments.

From the viewpoint of the anaesthetist, the usual criteria pertaining to all accidents apply in the first place. The possibility of additional injuries, especially head or thoracic injuries, are considered with regard to their effects on the outcome of general anaesthesia. Such injuries will probably have received appropriate attention before the patient is seen by the anaesthetist, but signs of progressive increase in intracranial pressure, atelectasis or pneumothorax must be borne in mind. Atelectasis can develop quite rapidly, especially in the partially dehydrated emphysematous or bronchitic patient, due to difficulties in expelling glutinous mucus.

If the patient is considered unfit for general anaesthesia then local anaesthesia can be used, although spinal anaesthesia should not be the first choice in patients over 60 years because of the possibility of producing bladder or prostatic problems.

Many old people are found to be in a state of dehydration and this requires attention before operation. The common signs are thirst, dry mouth, flaccid subcutaneous tissue, rapid pulse of poor volume, low blood pressure and poor urinary output. Blood urea and electrolytes, haemoglobin and packed cell volume should be obtained and, if necessary, estimated regularly. Saline, dextrose–saline or dextran solutions are given but care must be taken not to overload the circulation. A dehydrated elderly patient is a serious surgical and post-operative risk and adequate time should be allowed, after commencing treatment, for the fluid balance of the body to readjust.

If present on admission, shock will have been treated by the surgical team. However, it must not be forgotten that injections intramuscularly or subcutaneously to a shocked patient may have poor absorption and, in consequence, little effect. Thus the dose is sometimes repeated fairly soon thereafter. When the shock is alleviated the greatly improved circulation carries a double dose of depressant analgesic into the body with greatly increased effect and side-effects.

In shock it is much safer to give small doses of the chosen analgesic in a diluted form intravenously and to repeat, as necessary, at 15–20 min periods until the desired pain relief and sedation have been achieved. This periodicity allows time for any untoward effects, such as respiratory depression, to become manifest. The alleviation of pain is an important step in the reversal of the state of shock, but must be carried out with care and constant observation.

A history of previous disabilities or illnesses should be noted and a list of current medications obtained. Under the stress of an accident, or merely from diminishing faculties, the patient often forgets important information, and it is wise to question relatives or friends as well.

Cardiovascular system

Dyspnoea on mild exertion, orthopnoea and especially nocturnal dyspnoea sound a warning of cardiac problems and an ECG should be taken, even if cardiac arrhythmias are not clinically obvious. Operation should be postponed if the signs of heart failure are found, and the patient sedated and given analgesics while efforts are made to treat the cardiac problem. Extra care is required during premedication and anaesthesia if the patient is on digoxin, propranolol or other related drugs. For example, atrial fibrillation well controlled on digoxin, with an apical pulse of 60/min, may be found in a patient with a femoral neck fracture. But, this patient's myocardium may not respond to the acceleratory effect of atropine, and will then be in danger of excessive bradycardia developing from the effects of the anaesthetic such as halothane. It is well to allow time and therapy to correct any drug effects before surgery, but reasonable and satisfactory digitalization should not be stopped.

Hypertension may well be an additional hazard and the patient may be on hypotensive therapy. This therapy should not suddenly be curtailed, but care must be taken that other drugs are not given which increase the hazards of loss of blood pressure control during the anaesthetic. If the patient is being treated, or has been treated within the previous two weeks, with reserpine, monoamine oxidase inhibitors, guanethidine, tricyclic anti-depressants or chlorpromazine, careful consideration should be given to stopping these drugs; their elimination will occur while substitution therapy of a safer type is made. If this is not possible the premedication should be such that the risks of marked changes in blood pressure before and during anaesthesia are reduced. Droperidol 5.0–10 mg and phenoperidine 1.0–1.5 mg on average are an excellent premedication given intramuscularly 1 h before operation in this respect. Monoamine oxidase inhibitors reduce the excretion time of phenoperidine and pethidine.

The respiratory system

Chronic bronchitis, emphysema and bronchial asthma are the more common respiratory problems which can hinder satisfactory ventilation in the elderly with femoral neck fractures. Bronchiectasis may also be present. Acute pulmonary conditions preclude operation until they have been satisfactorily treated and pulmonary function studies may be needed. These include vital capacity, forced expiratory volume in one second and blood gases. Morphine and allied substances act as a respiratory depressant and reduce vital capacity. Chronic bronchitis presents a special problem in old people with hip injuries. If bed rest and immobility are prolonged, even for a few days, there is a real danger of progressive basal congestion of the lungs unless adequate treatment is given. Broad spectrum antibiotics, mucolytics, as much postural drainage with gentle percussion of the chest as the hip condition will allow and bronchodilators are used. Isoprenaline by nebulizer, or as 5.0 mg of the sulphate sublingually, are effective; salbutamol can be substituted for isoprenaline. Most of the patients with cardiovascular and respiratory dysfunction will prefer to be propped up in bed. Bronchial suction can also be performed in this position under local anaesthetic spray.

Diabetes mellitus

If surgery is delayed the pre-operative regime should include carbohydrate and insulin. Hypoglycaemia must be avoided, and it is better to risk hyperglycaemia during the operative period. Tests for glycosuria and ketonuria are performed and blood sugars estimated; a fasting blood sugar should not exceed 8 mmol/l (140 mg %) over the age of 50 years. It is usual to set up a 5% dextrose/saline drip before emergency surgery, and if insulin is indicated the soluble variety should be used because of shorter action and better control. Dietary controlled diabetics may be upset by surgery and hyperglycaemia and glycosuria persisting beyond the first post-operative day requires insulin for a short period. Oral hypoglycaemic drugs usually act for 12–16 h, but chlorpropamide can act for up to 60 h and should be stopped 24 h before surgery. If hypoglycaemia threatens, 25% glucose is given intravenously in 25 ml solution. Normal diets should commence as soon as possible after surgery, and a constant infusion of 5% glucose guards against hypoglycaemia.

The screening of elderly patients by random blood samples (mid-morning) should be carried out and glucose levels above 10 mmol/l (180 mg/100 ml) merit a glucose tolerance curve. Urine testing is highly unreliable as a screening test in old people as a raised renal threshold for glucose is commonly found.

Steroid treatment

Steroid treatment, either currently or within the previous six months, make it advisable to administer hydrocortisone hemisuccinate 100 mg i.m. both with the premedication and post-operatively, and the dose may be repeated for three days, if indicated. Patients receiving routine doses of prednisolone or equivalent steroids not exceeding 7.5 mg per day are not considered to be in danger during anaesthesia, but a single dose of 100 mg of hydrocortisone hemisuccinate i.m. is a wise precaution. Further doses can be given when indicated. It is not now considered necessary to perform a slow build-up and decline of therapy over several days as was formerly the custom.

PREMEDICATION

Many elderly patients, apparently quite frail, will prove surprisingly resistant to analgesic, sedative or central depressant drugs. The withholding of adequate amounts of pain-relieving drugs can lead to restlessness, agitation and thus deterioration in the general condition. The failure to provide pain relief out of consideration for the patient's age and apparent frailty is quite common, often being based on the incorrect assumption that respiratory depression is frequent after sedative and analgesic therapy in the aged.

Often the houseman or senior house officer is required to prescribe both the sedation and analgesic and in some cases the premedication; the latter at the wish of the duty anaesthetist. Thus some knowledge of the commoner premedication drugs is needed (Table 10.1).

Morphine is the commonly used analgesic-sedative, dosage 8–20 mg of the sulphate, with 10 mg premedication dose. If shock is present,

TABLE 10.1 Commonly used drugs for premedication

		Compound	i.m. dosage (mg)	
I	Analgesia and sedation	Morphine	5–10	
		Omnopon	10	
II	Analgesics	Pethidine	50–100	
		Phenoperidine	0.5–2	
		Fentanyl	0.05–0.1 (i.v.)	
		Levorphanol	1–2 (i.v.)	
			1–4	
III	Sedation	Droperidol	5–10	Can be combined with groups I or II
		Diazepam	5–20	
IV	Anti-cholinergic	Atropine	0.6	Can be combined with groups I and II
		Hyoscine	0.2–0.4	

(i.v. = intravenous dose).

or in the very old or debilitated it is wise to give increments of 2.5 mg diluted in 5 ml of water i.v.; allowing about 10 min between doses, up to the required amount for pain relief (usually 5–10 mg). Respiratory depression may occur, and bronchial asthma and emphysema are contra-indications; also signs of increased intracranial pressure, hypothyroidism, severe liver disease, steroid therapy (for adreno-cortical insufficiency) and recent treatment with monoamine oxidase inhibitors preclude the routine use. Kidney disease slows the elimination of morphine.

Omnopon (*Papaveretum*) has similar effects to morphine, 20 mg omnopon being equivalent to about 13.5 mg of morphine. Omnopon is commonly prescribed in 10 mg doses, this is only equivalent to 6.7 mg morphine, which is reasonably safe in older patients.

Droperidol (*Droleptan*) is a non-hypnotic sedative and is non-depressing to respiration. It is anti-emetic, potentiates analgesic drugs, and helps greatly by reducing the mental reaction to stress. It is useful when spinal anaesthesia is contemplated. It should not be used in Parkinsonian patients. The dose is 5 mg i.v. or 5–10 mg i.m., followed by a small dose of morphia or omnopon. In the author's experience this has proved to be an excellent premedication for the aged.

Diazepam (Valium) has no analgesic properties, and is only slightly depressant to respiration and the cardiovascular system. It has no anti-emetic action. However, it is an effective sedative for the anxious and restless patient. Dosage is 5–20 mg i.m.

Levorphanol tartrate (Dromoran) 2.0 mg i.m. is a substitute for morphine, being more powerful and longer acting, but it does not have the sedating properties.

Perphenazine (Fentazin) 2.5–5.0 mg i.m. is a sedative, strongly anti-emetic and can be combined with an analgesic drug. It is not so effective for calming the apprehensive patient as droperidol.

Pethidine is not really advisable in the elderly as it frequently causes hypotension and circulatory effects due to myocardial depression and peripheral vasodilatation. Dosage 50–100 mg i.m. or 10–25 mg i.v. It tends to relax bronchospasm and so may be preferred for the asthmatic or chronic bronchitic patient, but it has a powerful respiratory depressant action.

Phenoperidine (Operidine) 0.5–2.0 mg i.m. or i.v. or *Fentanyl* (Sublimaze) 0.05–0.10 mg i.v. are more powerful substitutes for pethidine and have similar effects, more marked but of a shorter duration.

Atropine The former tendency to prescribe this drug in the premedication one hour before surgery is changing to giving it intravenously with the inducing agents, thus avoiding the uncomfortable 'drying up' effect on the bronchial mucus and salivary gland secretions. The partial blocking effect on the vagus produces an acceleration in the pulse rate of up to 20 beats/min. The adult dose is 0.6 mg whichever route is used. Atropine should not be given to hyperpyrexic patients or when there is already a tachycardia present for any pathological reason, especially in the case of heart disease.

Hyoscine (Scopolamine)

Has similar actions to atropine and is a more powerful drying agent, but has in addition a depressant effect on the central nervous system, producing drowsiness and amnesia which can be pleasant for the patient. However, some young and elderly patients may suffer excitement and restlessness and for this reason it is not considered to be suitable in these groups. Dosage is 0.3–0.6 mg in the adult, commonly given in the proportion of hyoscine 0.2 mg with omnopon 10 mg (or morphine 5–10 mg).

This short article covers the more usual findings in patients in this accident group, and the most straightforward means of dealing with them; it is of necessity only a brief summary of some of the conditions associated with advancing years and drug therapy under stress.

THE POST-OPERATIVE PROBLEM

BRONCHOPNEUMONIA

Bronchopneumonia in the elderly may not be accompanied by pyrexia and leukocytosis, but increasing confusion, apathy, hypotension and rapid pulse and respiration in the post-operative period should arouse suspicion. In the early stage physical signs of consolidation may be absent on chest examination, while X-rays may show only minimal congestive changes at the lung bases. Sputum, which may be difficult to obtain, and blood cultures should be taken for the identification of the bacterial pathogen. Treatment is usually empirical and as the most dangerous hospital pathogens are Gram-negative bacteria and penicillin-resistant staphylococci, the antibiotics given should be a combination of ampicillin and cloxacillin (or talampicillin and flucloxacillin), initially by injection. Later the antibiotics can be changed according to sensitivity results.

HEART FAILURE

Left ventricular failure can occur alone but often accompanies bronchopneumonia. An electrocardiograph is needed to exclude silent myocardial infarction. In acute heart failure an intravenous diuretic (e.g. frusemide, 10 mg) will produce a rapid response; a larger dose may produce dehydration in the elderly and should be used with care. A combination of pethidine (25 mg) and levallorphan (0.3125 mg) i.v. or i.m. will allay anxiety and distress. Rapid digitalization is not usually necessary but can be initiated using smaller doses than in younger patients, e.g. digoxin 0.0625 mg (Lanoxin) three times daily, reducing to once daily.

Bronchopneumonia, left ventricular failure and pulmonary embolism may present difficulties in differential diagnosis and it is sometimes necessary to institute treatment for all three pending the return of investigatory results.

DEEP VEIN THROMBOSIS AND PULMONARY EMBOLISM

The most serious complication following a femoral neck fracture is pulmonary embolism, a sequel to deep vein thrombosis.

For many years the local signs in the legs, a spike of temperature, a pulmonary embolus, or the post-mortem findings were the only ways of diagnosing a deep vein thrombus. Other more sophisticated methods of diagnosis are now available.

Phlebography

Evans and Negus (1971) concluded that the best method of diagnosing a deep vein thrombosis was by phlebography. The only drawbacks were that it required skilled medical personnel to carry it out and that the calf sinusoids were not always fully demonstrated. Often it can be used after simpler techniques (ultrasound or radio-iodinated fibrinogen uptake) to give more definitive evidence of the thrombus especially its exact site, extent and fixity.

Phlebography has shown that 60% of venous thromboses occur in the calf, 25% in the thigh and 6% in the iliac veins and inferior vena cava (Gibbs, 1957). However, where the risks of embolism are highest, the incidence of thrombosis is low. Gibbs (1957) in a post-mortem study of 34 cases of pulmonary embolism found that in 23 cases the embolus had arisen from the femoral vein, the external iliac vein or the inferior vena cava. Mavor and Galloway (1969) found that two-thirds of all

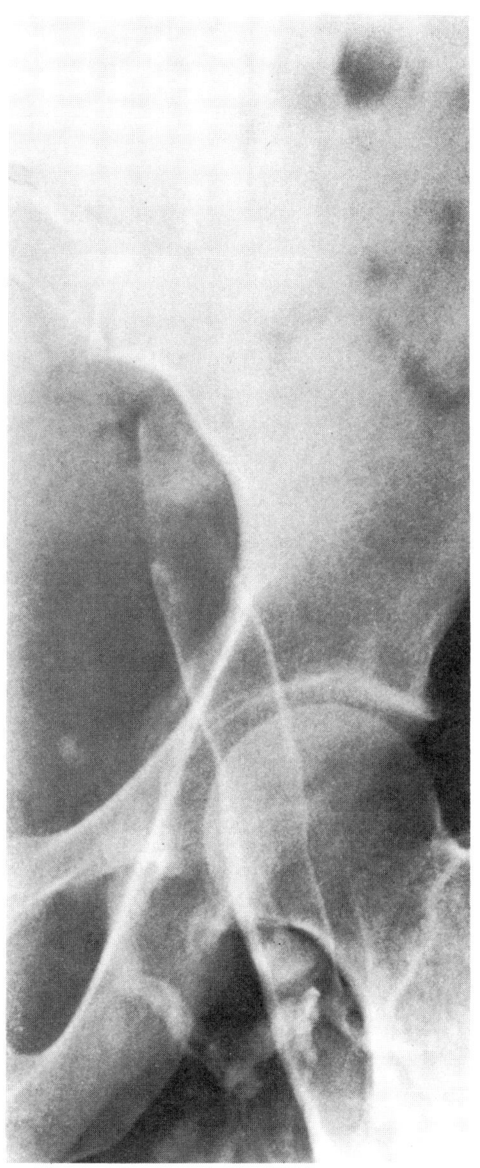

FIG. 10.1 A venogram showing the outline of the femoral and external iliac veins which are occluded with a thrombus. (By kind permission of Dr D. Tibbutt.)

cases of pulmonary embolism were derived from the ilio-femoral segment. Kemble (1971) reported that in 85 patients undergoing hip operations, 35% developed a deep vein thrombosis, with almost all (90%) occurring in the operative leg.

Phlebography has also shown that when the clinical signs are mild, the accuracy of clinical diagnosis is only about 50% (Flanc *et al.*, 1968) (Fig. 10.1).

^{125}I-labelled fibrinogen uptake

Negus *et al.* (1968) showed a 93% correlation between the results of phlebography and this method, which is simple to use. Care should be taken in the interpretation of results if the patient has had signs for more than five days; and it is not effective in diagnosing a thrombus in the femoral or iliac veins. A further disadvantage is that fibrinogen is taken up by healing wounds.

Ultrasound

Ultrasound is a simple screening test but will not detect minor calf vein thromboses, or if the vein is only partially occluded, the thrombus may be overlooked (Evans, 1970). Also if there is a good collateral flow around the obstruction the thrombus may not be found without careful siting of the transducer.

Therapy

Sevitt and Gallagher (1959) found that only 2 out of 150 patients with femoral neck injuries and hip fractures died from pulmonary embolism when anticoagulant therapy was instituted as a routine compared with 15 in a similar number of controls, not anticoagulated. Hamilton *et al.* (1970) studied 76 patients with femoral neck fractures using phlebograhic methods to detect the incidence of thrombosis. Their analysis showed that the incidence of this complication was significantly less in the anticoagulant group (19%) compared to the untreated controls (48%).

The most important aspect of therapy is to prevent a pulmonary embolus; although late complications of deep vein thrombosis such as persistent leg swelling, ulceration and other trophic changes, varicose veins, eczema and chronic venous insufficiency demand adequate treatment of the initial thrombus.

Oral anticoagulants are not effective until 24–48 h after oral administration so it is customary to cover the initial period with heparin 5 000–10 000 units i.v. every 6 h. Warfarin, 15 mg initially, with a dosage schedule to keep the prothrombin time to around 20% has been shown to be effective in reducing the incidence of pulmonary embolism after hip surgery (Muckle *et al.*, 1974). Anticoagulants are continued for 10–12 weeks.

Fibrinolytic agents (such as Streprokinase and Urokinase) are effective when the thrombi have been present for less than 96 h. Kakkar

(1971) advises a loading dose of 500 000 units of streptokinase over 30 min followed by a maintenance dose of 600 000 units every 6 h; the dose being dissolved in normal saline and given as a slow infusion. It can be given in high dosage in the region of the thrombus (Mavor *et al.*, 1969).

Many other forms of therapy are advocated including defibrinating agents (ancrod, Reid and Chan, 1968); subcutaneous heparin, 5000 units by deep subcutaneous injection, twelve hourly until full mobilization; and plasma expanders such as dextran 70 given both during and on alternate days after surgery.

In conclusion, the incidence of deep vein thrombosis can be reduced by early mobilization, passive compression on the limb from elastic supports and intermittent compression to the calves from pneumatic bags or galvanic stimulation. However prophylactic oral anticoagulants probably remain the most effective method.

Pulmonary embolism

This is referred to as massive when half of the pulmonary tree is blocked compared to the minor form which usually has repetitive embolization. Both may be fatal or cause chronic pulmonary hypertension. One-third of massive emboli are preceded by minor emboli.

Minor embolism presents with haemoptysis and pleurisy; major

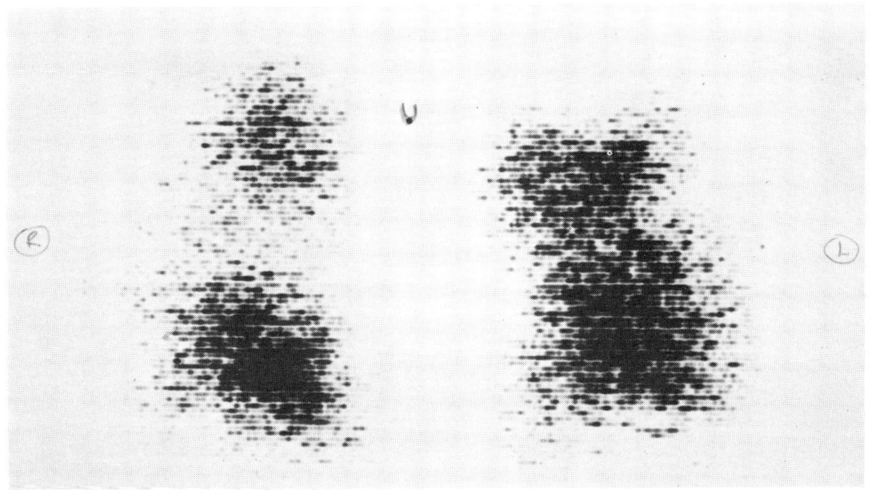

FIG. 10.2 A lung scan shows diminished isotope uptake in the left upper lobe and right middle lobe due to emboli. (After Dr D. Tibbutt.)

embolism is heralded with collapse, chest pain, hypotension, dyspnoea and a rapid pulse. The ECG patterns are complex and reflect right ventricular strain, but many patients with minor embolism and 9% with major embolism do not show ECG changes. The chest X-ray may show oligaemia in the lung fields and a pear-shaped hilum. Opacities, linear atelectasis, pleural effusion and elevation of the diaphragm may be seen. Lung scintillation scans (Fig. 10.2) aid diagnosis; but pulmonary arteriography is probably the treatment of choice (Fig. 10.3).

Bypass embolectomy is used for patients showing rapid deterioration or when medical therapy has failed. Thrombolytic therapy with fibrinolytic agents can be dramatic (Fig. 10.3). For minor embolism anticoagulant therapy with heparin and warfarin is the treatment of choice. However, the treatment of this condition requires expert advice.

FAT EMBOLISM

Fat embolism is defined in histological terms as the blockage of blood vessels by fat globules of 10–40 μm. Severe and even fulminating fat embolism has been described in patients with subcapital fractures treated by Thompson arthroplasty (Sevitt, 1972; Dandy, 1971–72).

Clinically fat embolism complicates 5% of all long bone fractures; severe cases have a rapid onset with coma, pyrexia, rapid pulse and respiratory rate and a petechial rash characteristically located in the shoulders, lower neck and upper chest. Hypoxaemia can be severe, and with a PO_2 of 50 mm Hg or less there is cyanosis, tachypnoea and other signs of respiratory distress. Pre-existing pulmonary disease, especially in the elderly, may aggravate the hypoxia; while collateral channels formed during chronic lung disease may facilitate the transit of emboli through the pulmonary circulation.

The exact relationship between fat embolism and hypoxia is difficult to deduce. Many patients with fractures have hypoxaemia on admission to hospital with PO_2 of about 60 mm Hg (Tachakra *et al.*, 1973). Collins (1969) found that the arterial PO_2 fell below 80 mm Hg in one-third of 33 subjects studied with comminuted femoral fractures.

FIG. 10.3 A pulmonary angiogram showing (*a*) diminished pulmonary markings in both lungs following a major occlusion of the pulmonary vessels. In (*b*) there is a return of blood flow as indicated by the pulmonary markings extending to the periphery of the lung fields. This marked improvement follows streptokinase therapy. (After Dr D. Tibbutt.)

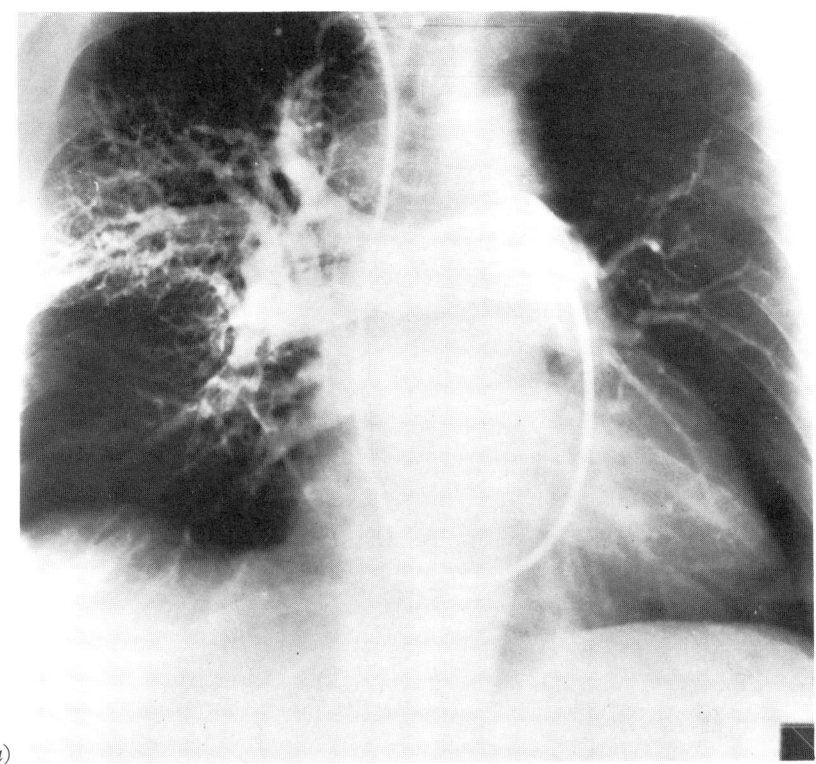

(*a*)

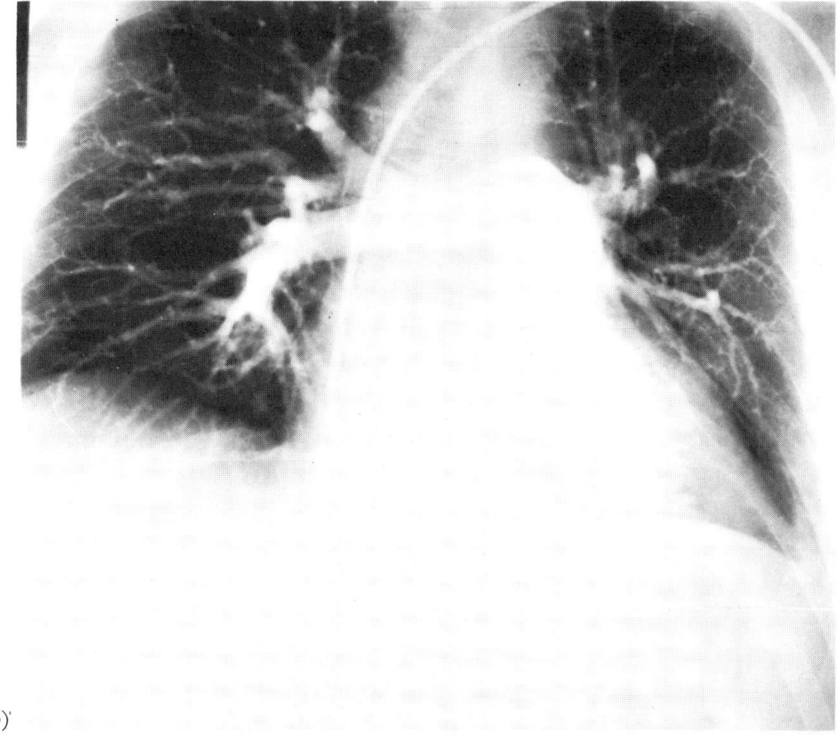

(*b*)

A second phase of hypoxaemia can occur during the second week after injury and this may be due to a second series of fat emboli (Sevitt, 1973). Tachakra and Sevitt (1975) postulated that the time relationship of hypoxaemia to the fracture was consistent with the rapidity with which fat emboli accumulated in the lung.

At present oxygen is the major therapeutic tool of proven worth in fat embolism (Sevitt, 1973). The administration of oxygen requires close co-operation with the anaesthetists and blood PO_2 and PCO_2 are estimated regularly. Heparin, dextran, clofibrate and steroids have all been tried in this condition.

ANAEMIA

About 10% of elderly people are anaemic with low serum iron. The classical presentation of iron deficiency anaemia as fatigue, breathlessness, angina, dizziness, dysphagia and palpitations may not be found in the aged who often present with heart failure, that is ankle oedema, basal lung crepitations and a functional systolic murmur.

On admission the patients' haemoglobin is checked and a haemoglobin below 11 g requires investigation for nutritional deficiencies and insidious blood loss. Post-operatively a check haemoglobin is carried out on the second day and any anaemia corrected with iron tablets or packed blood cells. Anaemic patients do badly after surgery and risk cardiac failure, bronchopneumonia, wound infection and delayed healing.

ELECTROLYTE DISTURBANCES

Such disturbances are not common after femoral neck surgery but the routine serum levels obtained require interpretation bearing in mind that serum values differ slightly in old age, for example the blood urea in the elderly can sometimes reach 18–20 mmol/l without any other indications of renal disease. Also apparently normal old people can have low potassium and sodium levels without overt causes. The administration of diuretics may aggravate electrolyte loss.

Electrolyte disturbances may present as apathy, nausea, anorexia, vomiting, excitation, depression, convulsions and coma in the elderly; it is easy to ascribe such signs to other causes while the basic electrolyte imbalance goes unchecked.

INCONTINENCE

This has many causes and it is important to eliminate such simple factors as diuretics, urinary infection and constipation before adding to patient morbidity by the premature use of a catheter. Many senile patients are incontinent because of defective frontal lobe cerebration but in others the conscious level may be impaired from head injury or metabolic factors such as uraemia or hypoglycaemia.

Incontinence may be an overflow phenomenon of acute retention, and in elderly men a history of prostatism should be sought and prostatic examination carried out. An enlarged prostate may cause only temporary trouble while the patient is recumbent in bed and the urinary difficulties end on mobilization. However, when retention is proven, the bladder must not be allowed to distend but should be drained with either an urethral or suprapubic catheter.

Catheterization should be carried out under strict aseptic conditions and the period the indwelling catheter remains *in situ* depends upon the previous history, prostatic size and general condition of the patient. One must also beware that some drugs (including certain antidepressants) can induce bladder atonia and retention. Drugs such as carbachol can be used to stimulate the bladder if there is no evidence of obstruction.

In all patients undergoing hip surgery the previous urinary function requires assessment paying due attention to any history of prostatism, cystitis, renal pain and stress incontinence; the clinical examination should include a prostatic and neurological examination. In this way any post-operative urinary complications can be anticipated and action taken to prevent their occurrence.

PRESSURE SORES

These are multifactorial in origin. Impaired movement due to lowered level of consciousness, paralysis, extrapyramidal rigidity, general weakness, apathy and pain must be counteracted by intelligent anticipation and a two-hourly change of position. All conditions which might decrease local or general circulation should be treated actively, especially local infection which can imperil tissues with poor vascularity. The best way to prevent pressure sores is to get the patient back to the vertical position with rapid mobilization.

The projection of bony points causes a disproportionate amount of body weight to be carried on the tissues of the heels, trochanters, ischial and scaral regions. Fat is no protection since under normal conditions it 'flows' out of the way. Erythema and oedema appear within hours, and will subside within a day if the pressure is relieved. However, should blistering occur then the affected area will not heal for two weeks. When the erythema does not fadc as the pressure is relieved and a coagulum has formed then the area will take three to four weeks to heal. Full thickness skin loss can involve fat and muscle with, in severe cases, a periosteal reaction.

Pressure sores are prevented by good nursing care with strict attention to detail such as a two-hourly cycle of turning, clean and crinkle-free sheets, and the application of bland ointments to the pressure areas. The treatment of an early sore consists of sitting the patient out of bed or by the use of a small blanket of sheep's wool. When a small ulcer has developed a swab is sent to bacteriology, and checks made on haemoglobin, albumin, urea and glucose blood levels. The raw area is gently cleaned with warm sterile saline or a mild antiseptic dressing or antibiotic spray. Ultraviolet light is also said to aid healing. If the skin is lax and necrosis is deep then excision of the area can be carried out or a graft or flap transposition used.

Other general measures which can be employed are ripple beds, heel and sacral rings, and foam or air mattresses.

THE GERIATRIC PROBLEM

Morbidity and mortality are high in femoral neck fractures and these sombre facts necessitate a critical assessment of the multiple clinical problems of the aged. Although many elderly people fall because they have sustained a fractured neck of femur, it is important to recall that others are injured during a falling episode from medical causes, and the same medical disability can affect prognosis, operative success and the whole course of rehabilitation. Thus it is necessary to identify critically the aetiological factors involved in falling, although more than one medical condition may be involved.

AETIOLOGY OF FALLS IN THE ELDERLY

Conditions which produce a temporary decrease in cerebral arterial perfusion are common in old age. Such transient ischaemic attacks (TIAs) are usually associated with arteriosclerosis of the carotid and vertebral arteries. Platelet emboli originating on an atheromatous plaque in the carotid vessels may produce a transient focal neurological deficit, either directly or through vasospasm. Cerebral blood flow may be affected by increased blood viscosity (for example, polycythaemia), anaemia and hypoglycaemia.

When there is occlusion of the internal carotid the results may vary from severe impairment in the affected hemisphere to only mild, transient symptoms, depending on the rapidity of occlusion and the efficiency of the cross circulation through the circle of Willis. While both extracranial and intracranial arteriosclerosis are concerned with the evolution of strokes, the internal carotid as a site of cerebral infarction is commonly overlooked. Large platelet emboli are undoubtedly involved in the production of some strokes.

Arteritis must be eliminated particularly if a history of vague ill-health and raised ESR precede the stroke.

Thus in any patient with a femoral neck fracture it is worth recalling the following conditions which may be directly associated with it:

(a) Carotid artery syndromes with the classical symptoms of hemiplegia, hemianaesthesia, monocular blindness and homonymous hemianopia. Ischaemia in the dominant hemisphere may cause dysphasia and lack of understanding.

(b) Vertebral artery syndromes. Cervical spondylosis is important in the production of circulatory problems in the vertebro-basilar system. Visual symptoms are common; while vertigo with diplopia or deafness may be confused with Menière's syndrome. Drop attacks are due to ischaemia of the midbrain's ascending reticular formation, and bruises and abrasions on the forehead, knees and hands may point to the vertebro-basilar origin of these falls.

(c) Emboli. Platelet emboli occur from atheromatous plaques in the main vessels, especially the extracranial vessels. Emboli may originate in the heart, the most common cause being post-rheumatic valvular disease and myocardial infarction. Septic emboli from bacterial endocarditis and fat emboli (the latter may direct the unwary into a search for a subdural haematoma) are sometimes found.

(d) Subdural haematoma. This can occur with minimal trauma in patients with cerebral atrophy. Headache and agitated confusion are presenting symptoms and neurological signs including hemiplegia develop.

(e) Cerebral haemorrhage rarely presents with concomitant injury to the femoral neck, but when the combination does occur the cerebral problem may overshadow and delay the diagnosis of the fracture, particularly when found on the same side as the hemiplegia.

(f) Postural hypotension may be part of cardiovascular disease, spinal cord lesions (e.g. trauma, transverse myelitis), peripheral neuropathy (due to diabetes mellitus, carcinoma, drugs) and hypovolaemia and hypokalaemia due to diuretics, inadequate intake and endocrine disturbances.

(g) Drug effect. Sedatives, tranquillisers, anti-parkinsonian, antidepressant, ganglion and peripheral autonomic blocking agents, laxatives and trinitrin can all produce falls, particularly in the aged at risk from other causes of postural hypotension.

(h) Hypoxia from several causes; vasodilatation and decreased circulating blood volume (for example on rapid rising from the recumbent position) can all contribute to producing postural hypotension.

Certain other medical problems may be found in the aged with femoral neck fractures.

Cardiac dysfunction

Cardiac pain is uncommon in the elderly, possibly due to degeneration of the afferent neurones. Angina may not occur on effort. Myocardial infarction may be silent and manifest by acute confusion, rapidly developing breathlessness, hypotension and dysrhythmia. Recurrent unexplained falls can be the result of paroxysmal dysrhythmias, Stokes Adams attacks, supraventricular tachycardia, and atrial flutter and fibrillation.

Thus patients with cardiac disease are liable to have a femoral neck fracture and rehabilitation may be limited by incipient or overt heart failure. In this context it must be remembered that fatigue is more common than breathlessness as a symptom of heart failure in old age. Undiagnosed anaemia frequently contributes to heart failure. Continuous ECG monitoring may help in the diagnosis of paroxysmal dysrhythmias, and a routine ECG is required on all elderly patients with femoral neck injuries.

Digoxin toxicity occurs in the elderly and is associated with impaired renal function; hypokalaemia is a contributory factor in patients on diuretics. Apathetic thyrotoxicosis, without classical signs and symptoms, may present with atrial fibrillation with a poor response to digoxin.

Thyroid disease

Almost 5% of geriatric patients have thyroid disease. Hypothyroidism may present in many ways including depression, dementia, anaemia, heart failure and ataxia. The assessment of this condition may be difficult, and since many elderly patients have swollen legs, delayed tendon reflexes may be difficult to elicit. Because of the frequent alterations in thyroxine-binding globulin levels and low T_3 estimations in the aged-ill it is essential to measure serum thyroid stimulating hormone (0–4μ μl^{-1} which is raised in myxoedema. L-thyroxine is the treatment of choice but the initial dose should be small, 0.05 mg daily, and most elderly patients are euthyroid on 0.2 mg daily. Angina and myocardial dysfunction can be aggravated by too energetic treatment.

Hyperthyroidism is found in about 2% of geriatric admissions. The presentation may be insidious with weight loss, myopathy and cardiac effects. The diagnosis is confirmed by a raised T_3 serum level and ^{131}I is the treatment of choice in the elderly, but antithyroid drugs can be used.

Diabetes mellitus is discussed under pre-operative assessment.

Epilepsies

Although many elderly patients with epilepsy have suffered from attacks for many years, the first attack in late adult life may be associated with arteriosclerosis or a space occupying lesion in the skull.

Not only are epileptic patients more liable to falling episodes, but the long-term ingestion of phenobarbitone and phenytoin can lead to osteomalacia by interfering with vitamin D metabolism.

Parkinsonism

The classical triad of tremor, rigidity and bradykinesia are found in the young-elderly, but in the over 75 years the so-called arteriosclerotic parkinsonism predominates. Tremor is minimal or absent in the latter and the immobility of the patient may be cursorily dismissed as senility. Rigidity may be more evident lying down and more severe in the legs than arms. In mild forms it can be overcome voluntarily and the doctor's initial suspicion allayed; in such instances the patient's attention should be distracted by concentration on deliberate movements in the other limb. Elicited in this way, rigidity is a common sign in older patients with femoral neck fractures. Depression may be common and drug induced parkinsonism (especially with phenothiazines, butyrophenones, rauwolfia alkaloids and methyl dopa) should not be forgotten.

Apart from a predisposition to falls and fractures, this syndrome is accompanied by increased morbidity and mortality. Pneumonia, collapse and consolidation of pulmonary segments due to poor cough, tendency to aspiration and immobility are common. Pressure sores are frequent and their prevention requires meticulous nursing care.

Ataxia

Walking is often considered to be automatic but it is a learned process and depends on stored memory patterns. Standing and walking are dependent on the integrity of special senses, cerebrum, basal ganglia, cerebellum, spinal cord, peripheral nerves and skeletal muscle. A detailed list of the conditions which affect these structures and cause ataxia is beyond the scope of this article. However, one should not forget that apraxia for walking is not uncommon in the aged and explains the difficulty in mobilization after a fracture. Such apraxia may follow a hemiplegia. Following prolonged confinement to bed, some elderly patients show a different postural problem in that they tend to lean backwards when walking is attempted. The picture of an old lady, supported by a physiotherapist on each side, leaning further and further backwards while her legs progress inadequately forwards, must have been experienced by all who have been involved in the rehabilitation of the elderly. The wide-based, swaying gait, intention tremor and hypotonia of cerebellar disease should be sought when ataxia is pronounced; myxoedema and a primary carcinoma must not be forgotten in the differential diagnosis of cerebellar disease.

Dementia

Toxiconfusional state (delirium) needs to be distinguished from dementia; the former is usually of acute onset and the patient is both disturbed and disturbing in a positive way. Dementia is essentially a negative disturbance with gradual onset and developing apathy, although in the earliest stages restlessness and agitation may be found.

Ten % of the over 65s suffer from some degree of dementia. Treatable conditions which resemble dementia are myxoedema, B_{12} deficiency, depression, normal pressure hydrocephalus and cerebral tumour; while trauma, infection, cerebral hypoxia, hypoglycaemia, alcohol, drugs, dehydration, uraemia, hepatic failure, arteritis and distant primary carcinoma incompletely express an extensive list of disorders which must be considered when dealing with the so-called demented patient on an orthopaedic ward. The true dementia can only be supported by attention to physical, and if possible, mental fitness with social support in the normal home situation whenever this is feasible.

Special senses

Diseases of the special sense especially perceptive deafness, senile cataract and senile macular choroidal degeneration can produce falls and femoral neck injuries.

Delayed recovery

Patients may present at follow-up clinics with a variety of complaints, the chief being pain in the hip region (sometimes radiating to the knee) and stiffness. Latent infection, irritation by screws, plates and wires, and early osteoarthrosis must be excluded. Physiotherapy to mobilize the joint, analgesics, and walking aids such as quadropod frames or sticks help ambulation in geriatric patients. If there is a leg length discrepancy then this should be corrected by a shoe-raise.

There should be programmed after-care which should be planned from admission. Regular case conferences with information from medical and nursing staff, physiotherapists, geriatric health visitors and medical social workers will ensure definition of the many problems, rehabilitation and structuring of their solutions. A planned withdrawal of facilities should develop as the patient is gradually integrated into the previous environment. The involvement of relatives in hospital care and then graduated discharge from care may be more suitable than the sudden loss of all support. Floating bed admissions, intermittent and holiday admissions associated with day hospitalization may provide continuing care.

The multiple problems involved necessitate a full assessment of all physical, mental, social and functional aspects of the elderly patient. The present tragic picture of high mortality, poor functional recovery and general deterioration following fracture of the femoral neck in the elderly is due to a failure to appreciate the total problem. The answer is not purely mechanical fixation but requires re-orientation and re-education of all staff dealing with the initial problem. A greater degree of involvement of, and co-operation with, the staff of the Geriatric Department is needed at all levels.

REFERENCES

PRE-AND POST OPERATIVE PROBLEMS

COLLINS, J.A. (1969). *J. Surg. Res.* **9**, 685.
DANDY, D.J. (1971–72). *Injury* **3**, 85.
EVANS, D.S. (1970). *Br. J. Surg.* **57**, 726.
EVANS, D.S. and NEGUS, D. (1971). *Br. J. Hosp, Med.* **6**, 729.
FLANC, C., KAKKAR, V. and CLARKE, M.B. (1968). *Br. J. Surg.* **55**, 742.
GIBBS, N.M. (1957). *Br. J. Surg.* **45**, 209.
HAMILTON, H.W., CRAWFORD, J.S., GARDINER, J.H. and WILEY, A.M. (1970). *J. Bone Jt. Surg.* **52B**, 268.
KAKKAR, V.V. (1971). *Br. J. Hosp. Med.* **6**, 741.
KEMBLE, J.V.H. (1971). *Postgrad Med. J.* **47**, 775.
MAVOR, G.E. and GALLOWAY, J.M.D. (1969). *Br. J. Surg.* **56**, 45.
MAVOR, G.E., OGSTON, D., GALLOWAY, J.M.D. and KARMODY, A.M. (1969). *Br. J. Surg.* **56**, 571.
MUCKLE, D.S., FORNEY, H.J. and BENTLEY, G. (1974). *Acta Orthop. Scand.* **45**, 412.
NEGUS, D., PINTO, D.J., LE QUESNE, L.P., BROWN, N. and CHAPMAN, M. (1968). *Br. J. Surg.* **55**, 835.
REID, H.A. and CHAN, K. E. (1968). *Lancet* **i**, 485.
SEVITT, S. (1972). *Lancet* **i**, 848.
SEVITT, S. (1973). *Br. J. Hosp. Med.* **9**, 784.
SEVITT, S. and GALLAGHER, N. (1959). *Lancet* **ii**, 981.
TACHAKRA, S.S., EVANS, R.F. and SEVITT, S. (1973). *Br. J. Hosp. Med.* **9**, 784.
TACHAKRA, S.S. and SEVITT, S. (1975). *J. Bone Jt. Surg.* **57B**, 197.

GERIATRIC MEDICINE

ADAMS, G.F. (1974). *Cerebrovascular Disability and the Ageing Brain*, Churchill Livingstone, Edinburgh and London.
ALLISON, R.S. (1962). *The Senile Brain*, Edward Arnold, London.
BIRREN, J.E. (1964). *The Psychology of Ageing*, Prentice-Hall, New Jersey.
BROCKLEHURST, J.E. (1973). *Textbook of Geriatric Medicine and Gerontology*, Churchill Livingstone, Edinburgh and London.
FERGUSON ANDERSON, W. and JUDGE, T.G. (1974). *Geriatric Medicine*, Academic Press, London and New York.

MATTHEWS, W.B. (1973). *Practical Neurology*, Blackwell, Oxford.

PEARCE, J. and MILLER, E. (1973). *Clinical Aspects of Dementia*, Baillière Tindall, London.

POST, F. (1965). *The Clinical Psychiatry of Late Life*, Pergammon Press, Oxford.

TOOLE, J.F. and PATEL, A.N. (1974). *Cerebrovascular Disorders*, McGraw-Hill, New York.

WEED, L.L. (1971). *Medical Records, Medical Education and Patient Care*, The Press of Case Western University Cleveland, Ohio.

WELLS, C.E. (1971). *Dementia*, Blackwell, Oxford.

INDEX